D1037118

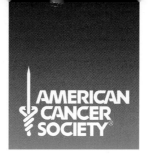

AMERICAN CANCER SOCIETY'S GUIDE TO

Complementary
and
Alternative
CANCER METHODS

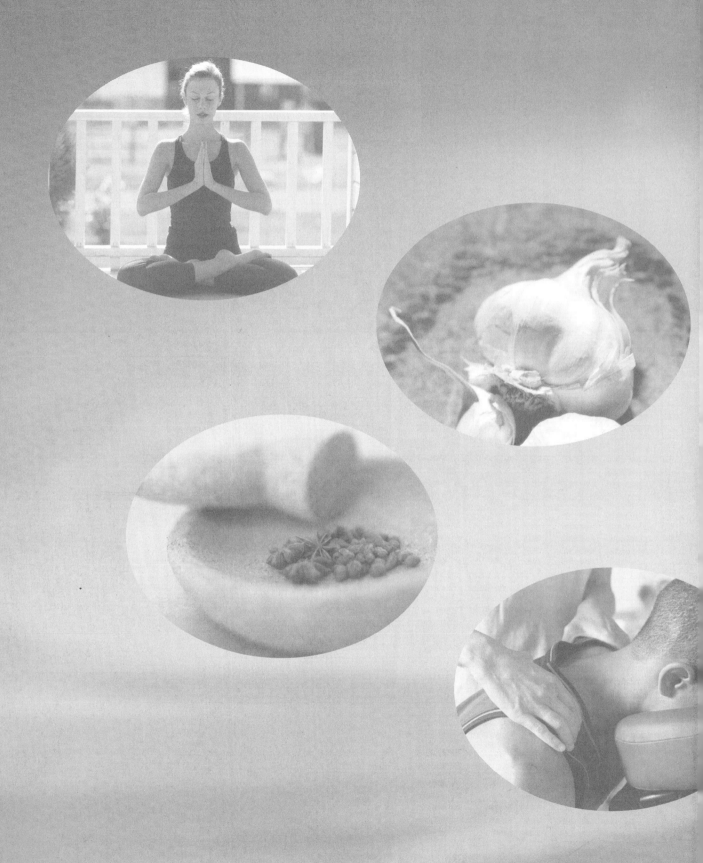

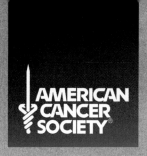

AMERICAN CANCER SOCIETY'S GUIDE TO

Complementary
and
Alternative
CANCER METHODS

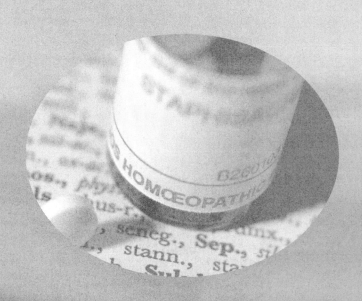

American Cancer Society
Health Content Products
1599 Clifton Road NE
Atlanta, Georgia 30329, U.S.A.

5   4   3   2   1   00   01   02   03   04   05

Library of Congress Cataloging-in-Publication Data

Guide to complementary and alternative cancer methods.
    American Cancer Society guide to complementary and alternative cancer methods.
        p. cm.
    Includes bibliographical references and index.
    ISBN 0-944235-29-8 — ISBN 0-944235-24-7 (softcover)
     1. Cancer—Alternative treatment. I. American Cancer Society.

    RC271.A62 G85 2000
    616.99'406—dc21   00-010596

A note to the reader

*This information may not cover all possible uses, actions, precautions,
side effects, or interactions, is not intended as medical advice, and
should not be relied upon as a substitute for consultation with your
doctor who is familiar with your medical needs. For more information,
contact your American Cancer Society at 1-800-ACS-2345.*

Printed in the United States of America
Set in Frutiger
Designed by Shock Design, Inc.

Table of Contents

Contributors List

Senior Editor
Katherine Bruss, PsyD

Editors
Christina Salter, MA
Esmeralda Galán

Contributors
Steve Frandzel
Dennis Connaughton
Stuart J. Birkby
Dorothy Breckner
Katherine Bruss, PsyD
Lynne Camoosa
Carol Carter
Jeff Clements
Suzy Crawford
Peter Dakutis
Tom Gryczan, MS
Christina Salter, MA
Melissa Kulick, PhD
Steve Lewis
Jennifer Miller
Ryan Siemers, MPH
Leah Tuzzio
Lynn Yoffee

Publishing Director
Emily Pualwan

Production Manager
Candace Magee

Editorial Review Board

Terri Ades, RN, MS, AOCN
Director, Health Content Nursing Staff
American Cancer Society
Atlanta, Georgia

Richard H. Lange, MD, FACP
Honorary Attending Staff
Ellis Hospital
Schenectady, New York

Mary Ann Richardson, DrPH
(Former Director of UT-CAM)
Program Officer, Division of
*   Extramural Research*
NIH National Center for
*   Complementary and Alternative*
*   Medicine*
Bethesda, Maryland

John J. Lynch, MD, FACP
Associate Medical Director
Washington Cancer Institute &
*   Washington Hospital Center*
Washington, D.C.

Muriel J. Montbriand, DrPH, RN
Research Associate
Applied Research/Psychiatry
College of Medicine
University of Saskatchewan
Saskatoon, Saskatchewan, Canada

Connie Henke Yarbro, RN, MS, FAAN
Clinical Associate Professor
Division of Hematology/ Oncology
Adjunct Clinical Assistant Professor
School of Nursing, University of
*   Missouri-Columbia*
Columbia, Missouri

William T. Jarvis, PhD
Professor of Public Health and
*   Preventive Medicine*
Loma Linda University School of
*   Medicine*
Loma Linda, California

Freddie Ann Hoffman, MD
(Formerly of the US Food and
*   Drug Administration)*
Senior Director, Medical and Clinical
*   Affairs—Complementary Medicine*
Consumer Healthcare Research &
*   Development, Warner-Lambert, Co.*
Morris Plains, New Jersey

(Note: Participation as a reviewer does not imply
endorsement by the US Food and Drug
Administration or any other body.)

Ted Gansler, MD, MBA
Director, Health Content
American Cancer Society
Atlanta, Georgia

Abby S. Block, PhD, RD
Nutrition Consultant in Private Practice
New York, New York

MaryBeth Augustine, RD, CDN
Nutritionist Counselor
Integrative Medicine Service
Memorial Sloan-Kettering Cancer Center
New York, New York

Carol A. Balmer, PharmD
Associate Professor
University of Colorado School of
*   Pharmacy*
Department of Pharmacy Practice
Denver, Colorado

Dan Nixon, MD
President, American Health Foundation
New York, New York

Daniel D. Anthony, MD
Associate Professor of Pharmacology,
*   School of Medicine*
Ireland Cancer Center
Case Western Reserve University
Cleveland, Ohio

Susan Paulsen, PharmD
University of Colorado
Health Science Center
School of Pharmacy
Denver, Colorado

LaMar McGinnis, MD
Medical Consultant
American Cancer Society
Atlanta, Georgia

David Rosenthal, MD
Director of Harvard University Health
*   Services*
Professor of Medicine at Harvard
*   Medical School*
Cambridge, Massachusetts

William Faire, MD
Baumritter Ancell Chair of Urologic
*   Oncology*
Memorial Sloan-Kettering Cancer
*   Center*
New York, New York

Foreword

Many factors have created the need for a book such as this. Over the past two decades, an increasing number of the people are using methods to maintain or improve health and well being. The public is spending more money for these methods, and the current estimate is that this has become a multi-billion dollar industry. A large percentage of the public's practice and use of these methods is focused in the cancer field, for reducing one's risk of developing cancer, improving the quality of life while undergoing treatment of cancer, or hoping that a different approach may treat or cure the cancer. Major cancer centers throughout the United States and in Europe have begun "integrated cancer programs." These are programs aimed at education, research, and clinical investigation of complementary and alternative therapies used alongside conventional therapies.

One of the most important messages for patients and the general public is to share with their doctor, their specialist, and their oncologist what they are doing in addition to the prescribed medications. What nutritional supplements are being taken or what form of relaxation or physical activity is making them feel better? A decade ago, there was very little sharing of this information with the treating physicians. Despite the fact that more than half of people with cancer participated in complementary therapies, they were not sharing this information with their oncologist for fear of a negative response. Recent physician surveys have shown that with the development of integrated cancer centers and positive outcome studies using complementary therapies, there is currently a greater acceptance by the medical community. In addition, numerous medical schools have incorporated the study of complementary and alternative medicine (CAM) into the curriculum.

The ACS Guide to Complementary and Alternative Cancer Methods is timely. It has been written to help the public, the consumer, patient, and family better understand this rapidly expanding industry and recognize the issues that accompany these methods. There are many questions raised. For example, what is the difference between "complementary" and "alternative" therapies? What is "evidence based" or "scientifically proven;" what is "unproven methods" or quackery?" The first approach to a better understanding of the issues is an appreciation of the terminology. Affirming or agreeing upon an offered definition will prevent existing confusion. As consumers access information from the media, whether it is newsprint, publication, television or the Internet, there must be uniform understanding of the meaning of CAM.

With agreed upon terminology, it is now possible to move ahead and categorize the various components of an integrated cancer program. This guide will assist the reader in understanding the therapeutic methods that focus on the mind, body, and spirit, and the role of the "placebo effect." The reader will have a better understanding of the issues related to the use of herbs, vitamins, minerals, and antioxidants. In the era of "Internet overload," the American Cancer Society wants to assure that the consumer is accessing the most reliable information.

David S. Rosenthal, MD

Director, Harvard University Health Services
Henry K. Oliver Professor of Hygiene, Harvard University
Professor of Medicine, Harvard Medical School
Past President, American Cancer Society
Chair of the American Cancer Society Advisory Group on Complementary and Alternative Medicine
Medical Director, Zakim Center for Integrative Medicine, Dana-Farber / Harvard Cancer Center

Introduction

Each year, Americans spend more than $34 billion on complementary and alternative treatment methods, and hundreds of these methods are marketed specifically to people with cancer. As part of its overall mission, the American Cancer Society (ACS) recognizes the enormous public interest in the growing area of complementary and alternative methods and is committed to providing the public with a reliable guide to selecting and using these treatment methods wisely.

The ACS is committed to studying the effects of complementary and alternative medicine among those living with cancer. Since 1914, the ACS has addressed the safety and effectiveness of cancer treatment. At that time, the ACS expressed concern over the claims of cancer cures and began gathering information on these therapies. The Society began publishing information in the 1950s about specific claims and criteria for assessing the merit of a cancer treatment or diagnostic test. This was based on concerns raised over the exploitation of people with cancer, especially those in the advanced phase of their illness. For example, in 1976 the ACS distributed a statement on laetrile, one of the few unproven therapies that went through the rigors of appropriate clinical testing (see Laetrile). It was found to be ineffective and unsafe. Yet, laetrile is still promoted and used today as an alternative therapy.

In 1990, the ACS commissioned a study of the prevalence and use of unproven therapies among more than 5,000 cancer patients. The study also polled 91 physicians regarding their perception of the use of unproven therapies. The study found 9% of the cancer patients had used an unproven therapy. Likelihood of use was directly related to increased income and education. Important differences were found between patients' and physicians' perceptions of use. For example, patients reported that physicians directed them to the unproven therapy, while physicians reported that they disapproved and were rarely supportive of the therapy. From this study, the Society concluded that more education was needed about unproven therapies for the health professional as well as the public. In 1996, the Society adopted the use of "complementary and alternative" terminology and defined the terms (see page 8).

The ACS believes that all cancer interventions must withstand the scrutiny of scientific evaluation before they can be recommended for the prevention, diagnosis, or treatment of cancer. The ACS urges individuals with cancer to remain in the care of physicians who use standard, conventional therapies for cancer and approved clinical trials of promising new treatments. The ACS also encourages patients to talk openly with their health care providers about any other therapy they are considering, and to seek information from unbiased and reliable sources. In this way, patients can make informed decisions about complementary and alternative methods.

The *American Cancer Society's Guide to Complementary and Alternative Cancer Methods* is designed to serve as a comprehensive, encyclopedic-type guide to the wide variety of treatment methods available. Each entry provides critical information, such as proponent's claims, what the method involves, historical background, recent research findings, and side effects and complications. The latest complementary and alternative treatment methods are included, as well as those that have been used for many years. Each method has been thoroughly reviewed by experts in the field from across the country. This information is presented to help each individual make an educated decision about the use of complementary and alternative treatments.

It is in the spirit of the longstanding ACS mission—to educate, advocate, research, and serve—that this book on complementary and alternative methods was born. This book is designed to provide clarity in the midst of a large amount of information and financial investment in the field of complementary and alternative medicine. The ACS does not promote any specific method. This book aims to provide readers with objective information based on scientific evidence contained in medical literature. It is the view of the ACS that until a method has been thoroughly researched and proven to be effective through rigorous scientific evaluation, any claims made by manufacturers or proponents cannot be relied upon.

This book will help you consider your options while working together with your health care team. Not everyone will have the same experience with these methods. This book is meant to present general information and is not designed to be a prescriptive guide or to replace any advice your health care providers may give. Resources listed at the end of the book are provided for your convenience. Inclusion in this book does not imply endorsement by the ACS.

The ACS supports the right of individuals with cancer to decide what treatment is best for them. The ACS also encourages people with cancer to use methods that have been proven to be effective or those that are currently under study in clinical trials. Unnecessary delays and interruptions in conventional therapies are detrimental to the success of cancer treatment. People are encouraged to discuss all treatments (conventional, complementary, or alternative) they may be considering with their physician and other health care providers. Open, trusting, non-critical communication is essential in making health care decisions. In this way, patients interested in complementary and alternative methods will be able to select those most likely to be safe and effective in relieving symptoms and improving their well being. They will also be able to avoid methods that are dangerous, likely to interfere with conventional treatments, and known to be ineffective.

Overview

Chapter 1

How to Use this Book

This book begins with a basic overview of complementary and alternative methods, including information on prevalence, safety issues, and guidelines for use. Specific entries for each method are listed. Methods are organized into the five categories listed below. Each method has been classified into one of the categories based on similar characteristics and how the treatment is administered or performed. Although classification was sometimes difficult, the categories were initially modeled after the classification system of the National Center for Complementary and Alternative Medicine, an office of the National Institutes of Health (NIH). Due to the large volume of entries, some reorganization was required.

Categories of Methods

Mind, Body, and Spirit Methods: This chapter includes methods that focus on the connections between the mind, body, and spirit, and their power for healing.

Manual Healing and Physical Touch Methods: Treatment methods in this chapter involve touching, manipulation, or movement of the body. These techniques are based on the idea that problems in one part of the body often affect other parts of the body.

Herb, Vitamin, and Mineral Methods: This chapter contains plant-derived preparations that are used for therapeutic purposes, as well as everyday vitamins and minerals. It is noted when there are instances where chemicals extracted from plants are used rather than the plant components.

Diet and Nutrition Methods: This chapter includes dietary approaches and special nutritional programs related to prevention and treatment.

Pharmacological and Biological Treatment Methods: This chapter provides information about substances that are synthesized and produced from chemicals or concentrated from plants and other living things. Extracted chemicals are not the same as the raw plant or plant in its natural state.

Methods within each chapter are listed alphabetically. Methods included in the book have been promoted for conditions related to cancer, its consequences, or effects related to treatment. There is also a resource guide at the end of the book that provides standards for finding reliable sources of information.

This book is intended to serve as a reference tool, not to be read from beginning to end. If you do not find a particular method in the section you would expect, please consult the index to see if it is included elsewhere. In some cases, methods have been grouped together into broader categories that you may not immediately consider. If, however, an entire chapter interests you, you may want to read through all of the entries contained in that chapter to gain a better understanding of that area of complementary or alternative care. Some methods contain only a few lines, or short paragraphs, because they have limited information, or are not widely available. In these cases, there was not enough scientific information to evaluate the evidence, so only a brief description is provided.

How the Research was Performed

The ACS advocates peer-reviewed scientific evidence to determine the safety and effectiveness of any treatment method. This is where the results of carefully designed studies are evaluated by unbiased experts in the field and published in scientific and medical journals. All cancer interventions must withstand the scrutiny of research based on the highest scientific and ethical standards before they can be recommended for the prevention, diagnosis, or treatment of cancer (see Chapter 2 for Evaluating Treatment). These same standards were used to gather scientific evidence on each treatment method and to evaluate its effectiveness for this book.

This first involved gathering literature widely available to the public, such as the latest books published on the subject, Internet Web sites, and recent nationwide magazine and newspaper articles found in the popular press. Searching these publications allowed the authors to gain insight into the enormous number of unconventional methods being marketed to the public and their claims.

Next we analyzed peer-reviewed medical journal articles and textbooks to determine if these claims could be supported by evidence. Medline, the National Library of Medicine's bibliographic database, was the vehicle our researchers used to retrieve scientific data. Medline is a database that contains bibliographic citations and author abstracts from approximately 3,900 current biomedical journals published in the United States and 70 foreign countries. The database contains approximately 9 million records dating back to journal articles published in 1966. A thorough review of the literature was conducted and a summary of the latest research is provided for each method.

Sample Book Entry

On the next page there is a sample book entry. The encyclopedic-type format allows a consistent presentation of information so the content can be quickly accessed from entry to entry.

Entry Name

The name that is most commonly used or most recognizable to the general public is listed at the top as the entry name.

Category of method appears down the side of each page for easy location reference.

Other common names
Other common names are listed in this section in order of usage.

Scientific/medical name
The Latin name or chemical name appears here where applicable. Not all entries will have a scientific or medical name.

DESCRIPTION
Here you'll find a brief definition of what the method is and/or contains as ingredients.

OVERVIEW
This summary provides an overview of whether or not the method is effective based on scientific findings, and if any serious side effects may occur.

How is it promoted for use?
Within this section are results promoters are claiming and how advocates claim this method works. Theories proposed for the effectiveness of the therapy are discussed. Claims about the method's value for conditions other than cancer may also be included.

What does it involve?
This covers what the treatment method involves, how often it is administered, and in what forms the treatment is provided.

What is the history behind it?
The background about how, when, and by whom the method was developed is discussed in this section.

What is the evidence?
This is where readers can find a summary of the findings of the latest peer-reviewed research that has been done on each treatment method. General conclusions can be found about the effectiveness of the method based on scientific data.

Are there any possible problems or complications?

This section notes anything people should be aware of or concerned about, such as side effects, drug interactions, contraindications, unsafe methodology, reports of death, or other adverse reactions.

References
A reference list of the resources used to compile each entry, specifically the most important peer-reviewed journal articles, can be found here. Readers may use this reference list, as well as the resource guide at the back of the book, to obtain more information.

Entry names appear at the bottom of each page to aid in searches.

Chapter 2

Description of Complementary and Alternative Methods

Although complementary and alternative methods have been around for many years, they have grown enormously in popularity during the past decade. In the 1990s, tens of millions of Americans began spending billions of dollars on complementary and alternative therapies for a wide variety of diseases, ailments, and medical complaints, including cancer. The growing popularity of complementary and alternative therapies has had an enormous impact on every aspect of health care in the United States, Europe, and elsewhere in the developed world. The rise of complementary and alternative medicine has had a particular influence on people with cancer. While accurate figures are difficult to obtain, it is estimated that as of the year 2000, up to 50% of people living with cancer had sought some type of complementary or alternative therapy.

The words *complementary* and *alternative* are often used interchangeably. However, there are very important distinctions between the two terms.

Complementary therapies are those that patients use **along with** conventional medicine. Many of these therapies have been shown to help relieve symptoms and improve quality of life by lessening the side effects of conventional treatments or providing psychological and physical benefits to the patient.

Alternative therapies are unproven treatments that patients use **instead of** conventional therapy in an attempt to prevent, lessen, or cure disease. Alternative therapies may be harmful in and of themselves or because they are used instead of conventional medicine, and thereby delay treatments that are proven to be helpful.

Until the late 1990s, the term alternative was generally used to describe most of the therapies that are not part of conventional medicine. When the NIH established a special department to evaluate complementary and alternative therapies, it was originally named the Office of Alternative Medicine (OAM). In 1999, recognizing the distinction between complementary and alternative therapies, the NIH renamed the office the National Center for Complementary and Alternative Medicine (NCCAM).

Evaluating Claims

Alternative medicine has many outspoken proponents as well as many vocal detractors. Physicians, by training, distrust medical claims that are not based on scientific evidence. However,

Commonly Used Terms

There is often confusion surrounding the use of different terms in the field. Here are some definitions of commonly used terms.

- **Proven treatments** refer to evidence-based, conventional, mainstream, or standard medical treatments that have been tested following a strict set of guidelines and found to be safe and effective. The results of such studies have been published in peer-reviewed journals — meaning that other physicians or scientists in the field evaluate the quality of the research and decide whether the article will be published. These treatments have been approved by the Food and Drug Administration (FDA).

- **Research or investigational** treatments are therapies being studied in a clinical trial. Clinical trials are controlled research projects that determine whether a new treatment is effective and safe for patients. Before a drug or other treatment can be used regularly to treat patients, it is studied and tested carefully, first in laboratory test tubes and then in animals. After these studies are completed and the therapy is found safe and promising, it is tested to see if it helps patients. After careful testing among patients shows the drug or other treatment is safe and effective, the FDA may approve it for regular use. Only then does the treatment become part of the standard, conventional collection of proven therapies used to treat disease in human beings.

- **Complementary** refers to supportive methods that are used to complement, or add to, conventional treatments. Examples might include meditation to reduce stress, peppermint tea for nausea, and acupuncture for chronic back pain. Complementary methods are not used to cure disease, rather they may help control symptoms and improve well being. Some methods, such as massage therapy, yoga, and meditation that are now called complementary have actually been referred to as "supportive care" in the past.

- **Integrative therapy** refers to the combined use of evidence-based proven therapies and complementary therapies. This is the term that many people in the field are using more frequently. In fact, integrative medicine services are becoming part of cancer centers and hospitals across the country.

- The terms **unproven or untested** can be confusing because they are sometimes used to refer to treatments with little basis in scientific fact, while they may also refer to treatments or tests that are under investigation. In general, adequate scientific evidence is not available to support the use of unproven or untested treatments.

- **Alternative** treatments are unproven because they have not been scientifically tested, or they were tested and found to be ineffective. Alternative treatments are used instead of conventional treatment. They may cause the patient to suffer either from lack of helpful treatment, delay in treatment, or because the alternative treatment is actually harmful.

- **Quackery** refers to the promotion of methods that claim to prevent, diagnose, or cure cancers that are known to be false or that are unproven. These methods are often based on the use of patient testimonials as evidence of their effectiveness and safety. Many times the treatment is claimed to be effective against other diseases as well as cancer.

- **Unconventional** is a term used to cover all types of complementary and alternative treatments that fall outside the definition of proven, conventional therapies.

- **Nontraditional** is used in the same way as unconventional to describe complementary and alternative therapies. However, some therapies that seem nontraditional to modern American or European physicians may have been used in certain cultures for thousands of years, such as traditional Chinese medicine or traditional Native American medicine (see Chinese Herbal Medicine and Native American Healing). These traditional native medicines are often used in complementary or alternative therapies.

- **Questionable** treatments are those that are unproven or untested therapies.

consumers, and people with cancer in particular, may be more accepting of word-of-mouth claims made by friends and others, reports found in reputable magazines, or even assertions made by advocates of alternative medicine over the Internet.

Promoters of alternative medicine may make claims about the effectiveness of these therapies ranging from the reasonable to the extraordinary. The most outlandish claim is that any alternative therapy can actually cure all people with cancer. Even conventional cancer therapies, such as surgery, chemotherapy, and radiation therapy, cannot guarantee a cure. If certain cancers are diagnosed early enough in their development, conventional therapies may completely remove or destroy the cancer. Many cancer specialists do not even like to use the term cure but prefer to say that a cancer is in remission. Alternative therapies cannot cure cancer, and any claims for a cure should be treated with skepticism.

The promise of a cure is often the main allure of alternative cancer therapies. Another appeal is the claim that the alternative therapy not only cures cancer or prolongs the survival time of a person living with cancer but also has no objectionable side effects. People should also be skeptical of these claims. Promoters usually have no evidence to back up these claims, except, perhaps, testimonials from some people who claim to have used the therapies. The reality is that some alternative therapies can actually cause serious side effects, including infections, heart problems, nutritional deficiencies, and harmful interactions with conventional cancer drugs and therapies (see Adverse Reactions, page 33).

Supporters of some alternative cancer therapies may claim that the treatments can reduce a person's risk of developing cancer, stop the progression of cancer once it has occurred, or stop cancer recurrences. These claims should be evaluated on the basis of the evidence presented to back them up. Is there solid scientific evidence based on clinical trials to support the claim or is the claim based solely on the word of the manufacturer, promoter, or certain people who have tried the therapy? Controlled human clinical trials of complementary and alternative cancer therapies are needed to evaluate these therapies. Animal and laboratory studies may show that a certain therapy holds promise as a beneficial treatment, but further studies are necessary to determine if the results apply to humans (see Evaluating Treatment, page 10).

Many complementary and alternative therapies designed to prevent cancer involve nutrition. There is a growing body of scientific evidence available to suggest that a diet high in fruits, vegetables, and whole grain products can help protect the human body against cancer. These foods contain vitamins and minerals necessary for normal growth and development, and overall health and well being. The ACS and many conventional physicians recommend that people get these essential vitamins and minerals from foods rather than from supplements. Supplements have not been proven to have the same cancer-protective effects as foods rich in vitamins, minerals, and other nutrients. Furthermore, foods provide nutrients in a complete package that may allow the vitamins and minerals to work together to help prevent cancer.

Other claims for complementary and alternative methods of cancer management may be that the therapies increase the functioning of the patient's immune system, inhibit tumor growth or spread, or destroy cancer cells. The immune system is the body's natural defense against infections and most cancers. It is a collection of cells and proteins that protects the body from invasion of bacteria, viruses, and fungi, and plays a role in controlling cancer and other diseases. Many diseases and other illnesses, such as colds and flu, can weaken the immune system. The stronger a person's immune system is, the better he or she is able to fight diseases, including cancer.

Because laws prohibit manufacturers and marketers of dietary supplements, such as vitamins, minerals, and herbal medicines, from claiming that their products can cure or prevent disease, many claim that the products "boost the immune system" to help the body fight disease naturally. This commonly used phrase leaves one to believe that the product will increase the function of the immune system. Yet these claims are often made without any evidence to back them up. All claims should be evaluated on the basis of available scientific evidence to support them. The same standard of proof should be held for claims that an herbal product or other type of complementary or alternative cancer therapy can inhibit the growth or spread of tumors or actually destroy cancer cells. In some cases, these claims may be based on solid evidence; in many other instances, they are not.

Proponents may claim that different methods have a direct effect on different types of cancer. For example, based on preliminary results from an animal study, ginseng is sometimes promoted as a herbal remedy for preventing lung cancer. Garlic is sometimes said to reduce the risk of stomach and colon cancers. Some claim that drinking green tea can help prevent prostate, stomach, and esophageal cancers. In many cases these claims are based on animal, laboratory, or population studies, but have not been confirmed to be effective in humans through controlled clinical trials.

Advocates of complementary and alternative cancer therapies sometimes claim that the therapies enhance conventional cancer treatments and decrease the side effects of conventional treatment. In the case of complementary cancer therapies, they often do. For example, a special diet prescribed by a dietitian or nutritionist may help a person living with cancer stay healthy even though he or she is experiencing vomiting and weight loss due to chemotherapy. Complementary therapies related to the mind, body, and spirit, such as prayer, meditation, and yoga may help relieve anxiety, depression, nausea, and pain resulting from conventional cancer treatments. While many complementary therapies have been shown to ease side effects and improve quality of life, they cannot change the course of the disease.

Consumers should be wary, however, about claims that alternative therapies can enhance cancer treatment or can detoxify, or flush out toxins from the body. If the scientific evidence were available to support these claims, the alternative therapies would become part of conventional medicine.

Evaluating Treatment

The beginning of the 20th century is widely viewed by medical historians as the turning point in cancer treatment. At that time, scientists began to look at life-threatening diseases, such as cancer, as solvable problems. Answers to puzzling medical questions were found, as scientists learned that mosquitoes were carriers of yellow fever, discovered a treatment for syphilis, and developed the first chemotherapy drug. Researchers and physicians began sharing knowledge with each other, and medical institutions became centers of research.

During these early years of cancer research, scientists began the long search to identify the cause of cancer, and soon realized there was no one single cause of the disease. Cancer is many diseases. Scientists also began investigating various treatment methods in the hope of finding methods that were safe and effective.

Today, researchers continue to search for causes of cancer and strive to find new and better ways to diagnose, treat, and, in some cases, even prevent the disease. What's different, however, is how they go about their work.

Most of what we know about cancer is the result of research, defined as a trained inquiry or experiment that follows what is known as the scientific method. Scientists ask a question, design experiments to answer that question, collect data, interpret the results, and apply those results to better our society.

Types of Research

- **In vitro research:** studies of human or animal cells growing in laboratory dishes or flasks.
- **In vivo research:** studies that use animals or humans.
- **Clinical research:** studies of human patients.
- **Epidemiological research:** the study of diseases in populations by collecting and analyzing statistical data.
- **Review studies** (meta-analyses): researchers combine and analyze the findings from several other studies.
- **Case control studies:** researchers compare data on people who have an illness with apparently similar healthy people matched by age, sex, and other factors, in order to define risk factors for an illness.
- **Population studies:** researchers look at disease incidence and death rates based upon an exact count of a given population in a specific geographic area.
- **Prospective studies:** researchers look at a group of people at a specific point (or points) in time and then wait to see who gets what diseases before making associations between lifestyle and risk of illness.
- **Retrospective studies:** researchers compare people with a disease or other condition to a similar group of people who aren't affected and then look back in time to see what differences in their lifestyles might have contributed to the different outcomes in their health status.

Epidemiological Research

In the field of cancer, epidemiologists look at how many people have cancer; who gets specific types of cancer; and what factors (such as environment, job hazards, family patterns, smoking, and diet) play a part in the development of cancer. This research is the source of many of our ideas about the causes of cancer, the factors that determine high risk for development of cancer, and methods for prevention of cancer.

It is important to note that epidemiological studies only point to an association between a factor and a disease. These studies *don't provide evidence* of cause and effect. For example, epidemiological studies show that a diet high in fruits, vegetables, and grains is associated with a lower risk of cancer, but the studies don't show how or why this type of diet lowers risk. To learn about cause and effect, researchers must conduct laboratory experiments on animals or isolated cells, or clinical trials.

Animal Research

Much of what is known about human physiology, such as organ functions, is based on research studies with suitable animal models. There is virtually no area of medicine that has not benefited enormously from appropriate animal model studies. Examples include the development of antibiotics, organ transplantation, smallpox, hepatitis, and polio vaccines, and cancer treatments such as those for childhood leukemia.

Animal research is crucial for understanding the biological processes involved in cancer, such as the causes of cancer and the development of chemotherapy drugs and regimens. All methods of treatment must first be tested in animals. Through research with animals, scientists can learn how to prevent cancer by identifying cancer-causing substances and the dietary factors that inhibit or encourage the growth of cancer. They can also study the effectiveness of new drugs and types of surgery, new ways to deliver radiation treatment, and other new treatments.

In early phases of research, test tube experiments can be done, and techniques involving human cell and tissue cultures continue to be developed. But treatments must also be tested on living systems, made of interrelated organs, to identify and evaluate proper doses and possible side effects in humans. Every drug must be tested on several species of animals before its proper dosage and side effects can be determined and before it can be tested with reasonable assurance of safety in humans. Risk assessment of new chemicals and occupational exposures are also most accurately tested in animal systems.

Computer models cannot predict the unusual effects of drugs upon organ systems, such as how the body will metabolize and clear both the drug and its metabolic product from the system, or whether or not the drug will actually have the power to produce the desired effect.

The ACS expects its research grantees to observe the traditional, compassionate ethics of animal experimentation. In addition, the ACS requires research grantees, individuals, and institutions, to be in compliance with the Federal Animal Welfare Act, which was amended in 1985. Among other regulations, this Act provides that these procedures are conducted under supervision of a licensed veterinarian. Most institutions also have their own review boards, which monitor all experiments using animals.

Clinical Trials and Informed Consent

Clinical trials provide scientific evidence about the effectiveness of a therapy in humans. While a therapy may have been shown to be effective in animals, it must be proven to be effective in humans.

In cancer research, a clinical trial is a study conducted with cancer patients, usually to evaluate a new treatment. Each study is designed to answer scientific questions and to find new and better ways to help cancer patients. For example, some clinical trials compare the best known conventional therapy with a newer therapy to see if one produces more cures and causes fewer side effects than the other. The search for good cancer treatments begins with basic research in laboratory and animal studies. The best therapies identified in basic research are studied in patients, hopefully leading to findings that may help many people. Not all clinical trials use new anti-cancer drugs. Now operations, new radiation techniques, and other new treatments such as immunotherapy and gene therapy are also studied in clinical trials.

Advances in medicine and science are the results of new ideas and approaches developed through research. New cancer treatments must prove to be safe and effective in scientific studies with a certain number of patients before they can be made widely available. Then they must withstand critical review by other scientists (known as peer-review) in order to publish results in peer-reviewed medical and scientific journals. Conventional treatments, the ones now being used, are often the basis for building new and better treatments. Many conventional treatments were first shown to be effective in clinical trials. Clinical trials show researchers which therapies are more effective than others. This is the best way to identify an effective new treatment. New therapies are designed to take advantage of what has worked in the past, and to improve on this base.

The gold standard of biomedical research is the randomized clinical trial. In a randomized clinical trial, patients are randomly assigned either to a group receiving the experimental treatment, or to a control group, which receives the conventional treatment. By comparing the effects of treatment on both groups, scientists can determine whether the experimental treatment is better than the conventional treatment

Clinical trials are carried out in steps called phases. Each phase is designed to find different information. Patients may be eligible for studies in different phases, depending on their general condition and the type and stage of their cancer.

The purpose of a **Phase I** study is to find the best way to give a new treatment and how much of it can be given safely. Physicians watch patients carefully for any harmful side effects. Even if a new treatment has been well tested in laboratory and animal studies, the side effects in patients are not completely predictable.

Phase II trials determine the effectiveness of a research treatment after safety has been evaluated in a Phase I trial. Patients are closely observed for an anticancer effect by careful measurement of cancer sites present at the beginning of the trial. In addition to monitoring patients for response, any side effects are carefully recorded and assessed.

Phase III trials require entry of large numbers of patients. Some trials enroll thousands of patients. The purpose of these studies is to compare a new treatment with the conventional treatment. One of the patient groups will receive conventional (the most accepted) treatment. The group that receives the conventional treatment is called the "control group." The second patient group will receive the new treatment being studied to see if this new treatment improves survival. All patients in Phase III trials are monitored closely for side effects, and treatment is discontinued if the side effects are too severe.

Informed Consent

An important part of clinical trials is a process called informed consent. In general, informed consent means that a physician or nurse must assure that the patient has been informed of the treatment or procedure and obtain the patient's consent before beginning diagnosis or treatment. In some cases, even a simple blood test or an injection requires written permission from the patient. In addition, medical care cannot begin unless the patient gives consent, as long as the patient is mentally and physically able to discuss his condition. If the patient is a minor, has a serious mental disability, or cannot communicate consent, then the parents, legal guardian, or person authorized by the court (usually a close family member who has reason to know what the patient would want) must give consent.

Informed consent laws apply to physicians and, increasingly, to nurses, and they vary from state to state. Some states have very specific laws governing particular situations (eg, the issues of treatment for breast cancer or for clinical trials). Some states call only for "reasonable" information, while others require "full and complete disclosure." The patient gives consent by signing a document that names the procedures to be performed. The language of the document may be very general, stating only that the patient has been informed of the risks of the treatment and what other treatments are available, or it may be very specific, outlining in detail what the risks and other options are. The patient may be signing for one specific procedure, or may give blanket approval for any procedures that the health provider decides are necessary.

The Placebo Effect

Placebos are sometimes used in clinical trials to test new medications or new treatments. A placebo is a substance or other kind of treatment that seems therapeutic, but is actually inactive. Even though placebos lack chemical or other value in and of themselves, they have a very real effect in 30% to 40% of patients.

In order to study the benefit of a new treatment when the effect of the new treatment is measured against no treatment, the study will involve two patient groups. Half the people in the study are given the actual medication, and the other half receive a current conventional treatment or placebo. A placebo is given only when there is no useful conventional treatment. If any treatments are available that might help a patient, these will be given instead of a placebo. The placebo looks, tastes, or feels just like the actual treatment. In a double-blind controlled study, neither the subjects nor the investigators know who receives which treatment. People who receive the placebo in medical studies play an important role because their reactions provide a base line against which the effect of the treatment being tested can be accurately measured.

Because people do not know when they are taking a placebo, and because they believe in the treatment and in their physician, 3 or 4 people out of every 10 will react to the placebo as though it were the active treatment. Their pain will lessen, or they will feel better generally. This change in signs or symptoms as a result of receiving a placebo is called a placebo response. Placebos can be so effective that they can actually produce unwanted side effects, including headaches, nervousness, nausea, and constipation.

A "placebo effect" is a change in a sign or symptom as a result of a nonspecific effect of a treatment or patient-physician interaction. A placebo effect can occur without the presence of a placebo. The relationship between a physician and patient can have a significant effect on the patient's symptoms. This effect occurs because the patient believes in the substance, the treatment, or the physician. The patient's mind somehow influences other physiologic systems in his or her body. Those systems act to bring about helpful results.

There is no question that the placebo effect is real. It has been the subject of many careful scientific tests. It is solid evidence that the mind can have a direct effect on the physical sensations we feel in our bodies.

Some scientific evidence suggests that the placebo effect may be due to the release of endorphins in the brain. Endorphins are the body's own morphine-like painkillers. However, science is just beginning to learn exactly how the placebo effect occurs.

Some scientists believe the effectiveness of many alternative therapies may simply be a placebo effect. The patient believed in the treatment and wanted it to work, and so it did. Or there was a belief that it did. If the positive effect remained and brought about long-lasting health, it would not be a placebo, but a new effective treatment.

Anecdotal Reports

Anecdotal stories from people who claim that a complementary or alternative method cured their disease can be quite powerful, especially for people with cancer. In recent years, a number of complementary and alternative methods for preventing or treating cancer have gained widespread attention, often on the basis of anecdotal reports and testimonial stories.

Television news shows, magazines, and even product advertisements, frequently carry compelling stories about children and adults with cancer who turned to a complementary or alternative method after a conventional treatment did not work; or they used a complementary or alternative method instead of conventional treatment. Because the person is alive to tell his or her story and appears to be restored to health, there is a strong implication that the complementary or alternative treatment is safe and effective, even if there is no scientific evidence to support the claim.

When it comes to anecdotal reports or personal testimonials about the effectiveness of complementary or alternative methods, it's important to remember that if something sounds too good to be true, it usually is. Sometimes the person providing the testimonial never had a biopsy to prove he actually had cancer. In such cases, a lump caused by some noncancerous condition may go away on its own shortly after the patient is treated with an alternative therapy. If the patient mistakenly believes the lump was cancerous, he will probably incorrectly attribute its disappearance to the treatment. In other cases, people treated with both conventional and complementary therapy may attribute benefit to the complementary therapy when the conventional treatment was really what helped them.

It's important to read the fine print describing how a product works rather than relying on one person's experience with the product. Claims about complementary or alternative methods that promise to instantly cure cancer, make tumors disappear, or prevent the disease from ever occurring are not based on scientific evidence and can be dangerous for people with cancer. Also note that patients harmed by alternative treatments are not selected by promoters for testimonials. For every claim of benefit, there may be many patients who get much worse. In contrast, conventional clinical trials determine and report how many patients are helped and harmed.

Research on Complementary and Alternative Methods

According to the National Center for Complementary and Alternative Medicine (NCCAM), complementary and alternative medicine needs to be investigated using the same scientific methods used in conventional medicine. The NCCAM encourages valid information about complementary and alternative medicine, applying the same rigorous research methods as the current standard in conventional medicine. This is because the research often involves novel concepts and claims, and uses complex systems of practice that need systematic, explicit, and comprehensive knowledge and skills to investigate.

Moving the field from alternative to evidence-based medicine will require the continued support of the NCCAM and the National Cancer Institute, the dedication of complementary and alternative medicine research centers, and the willingness of the oncology and complementary and alternative medicine communities to do the research.

History and Trends

According to a study published in the *Journal of the American Medical Association (JAMA)*, an estimated 42% of adult Americans—about 83 million people—used at least 1 of 16 complementary or alternative therapies the previous year, spending about $34 billion, most of it out-of-pocket. Moreover, the number of Americans using alternative therapies was up 38% compared to 1990 when a similar survey was conducted. It has also been reported that up to 50% of cancer patients in the United States use complementary and alternative medicine, spending more than $25 billion annually.

A recent *Consumer Reports* survey of 46,000 people found that 35% used complementary and alternative therapies. Although such methods have become popular, the survey reported that conventional medicine is still the treatment of choice. For example, prescription drugs were rated more effective than herbal remedies. They recommended that consumers consult a medical doctor for diagnosis and advice before seeking help from any alternative practitioner.

Clearly, health care consumers in America are turning to complementary and alternative medicine in record numbers, despite little or no evidence to support its use in many cases. That trend has been predicted to grow even more in the 21st century. Americans are flocking to complementary and alternative practitioners as never before, seeking treatments for chronic pain, anxiety, depression, insomnia, allergies, arthritis, Alzheimer's disease, and other long-term illnesses. The *JAMA* study showed that Americans now visit alternative practitioners more often than they see primary care physicians. In addition, herbal remedies and megavitamins are selling fast in health food stores and pharmacies, holding promises of relief from common complaints and long-term illnesses, despite being virtually unregulated for safety, effectiveness, quality, and actual content.

What is fueling this enormous appetite for the unregulated and largely unproven variety of treatments, practices, and products that make up alternative medicine? Ironically, the boon in alternative medicine may be based on the successes of conventional medicine. Primarily through the efforts of scientific medicine in the 20th century, the average life expectancy rose from 48 years in 1900 to 76 years by 2000. As more and more people live longer lives, chronic diseases and disorders, including cancer, have become more common. Conventional medicine is less effective in dealing with chronic illnesses than in extending life, and so many health care consumers with long-term complaints are turning to alternative medicine in hopes of obtaining relief.

Advances in modern technological medicine may also play a role. Many Americans see high-tech medicine as impersonal and expensive. And with increasing pressure to provide cost-effective care, physicians tend to spend less time with patients in an effort to see more people. On the other hand, many alternative practitioners spend an average of 30 minutes with their patients, or about four times the amount of time that physicians now spend with patients.

Several large surveys have reported that the holistic approach to medicine, which focuses on the whole body rather than focusing on the illness, is one of the main reasons Americans seek complementary and alternative therapies. Holistic medicine has roots in the centuries-old customs of traditional Chinese medicine, Ayurveda (traditional medicine from India), European folk medicine, and Native American medicinal traditions in North America (see Ayurveda, page 56). Proponents argue that modern scientific medicine tends to overlook the ancient healing traditions and their gentle methods of care.

Advocates of herbal therapies in the United States point to European countries as models Americans can emulate. European health care consumers, especially the elderly, have shown a strong preference for herbal medicines in treating chronic diseases. Germany, in particular, has a highly developed herbal industry, and the country represents the largest market for herbals in Europe. Moreover, the medical establishment in Germany, and the German government, support the use of many herbal remedies. At least 70% of general practitioners in Germany prescribe herbal medicines, and the public insurance system pays for most of the medicines. From 600 to 700 herbal remedies are now sold in Germany.

In 1978, the German government established a committee called "Commission E" to evaluate the safety and effectiveness of herbal medicines. The commission was made up of physicians, pharmacists, toxicologists, pharmacologists, lay people, and pharmaceutical industry representatives. Members of the committee examined information obtained from clinical trials and field studies, single case reports, information published in the scientific literature, and opinions from medical associations. If there were no controlled clinical trials available to confirm the absolute safety and effectiveness of a particular herb, the commission determined if there was "reasonable certainty" that the herb was safe and effective based on the other data it obtained. The commission functioned until 1993 and wrote a series of monographs on about 300 commonly used medicinal herbs. The monographs were originally published in the *German Federal Gazette* and then translated into English in 1998. Commission E concluded that roughly two-thirds of the herbs they reviewed were safe and effective based on the criterion of "reasonable certainty."

There is a shift in the United States toward greater acceptance of some complementary methods and more emphasis on research into the value of these therapies. John Dingell, chairman of the Committee on Energy and Commerce of the US House of Representatives, recognized the growing trend toward the use of complementary and alternative therapies by people living with cancer in the United States. He asked the federal Office of Technology Assessment (OTA) to draw up a report on the unconventional cancer therapies that were widely used in the United States, who was using them, and what legal and safety issues were involved in their use.

The 1990 OTA report identified the trend toward unconventional cancer therapies. They noted that the side effects of some conventional treatments, along with the uncertainty of long-term survival even after apparently successful treatment, may motivate people with cancer to seek treatments outside the conventional. The overt or implied promises of effective, natural, or nontoxic treatment through alternative methods also makes them appealing. The OTA, which has since been dismantled, also commented on the safety and effectiveness of the unconventional therapies:

> *The reliability of information on the effectiveness and safety of these [unconventional] treatments is questioned by most mainstream medical authorities, in part because most reports are anecdotal or represent unsupported claims of practitioners. Research and clinical studies of unconventional cancer treatments generally have not been well designed and have not met with the approval of academic researchers. Supporters of unconventional treatments tacitly approve these reports in the absence of anything better. Thus, one of the major rifts separating supporters of unconventional treatments from those in mainstream medical care and research is a distinct difference in what they accept as evidence of benefit.*

The establishment of the Office of Alternative Medicine (OAM) within the National Institutes of Health (NIH) was a major step by the US Government toward objective evaluation of complementary and alternative therapies of all sorts. The office was set up to investigate the most promising complementary and alternative medical practices and treatments using the same research standards used to determine whether conventional therapies should be given approval for public use. The OAM initially began with a $2 million budget for spending about $14.5 million annually on research. In 1999, when Congress elevated the OAM to the NCCAM, it increased the center's funding to $50 million annually.

In the 1990s, more than two dozen leading medical schools and hospitals in the United States established centers or departments to study complementary and alternative medicine, including Harvard University's Beth Israel Hospital in Boston, Columbia University in New York City, and Georgetown University in Washington, DC. And more than 27 medical schools began offering courses in complementary and alternative medicine. A number of medical centers around the country, including Stanford University Medical Center in northern California, Cedars-Sinai Medical Center in Los Angeles, and Memorial Sloan-Kettering Cancer Center in New York City, have opened integrative medicine programs or centers to offer patients massage, chiropractic, acupuncture, herbal therapies, and mind-body techniques.

The public fascination with complementary and alternative medicine is reflected in the number of books being published that provide information about unconventional therapies. In 1999, the Library Journal listed 144 book titles on complementary and alternative medicine out of 590 consumer health books published in just the first eight months of the year. The 1999 *Catalog of Integrative, Alternative, Complementary Health Books* listed more than 250 new or recently published titles.

Undoubtedly, the attitudes of those in conventional medicine toward alternative and complementary medicine are changing, but most still insist on objective, scientific evidence as the basis for judging complementary and alternative treatments. In an editorial accompanying the study that appeared in JAMA in 1998, editors of the journal argue that, "There is no alternative medicine. There is only scientifically-proven, evidence-based medicine supported by solid data, or unproven medicine for which there is no scientific evidence."

Chapter 3

How to Know What is Safe

*I*n 1937, more than 100 people, mostly children, died after taking Elixir Sulfanilamide, the drinkable form of a sulfa medicine. The liquid base of that medicine was diethylene glycol, a poisonous substance that can cause kidney failure and death. The liquid sulfa drug, manufactured in Tennessee and sold throughout the United States, had never been tested for safety. By law it didn't have to be tested, because at that time there were no government regulations that required tests for the safety of any drug sold in the United States.

The first comprehensive Food and Drugs Act of 1906, which Congress passed in reaction to risky and misleading practices in the food and drug industry, did not require testing of drugs for safety. It governed only the misbranding of drugs and the adulteration of food and drug products. In fact, the 1906 act did not even require manufacturers to report information about the safety and effectiveness of drugs.

Largely as a result of the liquid sulfa disaster, Congress passed the Federal Food, Drug, and Cosmetic Act of 1938 (FDC Act). This act required that manufacturers establish the safety of any product that was to be marketed across state lines. It also banned false and misleading labels on food, drugs, and medical devices. Unfortunately, however, Congress exempted any drug already on the market and covered under the 1906 act. Manufacturers, therefore, did not have to prove the safety of existing products, which remained for sale to unknowing consumers.

Another major public health crisis convinced Congress that even tighter regulation was required to protect the American public. Thalidomide, a drug manufactured in Germany, was widely distributed in Europe as a sedative. Of the many pregnant women who took it, nearly 4 out of 10 delivered disfigured babies. The babies were born with deformed limbs, or stumps, where arms and legs should have been. The resulting publicity was worldwide, as were demands for protection against harmful drug products.

Tennessee's popular Senator Estes Kefauver led the way. He chaired a committee that was investigating the American pharmaceutical industry. The committee produced a bill requiring proof that any drug marketed in the United States was not only safe, but also effective for its stated purpose. It passed Congress and became law, known as the Kefauver-Harris Amendments or the Drug Amendments Act of 1962. This law amended the FDC Act and applied to every "new " drug (a drug sold after 1962) and any drug sold after 1938. The FDA was given the authority to enforce the regulations and serve as a watchdog over the drug industry.

However, thousands of over-the-counter (OTC) drugs were already available for sale throughout the United States. In response to the Drug Amendments of 1962, the FDA established the Drug Efficacy Study Implementation (DESI) program. The DESI program reviewed those drug products that were approved between 1938 and 1962 solely on the basis of safety. As a result of this three-decade long process, more than 3,400 drugs with over 16,000 separate therapeutic claims were evaluated, using the criteria of "substantial evidence" for effectiveness. Only 12% of the drug products had acceptable claims. About 60% of the drugs were found to have at least one acceptable claim; however, 60% of the claims were rejected out of lack of evidence for effectiveness.

Drug Development in the United States

In the decades following the 1962 Drug Amendments, the FDA refined a regulatory scheme for both drug development and the marketing of foods in the United States. Drugs and foods are regulated in different ways by the FDA. Drugs must be shown to be both safe and effective before they are marketed to the public. Drugs must also undergo clinical trials that demonstrate their safety, effectiveness, potential interactions with other substances, and safe dosage for the specific clinical use. The FDA must review these studies and authorize the use of the drug. The FDA has the authority to prohibit interstate marketing of unsafe or ineffective drugs and to sanction manufacturers, promoters, and distributors who violate the law.

The requirements for marketing a drug in the United States are set out in the FDC Act. Under the FDC Act, a manufacturer must establish evidence of safety and effectiveness for what the FDA calls "new" drugs. The Act defines a new drug as "...any drug...the composition of which is such that the drug is not generally recognized, among experts qualified by scientific training and experience to evaluate the safety and effectiveness of drugs, as safe and effective for use under the conditions prescribed, recommended, or suggested in the labeling thereof."

The law specifies that a new drug cannot be approved by the FDA unless there is "substantial evidence" that it is safe and effective to diagnose, treat, cure, or prevent a specific disease or medical condition. Substantial evidence must be proven through well-controlled studies as described earlier. It must be conducted by qualified experts who, on the basis of the data, can fairly and responsibly conclude that the drug will have the effect it claims under the conditions of use prescribed, recommended, or suggested in the labeling or proposed labeling.

If the drug has never before been used in humans, animal studies are required prior to starting clinical (human) studies of the drug. To conduct a clinical research study on an unapproved drug, a company or individual researcher must submit to the FDA an Investigational New Drug (IND) application. If the IND application meets the FDA's requirements, experimental clinical research can begin. Small clinical trials are usually done initially and then one or more large, randomized clinical trials are conducted to demonstrate the drug's safety and effectiveness for its intended use (see Evaluating Treatment, page 10).

The law is designed to protect the consumer by making sure that a high standard of evidence has been met through an "adequate and well-controlled investigation." The FDA defines such a study as having these characteristics:

- It includes a clear statement of the objectives of the investigation and a summary of the proposed or actual methods of analysis in the protocol for the study and in the report of its results.
- It uses a design that permits a valid comparison with a control to provide a quantitative assessment of drug effect.
- Its method of selection of subjects provides adequate assurance that the subjects have the disease or condition being studied.
- Its method of assigning patients to treatment and control groups minimizes bias.
- Measures are taken to minimize bias on the part of the subjects, observers, and analysts of the data.
- Its methods of assessment of subjects' response are well-defined and reliable.
- There is an analysis of the results of the study adequate to assess the effects of the drug.

A key point to make about the standard of evidence is that anecdotal evidence (testimonials) from physicians or patients who have used the drug under study is not enough to meet the FDA's definition of safety and effectiveness. Ruling in a case involving the FDC Act, one judge put it this way:

> It is simply not enough to show that some people, even experts, have a belief in safety and effectiveness. A reasonable number of Americans will sincerely attest to the worth of almost any product or even idea. To remove the aberrations in uniformity, which can result from a well-staged "swearing match," the law requires more. Indeed, it has been heretofore held that the purpose of the normal inquiry is not to determine safety and effectiveness at all, but to ascertain the drug's general reputation in the scientific community for such characteristics. It is certain that a conflicting reputation is insufficient to establish general recognition. Therefore, what is required is more than belief, even by an expert; it is a general recognition based upon substantial scientific evidence as delineated in the regulatory guidelines.

The FDC Act recognizes different levels of safety risk for drugs that have a benefit in treating severe illnesses, such as cancer, but the benefits must outweigh the risks. For example, a number of cancer drugs have side effects so serious that the FDA would not approve them for use in treating less severe illness. However, because their benefits to cancer patients are considered greater than their risks, the FDA has approved them for use in treating cancer.

The FDC Act also allows researchers who have conducted animal studies and are involved in clinical trials to provide certain drugs that have not yet been approved by the FDA to patients who have life-threatening or other serious diseases that may be helped by the drug. As stated in the regulations, the purpose of this rule is "to facilitate the availability of promising new drugs to desperately ill patients as early in the drug development process as possible, before general marketing begins, and to obtain additional data on the drug's safety and effectiveness." The rule, which was written into the Act in 1988, permits eligible patients not enrolled in the clinical trials to receive drugs that are in phase III, or the final stage of study in the trials, or under certain circumstances, even drugs in phase II of the trials. The FDA requires manufacturers and researchers to provide a treatment protocol and experimental data on the drug before it grants approval to make the drug available to patients outside the trial. This is referred to as emergency (often referred to as compassionate) use of an investigational drug.

When the FDA finally approves a drug for marketing, it approves the product for specific uses or indications that were studied in the clinical trials. The approved indications for use must appear on the printed inserts packaged with the drug, along with the appropriate dose, route, and schedules, information on adverse reactions experienced during the drug's development, and any warning statements or contraindications for use. However, health professionals may prescribe the drug for other medical conditions if, in their professional opinion, the medical situation warrants it. This practice is referred to as *off-label* use of a drug, and it is done in cases in which there is sufficient scientific evidence to believe that the drug will be effective in treating the unapproved conditions.

Food Regulation

The regulations for foods differ significantly from those of drugs. Foods include conventional foods (those in conventional food form, such as cheese, processed foods, chewing gum, tea, sodas, etc.), food additives (items added to conventional foods, including colors, flavors, spices and preservatives), dietary supplements (see page 26), and "Foods for Special Dietary Uses" (eg, infant and enteral formulas, phenylketonuria diets).

Under the FDC Act and its various amendments, foods are required to be properly labeled, not adulterated or misbranded. In 1990, the Nutrition Labeling and Education Act (NLEA) required that the food label follow a specific format that provides nutrient content information for the consumer (see sample food label, page 25). The NLEA also authorized foods to carry nutrient content claims ("contains calcium," "fat free," or "lite"), and health claims. Health claims (eg, "folate may reduce the chance of pregnant women delivering an infant with neural tube defects") must be supported by evidence that is under "significant substantial agreement." These claims generally require information from in vitro, animal, and

All food labels must follow a specific format that provides standard nutritional content.

Nutrition Facts

Serving Size 24 pieces (30g)
Servings Per Container About 9

These listings show the average serving size and number of servings found in the package.

Amount Per Serving

Calories 130	Calories from Fat 40

% Daily Value*

Total Fat 4.5g	**7%**
Saturated Fat 1g	**4%**
Cholesterol 0mg	**0%**
Sodium 135mg	**6%**
Total Carbohydrate 23g	**8%**
Dietary Fiber Less than 1g	**3%**
Sugars 8g	
Protein 2g	

Vitamin A 0%	•	**Vitamin C 0%**
Calcium 0%	•	**Iron 4%**

The % value shows how the content of this food compares and fits into an average 2,000 calorie daily diet.

* Percent Daily Values are based on a 2,000 calorie diet. Your daily values may be higher or lower depending on your calorie needs:

	Calories	2,000	2,500
Total Fat	Less than	65g	80g
Sat Fat	Less than	20g	25g
Cholesterol	Less than	300mg	300mg
Sodium	Less than	2,400mg	2,400mg
Total Carbohydrate		300g	375g
Dietary Fiber		25g	30g

clinical studies to be submitted to the FDA, and the claims statements are preapproved by the FDA prior to the product being marketed.

Dietary Supplements

Another category of foods which has received a tremendous amount of attention over the past decade is dietary supplements. What exactly is a dietary supplement? If you take a vitamin pill regularly, you are taking a dietary supplement. That is, you are adding something to your diet of foods, most likely in an attempt to make up for a less-than-perfect diet, to promote good health, or to help speed healing when illness strikes.

The term *dietary supplement* includes vitamins, minerals, herbs, amino acids, and other products that are not already approved as drugs. Dietary supplements are sold in grocery stores, health food shops, drug stores, national discount chain stores, mail-order catalogs, and through television programs, the Internet, and direct sales. Vitamins are the supplements most often purchased in this country.

Dietary supplements as a category of foods were defined by the 1994 Dietary Supplement Health and Education Act (DSHEA). As a result of the DSHEA, dietary ingredients used in dietary supplements are no longer subject to the premarket safety evaluations required of other new food ingredients, such as "food additives," or for new uses of old food ingredients. However, they must meet the requirements of other safety provisions.

The DSHEA amends the adulteration provisions of the FDC Act. Under the DSHEA a dietary supplement is adulterated if it or one of its ingredients presents "a significant or unreasonable risk of illness or injury" when used as directed on the label or under normal conditions of use. A dietary supplement that contains an additional "new dietary ingredient" is said to be adulterated when there is inadequate information to ensure the new ingredient will not cause a significant or unreasonable risk of illness or injury. Supplement manufacturers must notify the FDA at least 75 days before marketing products containing new dietary ingredients by providing the agency with the documentation of safety.

Any interested party, including a manufacturer of a dietary supplement, may petition the FDA to issue an order prescribing the conditions of use under which a new dietary ingredient will reasonably be expected to be safe. The Secretary of the Department of Health and Human Services (DHHS) may also declare that a dietary supplement or dietary ingredient poses an imminent hazard to public health or safety. However, as with any other food product, it is a manufacturer's responsibility to ensure that the dietary supplement is safe and properly labeled before marketing.

The DHHS is currently writing regulations that will define the standards for manufacturing dietary supplements. Such regulations, called *Good Manufacturing Processes* (GMPs) will be more rigorous for dietary supplements than those applicable to conventional foods, but much less stringent than those for drugs. While drug GMPs are much stronger requirements, requiring consistency from batch to batch of product, GMPs for conventional foods deal mostly with tolerances for filth, pesticides, and other contaminants. GMPs for dietary supplements will be somewhere in the middle of these extremes. However, one major difference between drug and dietary supplements is that for drugs the FDA reviews the chemistry, manufacturing, and quality controls prior to marketing, which is not done for dietary supplements.

Under the DSHEA retailers and distributors of dietary supplements are permitted to make available third-party materials to help inform consumers about any health-related benefits of dietary supplements. These materials, which include articles, book chapters, scientific abstracts, or other third-party publications, cannot be false or misleading; cannot promote a specific brand of supplement; and must be displayed with other similar materials to present a balanced view. The literature must be displayed separately from the dietary supplements themselves and may not have other information attached, such as product promotional literature.

Dietary supplements can bear four types of claims: nutritional claims, claims of well being, health claims (see above), and structure or function claims. *Nutritional claims* are statements about the effects of dietary supplements, vitamins, and minerals on known nutrient-deficiency diseases (eg, "vitamin C prevents scurvy"). These statements are permissible—as long as these statements disclose the prevalence of the disease in the United States. Such claims are not required to be pre-approved by the FDA. Claims of *well being* are just that: they are claims such as "makes you feel better." These claims also are not preapproved by the agency. *Health claims*, which are authorized under the NLEA (see page 24) may make risk reduction claims, as described above. Such claims require testing and approval by the FDA.

The most controversial and confusing of the claims is the effect of the dietary supplement or ingredient to affect the *structure* or *function* of the body. In January 2000, the FDA published a ruling to clarify which kinds of structure or function claims would be acceptable and which would be unacceptable for dietary supplements. The changes expanded the number of acceptable structure or function claims and revised the definition of disease from a prior proposal. The DSHEA allows manufacturers to describe the product's effects on the mechanism of action (works as an antioxidant), cellular structure (helps membrane stability), on the body's physiology (promotes normal urinary flow), or on chemical or laboratory parameters (supports normal blood glucose). The rule permits claims of maintenance (eg, "maintains a healthy circulatory system"), other non-disease claims (eg, "helps you relax"), and claims for common conditions and symptoms related to life stages (eg, for symptoms of premenstrual syndrome [PMS[, menopause, adolescence, and aging). Serious conditions associated with aging (eg, osteoporosis), menopause, and adolescence will continue to be treated as diseases. Because these statements are not reviewed by the FDA prior to being sold to the public, manufacturers are required to include a disclaimer on the label: ***"This statement has not been evaluated by the Food and Drug Administration. This product is not intended to***

diagnose, treat, cure, or prevent any disease."

It is easy for consumers to misunderstand when interpreting exactly what structure or function claims really mean. Many people assume that a statement such as "maintains a healthy prostate gland" means that the herb has been proven to prevent or remove prostate diseases such as cancer of the prostate. In fact, no such evidence is required of the company selling an herb bearing this information on its package.

Manufacturers must ensure that the claims on the label (what is on the product and its immediate packaging materials) and in its labeling (all other materials accompanying the product, as well as advertising and promotion, including broadcast and print ads, catalogs, infomercials, and direct marketing materials) are "truthful and not misleading." While the product label is under the jurisdiction of the FDA, the labeling is regulated by the Federal Trade Commission (FTC). The FDA regulates the labeling of only prescription products. The FTC has published guidelines for advertisers that describe the principles it uses to evaluate substantiation of claims made for dietary supplements. The FTC evaluates the "totality" and "relevance" of the evidence.

Like most other food products, dietary supplement products must bear ingredient labeling. If a supplement product states that its ingredients are *USP*, that is, conforming to the specifications in the US Pharmacopeia, or other official compendium, then it is misbranded if it does not conform to those specifications. If not covered by a compendium, a dietary supplement must be the product identified on the label and have the strength it is represented as having.

Safety and Effectiveness

Do the terms *safe* and *effective* mean the same for foods and drugs? Drugs are those products that are intended to diagnose, prevent, treat, alleviate, or cure a disease and are required by the FDC Act to have documented safety and effectiveness prior to marketing. For drugs, safety is a relative term. Drugs are essentially considered unsafe until proven safe for a particular clinical indication. In contrast, foods, including dietary supplements, are assumed safe for the general population's use, or "Generally Recognized as Safe" or "GRAS." Under the 1994 DSHEA, "safe" means that the ingredients in a dietary supplement do not present a "significant or unreasonable risk" of causing illness or injury when the supplement is used as directed on the label or under normal conditions of use if there are no directions on the label. The Secretary of the DHHS may declare that a dietary supplement or ingredient presents an "imminent hazard" to public health or public safety.

The assessment of safety, however, is not straightforward. For approved drugs, adverse event (AE) reporting is required by the FDC Act. For foods, AE reporting by manufacturers is not a requirement. Consumers and health professionals are encouraged to report AEs to the MedWatch program (see Reporting Adverse Reactions, page 36). In addition, although the

FDA may be able to assess all of the AEs reported, unlike prescription drugs, there is no information as to how many individuals may have purchased the product and what their experience was. For example, if there are 10 AE reports for a particular dietary supplement, it is unknown if the incidence of the event represents 10 out of 100 or 10 out of 1 million users.

Regarding effectiveness, only those drug products that are approved for safety and effectiveness can claim effectiveness. Some drugs, such as those that were on the US market prior to the first comprehensive FDC Act passed in 1938, and homeopathic drugs (which have been deferred from the drug regulatory process), are *not approved* for safety or effectiveness. While these drugs may carry drug *claims*, they cannot advertise that they have been *approved* as safe or effective. While certain dietary supplements, such as the essential vitamins and minerals, may be *effective* in preventing a specific deficiency, the term *effectiveness* does not generally apply to food products. Even health claims, which are preapproved by the FDA, are usually couched in terms of prevention or risk reduction, rather than effectiveness. Regardless of what is claimed, the FTC requires proof in the form of adequate scientific studies.

Balancing Consumer Choice

Signs of Possible Fraudulent Products Include

- Claims that promote the supplement with such terms as *miracle cure, breakthrough,* or *new discovery.*
- Claims that the supplement has benefits but no side effects.
- Claims that the supplement can be used for a wide variety of unrelated illnesses.
- Claims that the treatment is safe and effective based solely on testimonials.
- Claims that the treatment is based on a secret ingredient or method.

In recent years, a number of legal challenges have been launched in the courts on behalf of people with cancer against laws and regulations designed to protect patients from untested drugs, such as the FDC Act. These cases charge that the laws limit cancer patients' access to complementary and alternative treatments and deny the patients freedom of choice in medical care. There are two opposing forces at work: those who defend the laws as consumer protection, and those who want to change the laws to allow consumers, such as cancer patients, freedom of choice. In general, the courts have not agreed with those arguing for freedom of choice in the unregulated use of complementary and alternative cancer treatments. Judges generally support the role of the current laws in protecting the public from drugs or treatments that might not be safe or effective. The thalidomide situation is a good example of the outcry from consumers for protection against unsafe products. Balancing freedom with protection poses difficult challenges.

There is a great need for public protection in this area. We are in a "let the buyer beware" mode when it comes to nutritional dietary supplements and herbal medicines. To this day, there is no requirement for proof of safety, accurate labeling, or proof of a health benefit for dietary supplements sold in the United States. Congress has seen the need to protect the public against harmful prescription medications, but this protection is not extended to dietary supplements sold directly to consumers.

In 1994, Congress attempted to pass such protective legislation. However, a multimillion-dollar effort by the food-supplement industry resulted in passage of a scaled-down DSHEA of 1994. That legislation protected thousands of vitamins, herbs, minerals, and any other food supplements already on the market from being reviewed. The regulation gives the FDA permission to stop production of a product only when the FDA proves that the product is dangerous to the health of Americans. Manufacturers still are not required to show that their products are safe or effective prior to marketing.

While Congress has limited the FDA's regulatory power over the dietary supplement industry, there are other government agencies that administer laws that apply to the sale of nutritional supplements and herbal remedies. The US Postal Service controls products marketed through the mail. From time to time, it has challenged products accompanied by remarkable claims of cures for cancer and other diseases. As described above, the FTC regulates the advertising of food, cosmetics, non-prescription products, and some other health-related goods and services that are sold across state lines. Many dietary supplements are sold over the Internet. Internet marketing is also regulated by the FTC in the same way as promotions through other advertising media. In addition to the federal government, individual states have regulatory powers through licensing laws. State boards can regulate the practice of the healing arts, including the licensing and scope of practice for health professionals, conventional practitioners and "alternative" practitioners. A few states have new laws regulating alternative and complementary therapies and their use by physicians.

But the public still has limited protection against the marketing of products that often promise much and produce little if any benefit. Indeed, some products marketed in health food stores have recently been removed from shelves only after serious harm and even death from those products were reported.

Until Congress passes useful legislation, the challenge to consumers is to determine which products are safe and which are not. The American Cancer Society (ACS) advises people living with cancer, and other health care consumers, to read labels carefully and consult with physicians before buying herbal medicines and food supplements. Just because a product is labeled "natural" does not mean that it is safe.

If a label on a dietary supplement makes a claim that the product can diagnose, treat, cure, or prevent disease, such as "cures cancer," the product is being sold illegally as a drug.

Botanicals as Medicines

In addition to vitamins and minerals, the term *dietary supplement* also includes botanical products. Botanicals include products such as garlic, ginger, ginkgo biloba, St. John's wort, and echinacea. It is estimated that 4 billion people, 80% of the world's population, presently use herbals as medicine for some aspect of primary health care. They have a long history of use in virtually every ancient culture. In many underdeveloped areas of the world, herbal remedies are the only medicines available to treat ailments of all kinds.

In the earliest days, herbs were chosen for medicinal purposes by what is now called the doctrine of signatures. If a plant's leaf was heart-shaped, for example, it would be used to treat heart ailments. If its flower was red, it would be used to treat blood problems, and so on. Today, of course, we know that the herb's chemical make-up, not its shape or color, makes it useful as a medication. Indeed, many chemicals taken from herbs have become modern drugs. At the beginning of the 20th century, the majority of the drugs used in the United States were from natural sources, including plants. Today about one in four drugs prescribed today came from plants. Although many chemotherapy drugs, such as paclitaxel (Taxol®) and vinblastine, are derived from plant sources, no raw herbal medicine has yet been approved in the United States by the FDA for use as a drug to treat cancer. However, the rawer forms of plants are being studied, and there are currently more than 100 Investigative New Drug (IND) applications that are studying plant and other natural products for drug indications.

Botanicals may be plants, either whole plants, or plant parts, including roots, stems, flowers, leaves, pollen, and juices. The term herbal refers specifically to the leafy part of a plant. Botanicals are made up of many chemicals, some helpful and others dangerous. In contrast, researchers and manufacturers who develop and produce conventional drugs from plant sources seek to purify the beneficial substances so the patient can avoid any harmful ones initially present in the plant material.

There are many forms in which botanicals are sold: dried, finely chopped, powdered, and in capsule or liquid form. Botanical products may include only a specific part of one plant or a mixture of many plants. They may be swallowed as tablets or capsules, brewed as teas, or applied to the skin as gels, salves, or perfumes, and added to bath salts or soaps and other cosmetics.

Botanicals are regulated by their "intended use," as determined from their label and labeling. This means, that the manufacturer's intent is determined through the claims made (or not made) about the product. Products that are intended to prevent or treat disease are classified as drugs. Cascara and Senna are examples of OTC botanical drugs that have been on the market prior to the 1938 FDC Act. Others are licensed biological products, such as the allergenic vaccines. Still others are being sold as devices, such as adhesives, poultices, and dental materials.

Botanicals are mostly sold as drugs in countries other than the United States. Although some countries have different regulatory requirements for botanicals that have been used traditionally as drugs in that country (eg, Traditional Chinese Medicine, German Commission E Monographs), newer botanicals are often required to undergo the same rigorous testing as other drug classes.

In the United States, botanicals are mostly sold as foods, including dietary supplements. They are self-prescribed by consumers. Self-medication can lead to problems. In other cultures, health professionals are trained in prescribing botanicals.

Many manufacturers of herbal products are conscientious about producing high-quality botanical products that are free of dangerous contaminants and contain exactly what the label lists. But other, less scrupulous manufacturers sell products that may contain little or none of the ingredients listed on the label or even too much of the ingredients. In one study of 64 ginseng products on the market, researchers found that 60% of these products contained cheaper herbs and were so watered down that they were virtually worthless. Labeling regulations, which were enacted on March 23, 1999, require the proper identification of ingredients contained in a product. However, if a botanical product is sold for considerably less money than a competing brand, it should be suspect and is probably made with inferior, lower quality ingredients.

Manufacturers are required to state on the label the part of the plant the ingredient comes from and list the ingredients in descending order (according to strength or potency) and by the ingredient's common name. Dietary ingredients that are not present in significant amounts do not need to be listed. Manufacturers must also put the company's name, address, product batch and lot numbers, and expiration date on the label. Different parts of a plant and different preparation methods can have different effects. For example, dandelion root is a laxative, while dandelion leaves contain a diuretic (increases urination). Consumers should read the product label to make sure they know the specific forms of the botanicals they purchase. Some botanicals do contain ingredients that can interact with conventional drugs, products or treatments, or may interact with other dietary supplement or food products.

Standardization

In an industry with rapidly growing numbers of products, the potential for a dietary supplement to lack quality control in manufacturing is high. The FDA, for example, found that some manufacturers were buying plant ingredients without testing to see if what they ordered was what they received and if the ingredients were free of contaminants.

The US Pharmacopeia (USP) establishes standards for the strength, quality, and purity of drugs and dietary supplements for human and veterinary use. The USP works closely with the FDA, the pharmaceutical industry, and health professions, to create reliable drug standards. Standards for vitamins and minerals have been included since 1994. In 1997, the USP began publishing standards for herbal products and continues to update and add more herbal standards yearly. The standards for these focus on the strength, quality, purity, packaging, and labeling of dietary supplements. The USP standards are published in the *United States Pharmacopoeia and the National Formulary* (USP-NF) which include over 37,000 drugs, dietary supplements, and dosage forms. Certain of these standards are legally recognized by the FDA and other regulatory agencies in the United States and throughout the world. A USP notation on the label of a dietary supplement indicates that the product complies with standards established by the USP.

The labels on vitamins and minerals may show the percentage of the daily value of the Recommended Dietary Allowance (RDA) per serving or per tablet for the vitamins and minerals the product contains. Recommended Dietary (Daily) Allowances were developed more than 40 years ago by the US Food and Nutrition Board to represent standards for the amounts of vitamins and minerals needed by a healthy person. They are the minimum amounts needed to prevent nutritional deficiencies and the diseases deficiencies can cause, such as rickets, scurvy, and beriberi. There is another standard used known as the upper tolerance intake (UTI) which represents the amounts of nutrients needed for optimal health. The UTIs are larger amounts than the standard RDAs. In addition, the National Academy of Sciences had developed a new standard known as dietary reference intakes (DRIs) that includes guidelines for the amounts of certain vitamins and minerals, such as selenium, vitamins C and E, and carotinoids (nutrients that are believed to play a role in preventing and treating cancer, such as beta carotene, lycopene, and lutein), needed for good health (see Beta Carotene, Selenium, Vitamin C, and Vitamin E). The DRIs include the Estimated Average Requirement, the Adequate Intake, the UTI, and the RDA.

The Commission on Dietary Supplement Labels established by the DSHEA of 1994 conducted a study of practices in the dietary supplement industry and provide recommendations to Congress and the Secretary of the DHHS on the regulation of label claims and statements for dietary supplements. In its final report to Congress in 1997, the commission emphasized the need for public access to the evidence manufacturers have to back up statements made on labels so consumers may make informed choices about using dietary supplements.

Adverse Reactions

More than 2,500 complaints of adverse effects of herbs have been reported to the FDA, and there have been 79 deaths reported from the use of botanicals. Many botanicals contain ingredients that can cause side effects, hazardous drug interactions, and allergic reactions. For example, ginkgo biloba, garlic, feverfew, vitamin E, and ginger can all thin blood and help prevent abnormal blood clotting, but if they are consumed by people who are also taking blood-thinning drugs, such as warfarin, heparin, or aspirin, the dietary supplements may cause excessive bleeding. St. John's Wort has recently been found to interfere with some prescription drugs, such as indinavir and cyclosporine. Taking combinations of dietary supplements could be even more dangerous by magnifying the effect of a single

Consumers should be aware of the ingredients in the herbal medicines and other dietary supplements they take and be wary of false claims. To help protect consumers, the FDA recommends that consumers

- Look for products with the USP notation, indicating that the manufacturer of the product followed standards set by the *US Pharmacopoeia* in formulating the product.
- Realize that the use of the term *natural* on an herbal product is no guarantee that the product is safe. Poisonous mushrooms are natural but not safe, for example.
- Take into account the name and reputation of the manufacturer or distributor. Herbal products and other dietary supplements made by nationally known food or drug manufacturers are more likely to have been made under tight quality controls because these companies have a reputation to uphold.
- Write to the manufacturer for more information than what is on the label of the supplement. Ask about the company's manufacturing practices and the quality-control conditions under which the product was made.

dietary supplement. In addition, if someone who is using medication to control diabetes takes ginseng supplements, his or her blood-sugar levels may fall dangerously low.

The possibility of drug supplement interactions is so high that cancer experts recommend that patients undergoing chemotherapy avoid taking dietary supplements at the same time. The same advice holds for patients receiving radiation therapy because some dietary supplements make the skin sensitive to light and cause severe reactions to radiation. A number of ingredients sold in supplements can produce severe changes in blood pressure and other dangerous interactions with anesthetics and, therefore, should not be taken before surgery. In fact, the American Society of Anesthesiologists advises that patients stop taking herbal medications at least two to three weeks before surgery to allow enough time for the herbals to clear from the body. If the patient does not have enough time to stop taking herbal medicines before surgery, he or she should bring the product to the hospital and show the anesthesiologist what it is.

The effects of dietary supplements also depend on the dose of the herb or vitamin. In this case, more is not better. The idea that if a little amount of a vitamin or mineral is good, then a megadose ought to do wonders is not valid. Orthomolecular therapy, the idea of using huge doses of vitamins to attack disease, has no scientific basis. In fact, large doses of some vitamins can have serious toxic effects. The American Psychiatric Association and the NIH have both warned against megadose therapies for the treatment of psychiatric diseases. Recent studies have suggested that high doses of beta carotene may be harmful to smokers. It is also thought that antioxidants may interact adversely with some chemotherapy drugs, although no definitive studies have been done to show the long-term effects of combining chemotherapy drugs and antioxidants in humans.

Many people are still convinced that megadoses of vitamin C can cure colds, although many good scientific studies have disproven that idea. One should be forewarned that megadoses of nutrients to treat or prevent illness can be harmful, even toxic. Too much vitamin C, for example, can interfere with the body's ability to absorb copper, an essential metal required in our body chemistry. Too much phosphorous has a negative effect on how well calcium is absorbed. Megadoses of the fat-soluble vitamins A, D, and K can easily reach toxic levels.

Because botanicals have an impact on a variety of systems in the human body, they present a potential danger by affecting the way drugs exert their activity on the body, either by increasing the drug's activity or by blocking it. Drug companies do not usually conduct research on such supplement-drug interactions, and herb manufacturers generally do not have the resources or the desire to do that type of research. So the consumer is left to search out information about possibly dangerous interactions on his or her own.

Guidelines for the Safe Use of Dietary Supplements

Rule One: Investigate before you buy or use. There are many resources in libraries and on the Internet. However, much of this information is produced by promoters and it contains biased or incorrect information (see Resource Guide). Rely on materials by a trained expert or government agency.

Rule Two: Check with your physician before you try a dietary supplement. He or she may or may not be thoroughly versed in all of the product areas, but hopefully your physician will prevent you from making a dangerous mistake.

Rule Three: Do not take any self-prescribed remedy instead of the medicine prescribed by your physician without discussing it first.

Rule Four: Introduce one product at a time. Be alert to any negative effects you experience while taking the product. Any product that produces a rash, or a feeling of sleeplessness, restlessness, anxiety, GI disturbance (nausea, vomiting, diarrhea or constipation), or severe headache, should immediately be stopped and the reaction should be reported to your physician.

Rule Five: Avoid any dietary supplements not prescribed by a licensed physician during pregnancy or if you are breast-feeding. Few, if any, of these products have been studied for safety, and their effects on the growing fetus are largely unknown.

Rule Six: Do not depend on any nonprescription product to cure cancer or any other serious disease. Regardless of the claims you might hear, "if it sounds too good to be true, it probably is."

Rule Seven: Never give a product to a baby or child under 18, without consulting your physician first. Their bodies metabolize nutrients and drugs differently from an adult's body, and the effects of the many products in children are not known.

Rule Eight: Always follow the dosage recommendations on the label. Overdosage could be deadly. Do not take a dietary supplement any longer than experts recommend.

Rule Nine: Try to avoid mixtures. The more ingredients, the greater the possibility for harmful effects.

Reporting Adverse Reactions

Health care consumers have an obligation to share information about any adverse reactions they may have with dietary supplements. If you or someone in your family suffer serious harm or illness you think is related to the use of a supplement, first call your physician or other health care provider. In addition to providing treatment, you or your physician can report the adverse reaction to the FDA by calling 1-800-FDA-1088 or going to the FDA's MedWatch Web site at http://www.fda.gov/medwatch/report/hcp.htm. You may also call the toll-free number yourself or go to the consumer page on the MedWatch Web site at http://www.fda.gov/medwatch/report/consumer/consumer.htm. In addition to reporting to the FDA, you should notify the manufacturer of the product listed on the label and the store where you bought the product.

When reporting to the FDA, you will be asked to provide

- The name, address, and telephone number of the person who got sick.
- The name and address of the physician who provided medical care.
- A description of the problem.
- The name of the product and the name of the store where it was purchased.

The MedWatch program is designed to gather information about and monitor medical products that cause serious adverse events. The FDA considers an adverse event serious if it causes death, a life-threatening situation, admission to a hospital or a longer-than-expected hospital stay, permanent disability, a birth defect, or medical or surgical care to prevent permanent impairment or damage.

In 1993, the FDA established the Special Nutritionals Adverse Event Monitoring System, which is administered by the Office of Special Nutritionals in the Center for Food Safety and Applied Nutrition at the FDA. The system maintains computer records of adverse events associated with the use of dietary supplements, infant formulas, and medical foods. MedWatch is one source of reports on adverse reactions to these special nutritionals. Other sources are letters and phone calls from consumers and health care professionals; FDA field offices; and other federal, state, and local public health agencies.

Chapter 4

Guidelines for Using Complementary and Alternative Methods of Cancer Management

A 54-year-old woman in Portland, Oregon was diagnosed with breast cancer and underwent surgery (a lumpectomy) to remove a tumor that had not spread to other parts of her body. However, because of a deep-seated disenchantment with conventional medicine, she refused conventional chemotherapy and radiation therapy after surgery. Instead, she turned to an alternative practitioner, a naturopath.

Naturopaths believe that a person's health can be maintained by avoiding things that are unnatural or artificial in the diet or the environment. They are licensed to provide primary care in Oregon and 10 other states. The natural remedies naturopaths offer include acupuncture, homeopathy, herbal medicines, and other dietary supplements. The Oregon woman's naturopath gave her a mysterious salve that, he said, would draw the cancer from her body. When that treatment failed, the alternative healer blamed the woman herself, charging she had given up on treatment. Without conventional treatment, the woman's cancer spread to her lymph nodes and then to her lungs and liver. She died a little more than a year after being diagnosed with breast cancer.

The greatest danger in alternative medicine for people with cancer lies in avoiding conventional therapy that has been shown to help treat cancer and prolong survival. Unnecessary delays and interruptions in conventional therapies are dangerous. According to recent statistics from the American Cancer Society (ACS), 96% of women diagnosed with localized breast cancer survive at least five years if they receive conventional medical care, which can include surgery, chemotherapy, and radiation therapy.

Many people with cancer use one or more kinds of alternative or complementary therapies. Often they are reluctant to tell their physicians about their decision. The best approach is to look carefully at your choices. There are many complementary methods you can safely use along with conventional treatment to help relieve symptoms or side effects, to ease pain, and to help you enjoy life more. Here is a partial list of some complementary methods that some people have found helpful when used along with conventional medical treatment:

- aromatherapy
- art therapy
- biofeedback
- massage therapy
- meditation
- music therapy
- prayer, spiritual practices
- tai chi
- yoga

Questions to Ask About Complementary and Alternative Methods

When evaluating any complementary or alternative method, ask yourself the following questions:

- What claims are made for the treatment: to cure the cancer? to enable the conventional treatment to work better? to relieve symptoms or side effects?
- What are the credentials of those supporting the treatment? Are they recognized experts in cancer treatment? Have they published their findings in trustworthy medical journals?
- How is the method promoted? Is it promoted only in the mass media (books, magazines, TV, and radio talk shows) rather than in scientific journals?
- What are the costs of the therapy?
- Is the method widely available for use within the health care community, or is it controlled with limited access to its use?
- If used in place of conventional therapies or clinical trials, will the ensuing delay in conventional treatment affect any chances for cure or advance the cancer stage?

In addition, use the checklist below to spot those approaches that might be open to question. If you are not sure, talk to your physician or nurse before moving ahead.

- Is the treatment based on an unproven theory?
- Does the treatment promise a cure for all cancers?
- Are you told not to use conventional medical treatment?
- Is the treatment or drug a secret that only certain people can give?
- Is the treatment or drug offered by only one individual?
- Does the treatment require you to travel to another country?
- Do the promoters attack the medical or scientific establishment?

Talking With Your Physician

About 60% of all people trying complementary or alternative therapies do not tell their physicians they are trying these treatments. Many patients feel uncomfortable asking their physician about complementary or alternative treatments. But most medical professionals understand that patients and caregivers want to do all they can to improve their quality of life or improve the quality of life for their loved ones. Although people may be reluctant to share their complementary or alternative therapy interests with their physician, it could be dangerous to the health of the person with cancer to withhold information.

The best approach is to look carefully at your choices. Talk to your physician about any method you are considering. Consider the risks and benefits of using any complementary or alternative methods and make an informed decision in an atmosphere of shared decision-making. There are many *complementary* methods you can safely use along with conventional treatment to help relieve symptoms or side effects, to ease pain, and to experience a better quality of life.

If you are considering using complementary or alternative therapies, here are some tips for your discussion with your physician:

- Educate yourself first. Before beginning a conversation with your physician, research the proven conventional treatment for your disease. It is important to be as informed as possible before the office visit. Then, find out as much as you can about the alternative method that you wish to discuss. Some questions for patients to ask their physician are: What do you know about this alternative? Can you give me additional sources of information? Do you know someone who tried the alternative method? What was their experience?

  When looking at information, particularly on the Internet, try to determine whether or not the information is provided by someone selling a product. If a product is being promoted for sale, then information will likely be slanted toward helping to sell the product. The objectivity and accuracy of the information may not be reliable.

- Be nonconfrontational. Let your physician know. Before beginning any alternative, tell your physician that you are thinking about taking an alternative therapy but that you want to make sure it does not interfere with the treatment he or she prescribes. Once the treatment is recorded in your medical record, your physician will be able to watch for potential drug interactions and/or harmful effects.

- Ask questions. It can be helpful to write down a list of questions for the physician and bring in any literature you want to discuss. Let your physician know you are an educated consumer, even though you may be apprehensive about what you are facing, you are seeking as much information as you can. Let your physician know you want him or her to be a supportive partner in your education and treatment process.

- Bring someone with you to the physician's office. A friend or relative can help you communicate with your physician and understand the information you are given. Support from your loved ones will not only help you communicate but can also help lessen the stress of making decisions alone.

- Understand your physician's perspective. If you take herbs or megadoses of vitamins or start a special diet, your physician needs to know. Some therapies are considered alternative because they have not been proven to be safe and effective in controlled scientific studies. People with cancer may run the risk of jeopardizing their primary treatment because of possible drug interactions or they may harm themselves with unsafe methods. You should realize your physician might not have heard of your particular alternative therapy. If he or she hasn't heard of it, don't become discouraged. Ask your physician to help you find out more about it.

- Don't delay or forego conventional therapy. If you are considering stopping or not taking current conventional treatment, please discuss the implications of this decision with your physician. You may be giving up the only proven treatment.

- Conventional cancer treatment involves much more than just removing and destroying tumors. Many treatments are available that can relieve pain and other symptoms of cancer. People, who choose alternative therapies only, forego the benefits of palliative and supportive care that can improve their quality of life.

- If taking dietary supplements, review usage. Any time you receive new medication or there is a change in medication or medical history, review the list of supplements you are taking with your physician or nurse. Also let your health care team know if you change or add any dietary supplements. By telling your health care providers about supplement use, your medical record can be used to analyze the risks, benefits, and interactions with medications.

- Ask about using complementary or alternative methods if you are pregnant or breast-feeding. Do not give herbal medicines to children.

- Ask your physician to help you identify possible fraudulent products.

- Follow up. On your next physician's visit, be sure to continue your conversation about the alternative therapy. Share with him or her any decision you have reached about using an alternative method. Your physician may or may not agree with your decision, but it's important that he or she know if you're planning to use alternative therapies so that he or she can provide you with the best possible care.

- Be open to change. Realize that new studies may yield new information about complementary and alternative methods of managing cancer that may change your treatment plan.

Not only do new studies yield new information about complementary and alternative methods of cancer treatment but conventional methods also change over time with new scientific discoveries. For example, 100 years ago, if a woman was diagnosed with breast cancer, she routinely underwent surgical removal of the affected breast, the underlying muscle, and the lymph nodes near the affected breast (a radical mastectomy) to prevent the cancer from spreading. Over the years, as researchers learned more about how cancer develops and patients sought treatment at earlier stages of disease development, surgeons began performing less extensive operations for early stage breast cancer. This change was based on large clinical trials of the effects of various types of surgery, from a lumpectomy (removing a small tumor from the breast only) to a radical mastectomy. Scientists also found that less extensive surgery combined with other treatment methods, such as chemotherapy and radiation therapy, could yield good results for the patient.

Preventing Cancer and Finding it Early

Some cancers are more easily prevented than others. For example, tobacco, alcohol, sun exposure, and diet are related to cancers of the skin, lungs, mouth, pharynx, larynx, esophagus, liver, bladder, kidney, pancreas, colon, and prostate. People can change their habits in these areas to lower cancer risk. Some cancers can be detected early. Regular screening examinations by health care professionals can result in the detection of cancers of the breast, colon, rectum, cervix, prostate, testis, oral cavity, and skin at earlier stages, when treatment is more likely to be successful. Self-examinations for cancers of the breast and skin may also result in detection of tumors at earlier stages.

The ACS offers seven broad recommendations to help reduce cancer risk or diagnose the disease early when it is most treatable.

1.   Choose most of the foods you eat from plant sources. The ACS urges all people, whether living with cancer or at high risk of developing cancer, to obtain vitamins, minerals, and other nutrients from food sources rather than from dietary supplements. The ACS publishes nutrition guidelines to advise the public about dietary practices that reduce cancer risk. These guidelines are developed by expert advisory committees and are based on existing scientific evidence that relates diet and nutrition to cancer risk in human population studies as well as in laboratory experiments.

➢   *Eat five or more servings of fruits and vegetables each day (see Table 1).*
- Include fruits or vegetables in every meal.
- Choose fruits and vegetables for snacks.

Table 1. What Counts as a Serving?

Fruits
- 1 medium apple, banana, orange
- ½ cup of chopped, cooked, or canned fruit
- ¾ cup of fruit juice

Vegetables
- 1 cup of raw leafy vegetables
- ½ cup of other cooked or raw vegetables, chopped
- ¾ cup of vegetable juice

Grains
- 1 slice of bread
- 1 ounce of ready-to-eat cereal
- ½ cup of cooked cereal, rice, pasta

Beans and nuts
- ½ cup of cooked dry beans
- 2 tablespoons of peanut butter
- ⅓ cup of nuts

Dairy foods and eggs
- 1 cup of milk or yogurt
- 1 ½ ounces of natural cheese
- 2 ounces of processed cheese
- 1 egg

Meats
- 2-3 ounces of cooked lean meat, poultry, fish

Source: US Department of Agriculture and US Department of Health and Human Services. Nutrition and Your Health: Dietary Guidelines for Americans, 4th ed. Home and Garden Bull 232. Washington, DC: Government Printing Office, 1995.

➤ *Eat other foods from plant sources, such as breads, cereals, grain products, rice, pasta, or beans several times each day.*
- Include grain products in every meal.
- Choose whole grains in preference to processed (refined) grains.
- Choose beans as an alternative to meat.

The scientific basis for these recommendations is very strong for cancers of many sites, particularly for cancers of the gastrointestinal and respiratory tracts. The evidence is particularly strong that increased consumption of fruits and vegetables reduces the risk of colon cancer. Of the many scientific studies on this subject, the great majority shows that eating fruits and vegetables (especially green and dark yellow vegetables and those in the cabbage family, soy products, and legumes) protects against colon cancer. Evidence is less strong for cancers considered hormonal, such as breast and prostate. Greater consumption of vegetables, fruits, or both together, has also been associated with a lower risk of lung cancer.

2. Limit your intake of high-fat foods, particularly from animal sources.

➤ *Choose foods low in fat.*
- Replace fat-rich foods with fruits, vegetables, grains, and beans.
- Eat smaller portions of high-fat foods.
- Choose baked and broiled foods instead of fried foods.
- Select non-fat and low-fat milk and dairy products.
- When you eat packaged, snack, convenience, and restaurant foods, choose those low in fat.

➤ *Limit consumption of meats, especially high-fat meats.*
- When you eat meat, select lean cuts.
- Eat smaller portions of meats.
- Choose beans, seafood, and poultry as an alternative to beef, pork, and lamb.
- Select baked and broiled meats, seafood, and poultry, rather than fried.

High-fat diets have been associated with an increase in the risk of cancers of the colon and rectum, prostate, and endometrium. The association between high-fat diets and breast cancer is much weaker. Whether these associations are due to the total amount of fat, the particular type of fat (saturated, monounsaturated, or polyunsaturated), the calories contributed by fat, or some other factor in the fats in food has not yet been determined. Because a gram of fat contains more than twice the calories of a gram of protein or carbohydrate (9 versus 4 kcal/gram), studies cannot easily distinguish the effects of fat itself from effects of the calories it contains.

3. Be physically active. Achieve and maintain a healthy weight.

➤ *Be at least moderately active for 30 minutes or more on most days of the week. Stay within a healthy weight range for your gender and height.*

Physical activity can help protect against some cancers, either by balancing caloric intake with energy expenditure or by other mechanisms. An imbalance of caloric intake and output can lead to being overweight and obese, and an increased risk for cancers at several sites: colon and rectum, prostate, endometrium, breast (among post-menopausal women), and kidney.

These findings are supported by animal studies and by epidemiologic studies demonstrating an association between physical activity and a reduced risk of developing some cancers. Activity simply may prevent obesity or it may act in other ways to reduce cancer risk. For breast and prostate cancer, physical activity may act through effects on hormone levels. For colon cancer, physical activity stimulates movement through the bowel, thereby reducing the length of time that the bowel lining is exposed to mutagens (agents that can change normal cells to cancer cells). Both physical activity and controlled caloric intake are necessary to achieve or maintain a healthy body weight.

4. Limit consumption of alcoholic beverages, if you drink at all.
Alcohol consumption increases the risk of cancers of the mouth, esophagus, pharynx, larynx, and liver in men and women, and of breast cancer in women. Cancer risk increases with the amount of alcohol consumed. For cancers of the mouth, esophagus, and larynx, risk increases substantially with intake of more than two drinks per day. A drink of alcohol is defined as 12 ounces

of regular beer, 5 ounces of wine, or 1.5 ounces of 80-proof distilled spirits. The combined use of alcohol and tobacco greatly increases the risk of these cancers compared to drinking or smoking alone. Many studies also have reported an increased risk of breast cancer in women who drink alcohol.

5. If you smoke or chew tobacco, stop. If you don't smoke or chew tobacco, don't start. Because cigarette smoking and tobacco use is an acquired behavior, one that the individual chooses to do, smoking is the most preventable cause of premature death in our society. Smoking accounts for at least 29% of all cancer deaths. Successful quitting is a matter of planning and commitment. There is no easy method to stop smoking. It involves developing a plan that addresses both the physical and psychological components of smoking. The plan can include a variety of options, such as using the nicotine patch or gum, joining a stop smoking class, going to Nicotine Anonymous meetings, or using self-help materials such as books and pamphlets.

6. Try to stay out of the sun as much as possible. It is impossible to completely avoid sunlight, but there are precautions you can take to limit your amount of exposure to harmful ultraviolet (UV) rays:

➤ *Limit direct sun exposure during midday.* The sun's ultraviolet rays are strongest during the midday hours (10 AM-4 PM), so exposure during these times should be limited.

➤ *Cover up.* When outdoors, wear darker clothing with tightly woven fabric to protect as much skin as possible, such as a long-sleeved shirt, long pants or skirt, and a hat with a 2-3 inch brim that shades the face, neck, and ears.

➤ *Wear sunglasses that block UV rays.* Check the label to be sure you buy sunglasses that block 99% to 100% of UV rays. Labels that say "special purpose" or "Meets ANSI UV Requirements" mean the glasses block at least 99% of UV rays. Those labeled "cosmetic" only block about 70% of the UV rays. If there is no label, don't buy the sunglasses.

➤ *Use a sunscreen with a SPF of 15 or higher and apply it properly.* The number of the SPF represents the level of sunburn protection provided by the sunscreen. It is important to remember that sunscreen does not provide total protection. For example, a SPF 15 blocks out 93% of the burning UV rays and a SPF 30 blocks out 97% of the burning UV rays. Products that are labeled "waterproof" provide protection for at least 80 minutes, while those labeled "water resistant" may provide protection for only 40 minutes. For maximum effectiveness, apply sunscreen 20-30 minutes before going outside. Reapply when swimming or perspiring and remember to use sunscreen lip balm for the lips. Medications can also make your skin more sensitive to the sun. Do not use sunscreens on babies younger than six months; use clothing, hats, and shading to protect them from the sun.

➤ *Consider your activity.* Be sure to consider your activity when thinking about sun protection and plan ahead. How long do you plan to be outside? What is the UV Index? Will you be at the beach or will you be hiking in the woods? Be sure to carry extra sunscreen with you, and put some in your car.

➤ *Avoid sunlamps and tanning booths.* The UV rays emitted from tanning beds can cause serious skin damage. Sunlamps are regulated by the FDA and there are specific guidelines for use.

7. Early detection is critical. The ACS recommends cancer-related checkups every three years for people aged 20-40, and every year for people age 40 or older. The cancer-related checkup should include health counseling and depending on a person's age, might include examinations for cancers of the thyroid, oral cavity, skin, lymph nodes, testes, and ovaries, as well as for some nonmalignant diseases.

Summary of American Cancer Society Recommendations for the Early Detection of Cancer in Asymptomatic People

SITE	RECOMMENDATION
Breast	Women 40 and older should have an annual mammogram, an annual clinical breast examination (CBE) by a health care professional, and should perform monthly breast self-examination. The CBE should be conducted close to the scheduled mammogram. Women ages 20-39 should have a clinical breast examination by a health care professional every three years and should perform monthly breast self-examination.
Colon & Rectum	Beginning at age 50, men and women should follow *one* of the examination schedules below: • A fecal occult blood test every year and a flexible sigmoidoscopy every five years.* • A colonoscopy every 10 years.* • A double-contrast barium enema every five to 10 years.* ** A digital rectal exam should be done at the same time as sigmoidoscopy, colonoscopy, or double-contrast barium enema. People who are at moderate or high risk for colorectal cancer should talk with a physician about a different testing schedule.*
Prostate	The ACS recommends that both the prostate-specific antigen (PSA) blood test and the digital rectal examination be offered annually, beginning at age 50, to men who have a life expectancy of at least 10 years and to younger men who are at high risk. Men in high-risk groups, such as those with a strong familial predisposition (ie, two or more affected first-degree relatives), or blacks may begin at a younger age (ie, 45 years).
Uterus	**Cervix:** All women who are or have been sexually active or who are 18 and older should have an annual Pap test and pelvic examination. After three or more consecutive satisfactory examinations with normal findings, the Pap test may be performed less frequently. Discuss the matter with your physician. **Endometrium:** Women at high risk for cancer of the uterus should have a sample of endometrial tissue examined when menopause begins.

Insurance Coverage

In response to growing patient demand for complementary and alternative therapies, more and more health insurance companies are beginning to cover at least some of the costs of complementary and alternative therapies and the services of alternative practitioners. By the year 2000, at least 30 major insurers, including about 15 Blue Cross plans, covered more than one complementary or alternative therapy. The most likely therapies to be reimbursed were acupuncture and chiropractic services. Insurers were also most likely to cover these services if the patient's physician prescribed the therapy.

The trend toward greater insurance coverage is also fueled by efforts on the part of managed care companies to control costs. Complementary and alternative therapies represent at least a potential cost saving for insurers, although actual cost-effectiveness studies are generally lacking. Naturopaths, acupuncturists, chiropractors, and other complementary and alternative therapists rely heavily on herbs and other dietary supplements to treat illnesses and medical complaints, and supplements are considered less costly than conventional drugs.

Among insurers and managed care companies that do offer coverage for nontraditional treatments, the amount of coverage varies widely. Some health maintenance organizations (HMOs) offer complementary and alternative methods as discounted services similar to the reduced-rate services offered for plastic surgery, eye care, and other services not fully covered by the HMO. Other managed care providers and insurers offer complementary and alternative methods as a carved-out benefit, for which the insured pays a premium. Other HMOs and managed care groups are adding alternative providers to their provider teams. And a growing number offer complementary services as a core benefit.

In 1995, Washington state passed a law mandating that all insurance carriers cover complementary and alternative medicine. The legislation requires insurers to provide patients with access to every category of provider. In line with the state law, Blue Cross of Washington and Alaska covers complementary and alternative therapies at 50% of the costs, with a limit of $500 per year. The plan includes a network of 400 alternative providers.

While insurance coverage for at least some of the costs of complementary and alternative methods is expanding, most of the costs are still paid out-of-pocket by consumers. Insurers, including Medicare, tend to grant coverage for treatments that they consider reasonable and necessary or medically necessary. To qualify, the treatment must be shown to be safe and effective. Complementary methods, such as meditation, biofeedback, acupuncture, and hypnosis may be covered because companies believe there is sufficient scientific evidence to indicate that these therapies help reduce pain and other side effects of treatment. *Insurers generally will not cover unproven therapies, however.*

As more controlled clinical trials are conducted to demonstrate the safety and effectiveness or danger and ineffectiveness of various complementary and alternative methods of cancer management, the safe and effective therapies will become part of conventional medicine and qualify for insurance coverage.

References

Albanes D. Energy balance, body size, and cancer. *CRC Crit Rev Oncol Hematol.* 1990;10:283-303.

Ames BN, Gold LS, Willett WC. The causes and prevention of cancer. *Proc Natl Acad Sci USA.* 1995;92:5258-5265.

Biesalski HK, de Mesquita BB, Chesson A, et al. European consensus statement on lung cancer: risk factors and prevention. *CA Cancer J Clin.* 1998;48:167-176.

Blumenthal M, ed. *The Complete German Commission E Monographs: Therapeutic Guide to Herbal Medicines.* Austin, Tx: American Botanical Council; 1998.

Brody JE. Alternative medicine makes inroads, but watch out for curves. *New York Times.* Apr. 28, 1998; sec F, pg 7, col 1.

Cassileth B. *The Alternative Medicine Handbook.* New York, NY: W. W. Norton & Co; 1998.

Cassileth B. Complementary and alternative cancer medicine. *J Clin Oncol.* 1999;17:44-52.

Cassileth B. Evaluating complementary and alternative therapies for cancer patients. *CA Cancer J Clin.* 1999;49:362-375.

Colditz GA, DeJong W, Emmons K, Hunter DJ, Mueller N, Sorensen G, eds. Harvard Report on Cancer Prevention. Vol. 2: Prevention of Human Cancer. *Cancer Causes Control.* 1997;(8 suppl l):sl-s5O.

Consumer Reports. The mainstreaming of alternative medicine. May, 2000.

Eisenberg DM, Davis RB, Ettner SL, et al. Trends in alternative medicine use in the United States, 1990-1997. *JAMA.* 1998;280:1569-1575.

Friedenreich CM, Rohan TE. A review of physical activity and public health: recommendations from the Centers for Disease Control and Prevention and the American College of Sports Medicine. *JAMA.* 1995;273:402-407.

Hill HA, Austin H. Nutrition and endometrial cancer. *Cancer Causes Control.* 1996;7:19-32.

Hunter DJ, Willett WC. Nutrition and breast cancer. *Cancer Causes Control.* 1996;7:56-68.

IARC Monographs on the Evaluation of Carcinogenic Risks to Humans. Vol. 44. *Alcohol Drinking.* Lyon, France: International Agency for Research on Cancer, 1988.

Institute of Medicine. *Weighing the Options: Criteria for Evaluating Weight-Management Programs.* Washington, DC: National Academy Press, 1995.

Kohlmeier L, Mendez M. Controversies surrounding the diet and breast cancer. *Proc Nutr Soc.* 1997;56:369-382.

Kolonel LN. Nutrition and prostate cancer. *Cancer Causes Control.* 1996;7:83-94.

Kurtzweil P. An FDA guide to dietary supplements. *FDA Consumer.* 1998;Sept-Oct; revised Jan 1999. Available at http://vm.cfsan.fda.gov/~dms/fdsupp.html.

Labriola D, Livingston R. Possible interactions between dietary antioxidants and chemotherapy. *Oncology (Huntingt).* 1999;13:1003-1008.

National Center for Complementary and Alternative Medicine. What is CAM? NIH Web site. Available at http://nccam.nih.gov/nccam. Accessed January 7, 2000.

McCann J. Texas center studies research alternative treatments. *J Natl Cancer Inst.* 1997;89:1485-1486.

Murphy GP, Morris LB, Lange D. *Informed Decisions: The Complete Book of Cancer Diagnosis, Treatment, and Recovery.* New York, NY: Viking; 1997.

Potter ID. Nutrition and colorectal cancer. *Cancer Causes Control.* 1996;7: 127-146.

Richardson MA. Research of complementary/alternative medicine therapies in oncology: promising but challenging. *J Clin Oncol.* 1999;17:38-43.

Richardson MA, White JD. Complementary/alternative medicine and cancer research: a national initiative. *Cancer Pract.* 2000;8:45-48.

Shepherd RJ. Exercise in the prevention and treatment of cancer: an update. *Sports Med.* 1993;15:258-280.

Spiegel D, Stroud P, Fyfe A. Complementary medicine. *West J Med.* 1998;168:241-247.

Steinmetz KA, Potter JD. Vegetables, fruit, and cancer. 1. Epidemiology. *Cancer Causes Control.* 1991;2:325-357.

Steinmetz KA, Potter ID. Vegetables, fruit, and cancer. II. Mechanisms. *Cancer Causes Control.* 1991;2:427-442.

The Alpha-Tocopherol, Beta Carotene Cancer Prevention Study Group. The effect of Vitamin E and beta carotene on the incidence of lung cancer and other cancers in male smokers. *N Eng J Med.* 1994;330:1029-1035.

Thun MJ, Peto R, Lopez AD. Alcohol consumption and mortality among middle-aged and elderly US adults. *N Engl J Med.* 1997;337:1704-1714.

US Congress, Office of Technology Assessment. *Unconventional Cancer Treatments.* Washington, DC: US Government Printing Office; 1990. Publication OTA-H-405.

Ward DE. *Reporting on Cancer: A Guide for Journalists.* Columbus, OH: The Ohio State University; 1994.

Willett WC. Micronutrients and cancer risk. *Am J Clin Nutr.* 1994;59:1162s-1165s.

Wolk A, Lindblad P, Adami HO. Nutrition and renal cell cancer. *Cancer Causes Control.* 1996;7:5-18.

World Cancer Research Fund and American Institute for Cancer Research. *Food, Nutrition and the Prevention of Cancer: A Global Perspective.* Washington, DC: American Institute for Cancer Research, 1997.

Zeigler RG, Mayne ST. Swanson CA. Nutrition and lung cancer. *Cancer Causes Control.* 1996;7:157-177.

Categories
of Methods

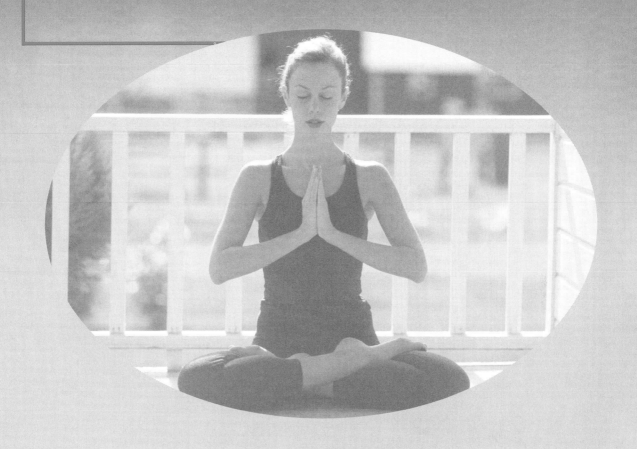

Chapter 5

Mind, Body, and Spirit Methods

This category includes methods

that focus on the connections between

the mind, body, and spirit, and their

power for healing.

Aromatherapy

Other common name(s)	Scientific/medical name(s)
Holistic Aromatherapy, Aromatic Medicine	None

DESCRIPTION

Aromatherapy is the use of fragrant substances distilled from plants, called essential oils, to alter mood or improve health. These highly concentrated aromatic substances are either inhaled or applied as oils during massage. There are approximately 40 essential oils commonly used in aromatherapy; among the most popular are lavender, rosemary, eucalyptus, chamomile, marjoram, jasmine, peppermint, and geranium.

OVERVIEW

There is no scientific evidence that aromatherapy is effective in preventing or treating cancer, but it can be used to enhance quality of life. Early clinical trials suggest aromatherapy may have some benefit as a complementary treatment in reducing stress, pain, and depression.

How is it promoted for use?

Aromatherapy is promoted as a natural way to help patients cope with chronic pain, depression, and stress, and produce a feeling of well being. There is some evidence suggesting this may be true. Proponents also claim aromatherapy can help relieve bacterial infections, stimulate the immune system, fight colds, flu and sore throats, improve urine production, increase circulation, and cure cystitis, herpes simplex, acne, headaches, indigestion, PMS, muscle tension, and even cancer. There is no scientific evidence, however, to support these further claims. Fragrances from different oils are promoted to have specific health benefits. For example, lavender oil is promoted to relieve muscular tension, anxiety, and insomnia.

There are two schools of thought as to how aromatherapy works. Scent receptors in the nose are known to send chemical messages through the olfactory nerve to the brain's limbic region, which influences heart rate, blood pressure, and respiration. Some say these connections explain the effects of essential oils' pleasant smells. Others say the oils are absorbed directly into the system through the skin.

What does it involve?

Aromatherapy is either self-administered or applied by a practitioner. Many aromatherapists in the United States are trained as massage therapists, psychologists, social workers, or chiropractors, and use the oils as part of their practices.

The essential oils, which are used individually or in combination, may be inhaled or applied to the skin. For inhalation, a few drops of the essential oil are placed in steaming water, diffusers, or humidifiers that are used to spread the steam/oil combination throughout the room.

Essential oils can be applied to the skin during massage, or they can be added to bathwater. For application to the skin, the oils are combined with a carrier, usually vegetable oil. Some people also apply drops of certain essential oils on their pillows.

What is the history behind it?

Use of aromatic, perfumed oils dates back thousands of years to ancient Egypt, China, and India. In Egypt, such oils were used after bathing and for embalming mummies. Thousands of years ago the Chinese compiled an encyclopedia of information on plants, herbs, and wood. In ancient India, aromatic massage was part of Ayurvedic medicine.

The Greeks and Romans used fragrant oils for both medicinal and cosmetic purposes. However, it was the medieval physician Avicenna who first extracted these oils from plants.

Rene Maurice Gattefosse, a French chemist, originated modern aromatherapy, and even the term itself. After burning his hand in a laboratory accident, he used lavender oil to soothe the pain. His hand healed quickly with no scar, and he attributed this outcome to the lavender oil. He published his first thesis on "Aromatherapie" in 1928 and a book under the same title in 1937. Aromatherapy was revived in the 1960s by French homeopaths Dr. and Mme. Maury. In the 1980s, aromatherapy began in the United States in California, and is fairly well established in England, France, Switzerland, New Mexico, and New Zealand.

What is the evidence?

There is no scientific evidence that aromatherapy cures or prevents disease, however, a few clinical studies suggest aromatherapy may be a beneficial complementary therapy. In Britain, there are reports of the successful use of aromatherapy massage as a complementary treatment for people with cancer to reduce anxiety, depression, tension, and pain. There are also reports that inhaled peppermint, ginger, and cardamom oil seem to relieve the nausea caused by chemotherapy and radiation, however, these reports have not been scientifically proven.

Clinical research on aromatherapy is in its infancy, however, early trials suggest aromatherapy may help patients cope with chronic pain, stress, and depression. A randomized clinical trial of patients with bald patches on their scalp or skin showed aromatherapy to be a safe and effective treatment for hair loss resulting from alopecia areata, a condition in which damage to hair follicles is caused by the patient's own immune system. Aromatherapy has not been evaluated as a treatment for hair loss related to cancer treatments. In another controlled clinical trial, inhaling the vapors from black pepper extract reduced the craving for tobacco, and improved participants' moods. In a third controlled trial, citrus fragrance used in 12 depressed patients made it possible to reduce the amount of antidepressant medicine needed for the treatment of depression.

Are there any possible problems or complications?

Essential oils should never be taken internally, as many of them are poisonous. Also, people should avoid exposure for a long period of time, because some may have allergic reactions to the oils.

References

Buckle J. Use of aromatherapy as a complementary treatment for chronic pain. *Altern Ther Health Med.* 1999;5:42-51.

Cawthorn A. A review of the literature surrounding the research into aromatherapy. *Complement Ther Nurs Midwifery.* 1995;1:118-120.

Cerrato PL. Aromatherapy: is it for real? *RN.* 1998;61:51-52.

Hay IC, Jamieson M, Ormerod AD. Randomized trial of aromatherapy. Successful treatment for alopecia areata. *Arch Dermatol.* 1998; 134: 1349-1352.

Komori T, Fujiwara R, Tanida M, Nomura J, Yokoyama MM. Effects of citrus fragrance on immune function and depressive states. *Neuroimmunomodulation.* 1995;2:174-180.

Nelson NJ. Scents or nonsense: aromatherapy's benefits still subject to debate. *J Natl Cancer Inst.* 1997;89:1334-1336.

Rose JE, Behm FM. Inhalation of vapor from black pepper extract reduces smoking withdrawal symptoms. *Drug Alcohol Depend.* 1994;34:225-229.

Mind / Body / Spirit

Art Therapy

Other common name(s)	Scientific/medical name(s)
None	None

DESCRIPTION

Art therapy is a form of treatment used to help people with physical and emotional problems by using creative activities to express emotions. It provides a way for people to come to terms with emotional conflicts, increase self-awareness, and express unspoken and often unconscious concerns about their illness.

OVERVIEW

Many clinicians have observed and documented significant benefits among people who have participated in art therapy. Art therapy has not undergone rigorous scientific study to determine its therapeutic value for people with cancer.

How is it promoted for use?

Art therapy is based on the idea that the creative act can be healing. According to practitioners, called art therapists, it helps people express hidden emotions, reduces stress, fear and anxiety, and provides a sense of freedom. Art therapists also believe the act of creating influences brain wave patterns and the chemicals released by the brain.

Art therapy has been used to treat burn patients, people with eating disorders, emotionally impaired young people, disabled people, the chronically ill, chemically addicted individuals, sexually abused adolescents, and others. Art therapy may also be used to distract patients whose illnesses or treatments cause pain.

Proponents use artwork as a diagnostic tool, particularly with children, who often have difficulty talking about painful events or emotions. Art therapists say that often children can express difficult emotions or relay information about traumatic times in their lives more easily through drawings than in conventional therapy.

What does it involve?

People involved in art therapy are provided with the tools necessary to produce paintings, drawings, sculptures and other types of artwork. Art therapists work with patients individually or in groups. The job of the art therapist is to help patients express themselves through their creations and to discuss patients' emotions and concerns as they relate to their art. For example, an art therapist may encourage a person with cancer to create an image of themselves with cancer, and in this way express feelings about the disease that may be difficult to verbalize or may be unconscious.

In another form of art therapy, patients view pieces of art, often in photographs, then talk with a therapist about what they have seen. A caregiver or family member can also gather artwork in the form of photographs, books or prints, and give the patient an opportunity to look at and enjoy the art.

Many medical centers and hospitals include art therapy as part of inpatient care. It can be practiced in many other settings, such as schools, psychiatric centers, drug and alcohol rehabilitation programs, prisons, day care treatment programs, nursing homes, hospices, patients' homes, and art studios.

What is the history behind it?

The connection between art and mental health was first recognized in the late 1800s. In 1922, a book entitled *Artistry of the Mentally Ill* aroused interest in the subject and caused the medical community to examine the diagnostic value of patients' creations. Some practitioners realized that art might be valuable for rehabilitating patients with mental illness.

In the 1940s, ideas from psychoanalysis and art were combined to develop art as a tool to help patients release unconscious thoughts. The creations of patients began to be considered as a type of symbolic speech. In 1958, an artist named Hana Kwiatkowska translated her knowledge as an artist into the field of family work and introduced methods of evaluation and treatment techniques using art therapy at the National Institute of Mental Health.

In 1969, the American Art Therapy Association was established. The organization now has over 4,000 members, and along with the Art Therapy Credentials Board, sets standards for art therapists and educates the public about the field. Registered art therapists must have graduate degree training and a background in studio arts and therapy techniques.

What is the evidence?

Numerous case studies have reported art therapy benefits patients with both emotional and physical illnesses. Case studies have involved many areas including burn recovery in adolescent and young children, eating disorders, emotional impairment in young children, reading performance, chemical addiction, childhood grief, and sexual abuse in adolescents. Some of the potential uses of art therapy to be researched include reducing anxiety levels, improving recovery times, decreasing hospital stays, and pain control.

Are there any possible problems or complications?

Art therapy is considered safe and may be useful as a complementary therapy to help people with cancer deal with their emotions. Although uncomfortable feelings may be stirred up at times, this is considered part of the healing process.

References

Alternative Medicine: Expanding Medical Horizons. *A Report to the National Institutes of Health on Alternative Medical Systems and Practices in the United States*. Washington, DC: US Government Printing Office; 1994. NIH publication 94-066.

Complementary and Alternative Methods. Art therapy. American Cancer Society Web site. Available at: http://www.cancer.org. Accessed January 24, 2000.

Ayurveda

Other common name(s)	**Scientific/medical name(s)**
Ayurvedic Medicine	None

DESCRIPTION
Ayurveda is an ancient Indian system of medicine that has an integrated approach to the prevention and treatment of illness, which tries to maintain or reestablish the harmony between the mind, body, and forces of nature. It combines a variety of interventions, such as changes in lifestyle, herbal remedies, exercise, and meditation.

OVERVIEW
Ayurveda is one of several ancient Asian healing systems that have recently gained popularity in the West. While the effectiveness of many aspects of Ayurveda has not been scientifically proven, some preliminary research suggests certain components may offer potential therapeutic value.

How is it promoted for use?
A central idea in Ayurveda is that illness results when a person's physical, emotional and spiritual forces are out of balance with each other and with the natural environment.

Practitioners claim certain combinations of Ayurvedic interventions, matched to a patient's unique physical and emotional needs and personal medical history, increase physical vitality, foster spiritual well being, bring individuals into harmony with the world, and even prevent and cure disease.

According to Ayurvedic theory, all diseases and other health problems result from imbalances in the body's fundamental forces and disharmony with the natural environment. One of the primary goals of Ayurveda is to restore this balance and invigorate the body's biological and spiritual forces. Practitioners of Ayurveda use a combination of therapies to restore physical and spiritual harmony by balancing energy forces.

What does it involve?
Practitioners of Ayurveda may combine dietary programs, herbal remedies, intestinal cleansing preparations, yoga, meditation, massage, breathing exercises, and visual imagery to treat their patients (see Massage, Meditation, Imagery, and Yoga). Ayurvedic herbal preparations often consist of complex mixtures of plants. An estimated 1,250 plants are used by practitioners. Some of the more controversial and less common practices of Ayurveda include bloodletting, bowel purging, and inducing vomiting.

To diagnose illness, Ayurveda practitioners closely observe a patient's tongue, nails, lips, and body's nine "doors": two eyes, two ears, two nostrils, mouth, genitalia, and anus. They also listen carefully to the lungs and pulse, and take a detailed history of the patient's life and health. Through these observations, practitioners claim to evaluate a patient's doshas. According to Ayurveda practitioners, doshas not only enable the various organs of the body to work together, they also establish a person's connection to the environment and the cosmos. Practitioners claim each person is dominated by one dosha, but is influenced to some extent by all three. The dominant dosha describes an individual's physical, emotional, and spiritual characteristics as well as his or her daily habits and lifestyle.

When formulating a plan of treatment, Ayurveda practitioners consider the state of a patient's doshas and the complex relationship between the doshas and other factors such as emotions, illness, physical activity, lifestyle, diet, relationships with other people, and even the four seasons, colors, and the time of day. Practitioners strive to harmonize all of these factors so that their patients can attain health and well being.

What is the history behind it?

Ayurveda is thought to have appeared in India nearly 5,000 years ago. It emerged from an ancient body of knowledge called the "Vedas," which is a Sanskrit word meaning "knowledge." From these Vedas, India developed its moral, religious, cultural, and medical codes. Many of the beliefs and practices of Ayurveda are similar to those of ancient Chinese medicine.

In India today, Ayurveda practitioners are trained by institutions in state-recognized programs. Some of these practitioners are now practicing and teaching Ayurveda in the United States. There are approximately 10 Ayurvedic clinics in North America.

What is the evidence?

Although Ayurveda has been largely untested by Western researchers, there is a growing interest in integrating some components of the system into modern medical practice. Some preliminary studies suggest Ayurveda may have potential therapeutic value.

According to a report of a panel convened by the National Institutes of Health (NIH), one clinical study showed that in 79% of cases, the health of patients with various chronic diseases improved measurably after Ayurvedic treatment. Laboratory and clinical studies have suggested that some Ayurvedic herbal preparations may have the potential to prevent and treat certain cancers, including breast, lung, and colon cancers. Randomized clinical trials in humans are needed to make conclusions about the role of Ayurveda in cancer prevention and treatment. The National Cancer Institute (NCI) has added several Ayurvedic herbal compounds to its list of potential anticancer agents and has funded a series of laboratory studies to evaluate two Ayurvedic herbal remedies (called MAK-4 and MAK-5). Their decision was based on preliminary laboratory studies indicating that the two medicines significantly inhibited growth of cancer cells from human and rat tumors.

In a controlled clinical trial of cancer patients in India, researchers found an Ayurvedic herbal mixture was just as effective as a conventional laxative for relieving constipation caused by narcotic pain medicine. In another controlled clinical trial, Ayurveda was found to be an effective treatment for patients with Parkinson's disease.

Are there any possible problems or complications?

Some aspects of Ayurveda, such as bloodletting and inducing vomiting, can be harmful. Many people with cancer already have low blood cell counts as a consequence of the disease itself, and removing additional blood can worsen fatigue and other symptoms. Inducing vomiting can cause imbalances of electrolytes (salt and minerals) in the blood. In addition, the potential interactions between Ayurvedic herbal preparations and conventional drugs and other herbal medications should be taken into consideration. Some of these combinations may be dangerous. Relying on this type of treatment alone, and avoiding conventional medical care, may have serious health consequences.

References

Alternative Medicine: Expanding Medical Horizons. *A Report to the National Institutes of Health on Alternative Medical Systems and Practices in the United States.* Washington, DC: US Government Printing Office; 1994. NIH publication 94-066.

An alternative medicine treatment for Parkinson's disease: results of a multicenter clinical trial. HP-200 in Parkinson's Disease Study Group. *J Altern Complement Med.* 1995;1:249-255.

Complementary and Alternative Methods. Ayurveda. American Cancer Society Web site. Available at: http://www.cancer.org. Accessed January 24, 2000.

Dev S. Ancient-modern concordance in Ayurvedic plants: some examples. *Environ Health Perspect.* 1999;107:783-789.

Ramesh PR, Kumar KS, Rajagopal MR, Balachandran P, Warrier PK. Managing morphine-induced constipation: a controlled comparison of an Ayurvedic formulation and senna. *J Pain Symptom Manage.* 1998;16:240-244.

Bioenergetics

Other common name(s)	**Scientific/medical name(s)**
Bioenergetic Therapy, Bioenergetic Medicine, Bioenergetic Analysis	None

DESCRIPTION
Bioenergetics is a complementary therapy that involves psychotherapy, relaxation techniques, and gentle touch to relieve muscle tension.

OVERVIEW
There is no scientific evidence that bioenergetics therapy is effective in treating cancer; however, some patients report it is useful as a relaxation method.

How is it promoted for use?
Proponents of bioenergetics believe the body "records" negative emotional reactions and stores them in the form of muscle tension and stiffness, poor posture, and low energy levels. To release these trapped emotions and return the body and mind to a balanced, healthy, peaceful state, patients must first release muscle tension and correct physical imbalances. Proponents further claim bioenergetics can offer relief from the side effects of cancer treatment, and even strengthen the body's ability to fight disease, although there is no scientific evidence to support this claim.

Bioenergetics practitioners claim they can "read" a patient's muscular movements, tone of voice, breathing, posture and emotions to determine his or her physical and psychological problems. They also believe disease is a part of the life process, and serious illnesses, including cancer are symptoms of underlying imbalances caused by factors such as poor diet, exposure to toxins, genetic history, and repressed emotions. They claim that by balancing electrical and energy disturbances within the patient and eliminating toxins, the body will heal itself (see Electromagnetic Therapy).

What does it involve?
Bioenergetics therapists use a combination of psychotherapy, gentle body movements, massage, deep breathing, and exercises that involve crying, screaming and kicking, in an effort to help patients "release" their emotional memories. The therapy may also incorporate aspects of traditional Chinese medicine, biofeedback, herbal medicine, homeopathy, and nutrition (see Acupuncture, Biofeedback, Chinese Herbal Medicine, and Homeopathy).

What is the history behind it?
Bioenergetics was developed by psychiatrist Alexander Lowen, MD in the 1950s. He based his work on Reichian therapy, which theorized that a person's repressed emotions are transformed into muscle tension and rigidity, which Wilhelm Reich, MD called "body armor." Dr. Lowen, who first earned a law degree in New York, became a therapist under Dr. Reich's training and then completed medical school at the University of Geneva in Switzerland. In 1956, Dr. Lowen created the Institute for Bioenergetic Analysis.

What is the evidence?
Some patients may feel more relaxed and at ease after a bioenergetics therapy session.

However, there is no scientific evidence that bioenergetics is useful in treating cancer or any other disease. No studies have been published in medical journals to show that it offers any long-term physical or psychological benefits.

Are there any possible problems or complications?

People with cancer and chronic conditions, such as arthritis and heart disease, should consult their physician before undergoing any type of therapy that involves herbs or manipulation of joints and muscles. Relying on this type of treatment alone, and avoiding conventional medical care, may have serious health consequences.

References

Alternative Medicine: Expanding Medical Horizons. *A Report to the National Institutes of Health on Alternative Medical Systems and Practices in the United States*. Washington, DC: US Government Printing Office; 1994. NIH publication 94-066.

Cassileth B. *The Alternative Medicine Handbook*. New York, NY: W. W. Norton & Co; 1998.

Biofeedback

Other common name(s)	Scientific/medical name(s)
None	None

DESCRIPTION

Biofeedback is a treatment method that uses monitoring devices to help people consciously regulate physiological processes that are usually controlled automatically, such as heart rate, blood pressure, temperature, perspiration, and muscle tension.

OVERVIEW

Biofeedback is one of several relaxation methods that has been approved by an independent panel, convened by the National Institutes of Health (NIH), as a useful complementary therapy for treating chronic pain and insomnia. There is no scientific evidence that biofeedback can influence the development or progression of cancer; however, it can help to improve the quality of life for some people with cancer.

How is it promoted for use?

Biofeedback is used to regulate specific physiological functions. Through changing heart rates, skin temperature, breathing rates, muscle control, and other physiological activity in the body, biofeedback can reduce stress and muscle tension from a variety of causes. It can promote relaxation, correct urinary incontinence, treat migraines, and less serious headaches. It helps people with Raynaud's disease (problems of blood circulation in the fingers and toes which makes them feel very cold) increase the temperature of their hands and toes. Through a greater awareness of bodily functions, it can regulate or alter other physical functions that may be causing discomfort. Biofeedback is useful also in retraining muscles after injury, or teaching new muscles to take over.

What does it involve?

Various monitoring devices are used to provide biofeedback information so the person can adjust his or her thinking and other mental processes in order to control bodily functions.

Under the guidance of a biofeedback therapist, the patient concentrates on changing a specific physiological process, such as heart rate, temperature, perspiration, blood flow, brain activity, or muscle tension. A monitor hooked via electrodes to the patient's skin measures changes in whichever function is to be altered. Tones or images produced by the monitor inform the patient when he or she achieves the desired results. The process is repeated as often as necessary until the patient can reliably use conscious thought to change physical functions.

There are at least five different ways to measure body functions for biofeedback purposes. An electromyogram (EMG) measures muscle tension. It is used to help heal muscle injuries, and relieve chronic pain and some types of incontinence. Thermal biofeedback provides information about skin temperature, which is a good indicator of blood flow. Several health problems are related to blood flow, such as migraine headaches, Raynaud's disease, anxiety, and high blood pressure. Electrodermal activity (EDA) shows changes in perspiration rates, which is used in treating anxiety. Finger pulse measurements are used to reflect high blood pressure, heart beat irregularities, and anxiety. Breathing rate is also monitored, which is used to treat asthma and hyperventilation, and to promote relaxation.

Biofeedback is often a matter of trial and error in that patients learn to adjust their thinking and connect alterations in thought, breathing, posture, and muscle tension with changes in physiologic functions that are generally controlled unconsciously.

What is the history behind it?

For centuries, followers of ancient eastern practices such as meditation and yoga have claimed they could control physical processes usually considered beyond the power of conscious thought. Studies on how biofeedback works were not conducted until the 1970s. Today, some physicians in the United States use biofeedback as a complementary therapy to promote relaxation, and treat headaches, migraines, and insomnia.

What is the evidence?

Although biofeedback has no direct effect on the development or progression of cancer, it can improve the quality of life for some people with cancer. Research has found that biofeedback can be helpful for patients in regaining urinary and bowel continence following surgery. In one randomized clinical trial, relaxation therapy was more effective than biofeedback in reducing some side effects of chemotherapy.

After examining data on biofeedback, an NIH panel found the technique is moderately effective for relieving many types of chronic pain, particularly tension headaches, and that it alleviates some types of insomnia. The panel also found that biofeedback was better than relaxation therapy for treating migraine headaches. The effects of biofeedback vary significantly from person to person.

Are there any possible problems or complications?

Biofeedback is considered a safe technique. It is noninvasive and requires little effort. It does, however, require a trained and certified professional to control monitoring equipment and interpret changes. Battery operated devices sold for home use have not been found to be reliable.

References

Burish TG. Effectiveness of biofeedback and relaxation training in reducing the side effects of cancer chemotherapy. *Health Psychol.* 1992;11:17-23.

Cassileth B. *The Alternative Medicine Handbook.* New York, NY: W. W. Norton & Co; 1998.

Mathewson-Chapman M. Pelvic muscle exercise/biofeedback for urinary incontinence after prostatectomy: an education program. *J Cancer Educ.* 1997;12:218-223.

National Center for Complementary and Alternative Medicine. Fields of practice: mind-body control. National Institutes of Health Web site. Available at: http://nccam.nih.gov/nccam/ what-is-cam/fields/mind.shtml#biofeedback. Accessed October 27, 1999.

NIH panel endorses alternative therapies for chronic pain and insomnia. CAM Newsletter; December 1995. National Institutes of Health Web site. Available at: http://altmed.od.nih.gov/nccam/cam/1995/dec/4.htm. Accessed October 27, 1999.

NIH Technology Assessment Panel. Integration of behavioral and relaxation approaches into the treatment of chronic pain and insomnia. *JAMA.* 1996;276:313-318.

Breathwork

Other common name(s)	Scientific/medical name(s)
None	None

DESCRIPTION / OVERVIEW

Breathwork is the general term used to describe a variety of breathing techniques that are implemented in many relaxation exercises and spiritual healing methods. Focused, deep breathing exercises, such as exaggerating the way you naturally inhale and exhale, is said to promote relaxation, awareness, and emotional release. Shallow breathing is an indicator of stress, so the goal in breathwork is to take long, deep breaths. These breaths are said to be "cleansing," freeing both the body and mind from toxins that prohibit a healthy state. There is no scientific evidence to support this claim; however, breathwork may help in relaxation and stress reduction (see Imagery and Meditation).

Crystals

Other common name(s)	Scientific/medical name(s)
Crystal Healing	None

DESCRIPTION

Crystals such as quartz, malachite, and other gemstones are used for the purposes of healing physical and emotional conditions.

OVERVIEW

There is no scientific evidence that crystals are effective in treating cancer or any other disease. However, there are some anecdotal reports that crystals can be used as a method to promote relaxation and relieve stress.

How is it promoted for use?

Crystals are used to treat a wide variety of physical and emotional conditions including bursitis, headaches, indigestion, insomnia, hemorrhages, rheumatism, thrombosis, forgetfulness, anxiety, depression, Parkinson's disease, blindness, and cancer. Some people claim certain gemstones or crystals contain special energy that can be transferred to people to provide protection against disease, restore health, and provide spiritual guidance. There is no scientific evidence to support these claims.

Most supporters do not claim stones or crystals can cure illness directly. They say certain stones and crystals emit vibrations that can correct underlying problems. It is thought that illness occurs when an individual is misaligned with the divine energy (or light) believed to be the foundation of all creation. The application of stones or crystals within specific energy centers (chakras) creates a flow of energy that promotes healing by clearing, balancing, and re-energizing the body's energy fields (auras) (see Electromagnetic Therapy).

What does it involve?

Crystal therapists are said to intuitively determine where "blockages" of energy are located and then place particular stones or crystals on specific parts of the body. Different types and colors of stones or crystals are promoted to have different healing powers. For example, amethysts are thought to calm the mind, red-orange agates are thought to energize, and bloodstones are thought to purify the blood. Each one is chosen based on the individual's needs and energy fields.

Some people carry crystals in their pockets, wear them on a chain, or place them in the house to bring the power of healing within reach. Crystals are sometimes used along with other methods such as acupuncture, meditation, and polarity therapy (see these entries for more information).

What is the history behind it?

The use of crystals for healing dates back to the ancient Greeks and Hindus who believed there were large gems that gave light to another world under their known world. Ancient cultures believed that spirits lived inside crystals. The Old Testament in the Bible even suggests that God dwells in a stone. They also thought crystals created and gave off light. Crystals remain popular among some alternative therapy proponents today.

What is the evidence?

There is no scientific evidence that crystals are useful in promoting healing. Some crystals have the ability to bend light, which creates a rainbow effect. Phosphorescent crystals can hold light for a short period of time, but they do not have their own energy source or special powers. Some people believe that crystals or gemstones are helpful as a complementary treatment to promote relaxation and reduce stress. This may occur as a result of the "placebo effect" in which believing that something can or will happen generates a positive result.

Are there any possible problems or complications?

Crystals are considered relatively safe. However, relying on this type of treatment alone, and avoiding conventional medical care, may have serious health consequences.

References

Complementary and Alternative Methods. Crystal healing. American Cancer Society Web site. Available at: http://www.cancer.org. Accessed January 26, 2000.

Raso J. Dictionary of metaphysical healthcare. Quackwatch Web site. Available at: http://www.quackwatch.com. Accessed November 16, 1999.

Curanderismo

Other common name(s)	Scientific/medical name(s)
Curanderos, Latin American Healing	None

DESCRIPTION

Curanderismo is a form of folk healing which includes various techniques such as herbal medicine, healing rituals, elements of spiritualism, and psychic healing (see Homeopathy, and Spirituality and Prayer). It is a system of traditional beliefs that are common in Hispanic-American communities, particularly those in the southwestern United States.

OVERVIEW

There is no scientific evidence that curanderismo is effective in treating cancer or any other disease. However, there are some anecdotal reports curanderismo helps to improve symptoms, reduce pain, and relieve stress.

How is it promoted for use?

While some aspects of curanderismo are practiced at home, for mild cases of illness, most people seek out specially trained folk healers called curanderos. Curanderos believe their healing powers are gained through divine inspiration, are passed down from close relatives, or are learned through apprenticeships with experienced healers.

Proponents claim curanderismo can be

used to treat a wide range of physical complaints, including headache, gastrointestinal distress, back pain, and fever, as well as emotional problems such as anxiety, irritability, fatigue, and depression. However, there is no scientific evidence to support these claims.

Practitioners believe good health is achieved by maintaining a balance of hot and cold. In order to treat a person, curanderos often classify that person's physical activities, food intake, drugs consumed, and illnesses as hot or cold and treat the person to restore a balance of both. Proponents also claim folk illnesses such as mal de ojo (the evil eye), susto (fright), and empacho (blockage of the digestive tract) can be treated by curanderismo. In these cases, the curandero may perform barridas (ritual cleansing) to rebalance the body and soul of the sick person.

What does it involve?
Curanderismo techniques can involve the use of herbs, massage, manipulation of body parts, spiritual rituals, and prayer, either in combination or by themselves. The healing often involves others in the family and community.

For physical illnesses, patients are often given herbal mixtures or teas. One cure for a headache is to place a slice of raw potato over each temple. Dandruff is treated by rinsing hair with juice from the olivera plant, a type of cactus. To reduce the size of an overly large "energy field," the curandero may beat the air around the patient's head with a large feather, then roll an egg around the patient's face before cracking it open into a glass.

The treatments given by curanderos can vary widely depending upon the nature of the illness or complaint.

What is the history behind it?
Curanderismo evolved from the culture that grew out of the Spanish colonization of Mexico hundreds of years ago. It takes its name from the Spanish word "curar," meaning to heal. The tradition combines aspects of both Catholicism and the traditional folk medicine of the natives of Latin America.

Today, it is practiced in several Latin American countries as well as Mexico, Peru, and the United States. Because of its long history of cultural connection, curanderismo remains popular among some Mexican-American communities as an alternative form of medicine. Curanderismo has remained popular among some of these communities because it offers a spiritual treatment for problems which conventional medicine does not recognize such as evil spirits. Also, many people have turned to curanderismo after conventional treatments have failed to cure their disease or because they do not trust conventional methods.

What is the evidence?
There is no scientific evidence that curanderismo cures cancer or any other disease. However, some people report it helps to reduce pain, relieve stress, and promote spiritual peace. A study in 1977 which looked at the relationship between Mexican-American populations and folk medicine suggested that curanderismo should be looked at more closely by conventional medicine. Researchers proposed that a better understanding of folk medicine, such as curanderismo, might help physicians treat their patients more effectively and understand patient fears and beliefs. A more recent study found that patients often seek treatment by curanderismo alongside conventional medical treatment.

Are there any possible problems or complications?

There are no known harmful effects. However, some treatment by curanderos may involve the ingestion of unregulated herbs and teas. Relying on this type of treatment alone, and avoiding conventional medical care, may have serious health consequences.

References
Alegria D, Guerra E, Martinez C Jr, Meyer GG. El hospital invisible. A study of curanderismo. *Arch Gen Psychiatry.* 1977;34:1354-1357.

Allen H. Folk healer discusses art of 'curanderismo.' Yale Daily News Online. Yale University Web site. Available at: http://www.yale.edu. Accessed December 11, 1999.

Alternative Medicine: Expanding Medical Horizons. *A Report to the National Institutes of Health on Alternative Medical Systems and Practices in the United States.* Washington, DC: US Government Printing Office; 1994. NIH publication 94-066.

Ness RC, Wintrob RM. Folk healing: a description and synthesis. *Am J Psychiatry.* 1981;138:1477-1481.

Cymatic Therapy

Other common name(s)	Scientific/medical name
None	None

DESCRIPTION / OVERVIEW

Cymatic therapy is a form of sound therapy developed by Sir Peter Guy Manners, MD, DO, PhD, from England. Although no sounds can be heard by those treated with this method, hand-held instruments are used to transmit sound waves through the skin. According to practitioners, illness appears when the rhythms of the heart, brain, and other organs are not working harmoniously. The signals passed through these cymatic devices are supposed to restore synchronous rhythms and boost the body's regulatory and immunologic systems. There is no scientific evidence to support this claim (see Music Therapy).

Dance Therapy

Other common name(s)	Scientific/medical name(s)
Movement Therapy	None

DESCRIPTION

Dance therapy is the therapeutic use of movement to improve the mental and physical well being of a person. It focuses on the connection between the mind and body to promote health and healing.

OVERVIEW

There have been few scientific studies conducted to evaluate the effects of dance therapy on health, prevention, and recovery from illness. Clinical reports suggest dance therapy is effective in improving self-esteem and reducing stress. As a form of exercise, dance therapy can be useful.

How is it promoted for use?

Dance therapy is offered as a health promotion service for healthy people, and as a complementary method of reducing the stress of caregivers and people with cancer and other chronic illness. Physically, dance therapy can provide exercise, improve mobility and muscle coordination, and reduce muscle tension. Emotionally, dance therapy is reported to improve self-awareness, self-confidence, and interpersonal interaction, and is an outlet for communicating feelings. Some promoters claim that dance therapy may strengthen the immune system through muscular action and physiological processes and even help prevent disease. There is no scientific evidence to confirm the effects of dance therapy on prevention and recovery from illness, however.

Dance therapy is based on the belief that the mind and body work together. Through dance, it is thought people can identify and express their innermost emotions, bringing those feelings to the surface. Some people claim this can create a sense of renewal, unity, and completeness.

What does it involve?

Dance therapists help people develop a nonverbal language that offers information about what is going on in their bodies. The therapist observes a person's movements to make an assessment and then designs a program to help the specific condition. The frequency and level of difficulty of the therapy is usually tailored to meet the needs of the participants.

Dance therapy is used in a variety of settings with people who have social, emotional, cognitive, or physical concerns. It is often used as a part of the recovery process for people with chronic illness. Dance therapists work with both individuals and groups, including entire families.

What is the history behind it?

Dance has been an important part of self-expression, ceremonial and religious events, and health in most cultures throughout history. For example, medicine men of many Native American tribes used dance as part of their heal-ing rituals. The use of dance as a medical therapy began in 1942 through the work of Marian Chace. She was asked to work at St. Elizabeth's Hospital in Washington DC after psychiatrists found that their patients received therapeutic benefits from attending her dance classes. Another woman who was a dancer and mime, Trudi Schoop, volunteered to work with patients at a state hospital in California at about that time. In 1956, the American Dance Therapy Association was founded to establish and maintain high standards in the field of dance therapy. There are now more than 1,200 dance therapists in the United States and abroad. In 1993, the Office of Alternative Medicine of the National Institute of Health provided a research grant to explore dance therapy for people with medical illnesses.

A master's degree is required to be a dance therapist. Beginning level dance therapists who have at least 700 hours of supervised clinical training hold the title of "Dance Therapists Registered" (DTR). The title "Academy of Dance Therapists" (ADTR) is awarded to advanced level dance therapists who have completed 3,640 hours of supervised clinical work in an agency, institution, or special school with additional supervision from an ADTR.

What is the evidence?

Although anecdotal accounts provide support for the value of dance therapy, few experimental studies evaluating the effects of dance therapy on health have been published. Clinical reports suggest that dance therapy helps in developing body image; improving self-concept and self-esteem; reducing stress, anxiety, and depression; decreasing isolation, chronic pain, and body tension; and increasing communication skills and feelings of well being. Well-controlled research is needed, however, to confirm the effects of dance therapy on prevention and recovery of illness.

Some of the physical motions of dance therapy can be useful exercises that provide similar health benefits gained through exercise. Physical activity is known to increase special neurotransmitter substances in the brain (endorphins) which create a state of well being. And total body movement enhances the functions of other body systems, such as circulatory, respiratory, skeletal, and muscular systems. Dance therapy can help people stay physically fit and enjoy the pleasure of creating rhythmic motions with their bodies.

Are there any possible problems or complications?

People with cancer and chronic conditions such as arthritis and heart disease should consult with their physician before undergoing any type of therapy that involves manipulation of joints and muscles.

References

Alternative Medicine: Expanding Medical Horizons. A Report to the National Institutes of Health on Alternative Medical Systems and Practices in the United States. Washington, DC: US Government Printing Office; 1994. NIH publication 94-066.

Cassileth B. The Alternative Medicine Handbook. New York, NY: W. W. Norton & Co; 1998.

Cohen SO, Walco GA. Dance/movement therapy for children and adolescents with cancer. Cancer Pract. 1999;7:34-42.

Hanna JL. The power of dance: health and healing. J Altern Complement Med. 1995;1:323-331.

Faith Healing

Other common name(s)	Scientific/medical name(s)
Spiritual Healing	None

DESCRIPTION

Faith healing is founded on the belief that certain people or places have the ability to cure and heal—that someone or something can eliminate disease or heal injuries through a close connection to a higher power. Faith healing can involve prayer, a visit to a religious shrine, or simply a strong belief in a supreme being.

OVERVIEW

There is no scientific evidence that faith healing can cure cancer or any other disease. Even the "miraculous" cures at the French shrine of Lourdes, after careful study by the Catholic Church, do not outnumber the historical percentage of spontaneous remissions seen among people with cancer. However, faith healing may promote peace of mind, reduce stress, relieve pain and anxiety, and strengthen the will to live.

How is it promoted for use?

According to proponents, there is little that faith healing cannot do. They claim it can cure blindness, deafness, cancer, AIDS, developmental disorders, anemia, arthritis, corns, defective speech, multiple sclerosis, skin rashes, total body paralysis, and heal various injuries. Christian Scientists claim that illness is an illusion caused by bad thoughts which can be healed or made to leave the sick person's body by trained practitioners through prayer. However, there is no scientific evidence to support these claims.

What does it involve?

Faith healing is practiced either at a distance from, or in close proximity to, the patient. When practiced from afar, it can involve a single faith healer or a group of individuals praying for the patient. When near to the patient, as in revivalist tent meetings, the healer touches, or "lays hands on," the patient while invoking a supreme being. Faith healing can also involve a pilgrimage to a religious shrine, such as the French shrine at Lourdes, in search of a miracle. Christian Scientists train and use their own practitioners in order to heal sick persons through prayer.

What is the history behind it?

Faith healing is believed to have originated even before the earliest recorded history. In the Bible, both God and holy people are said to have the power to heal. In Medieval times, the "Divine Right of Kings" was thought to give royalty the ability to heal through touch. Through the years there have been numerous reports of saints performing miracle cures, up to and including the 20th century. Today, several religious groups, including Christian Scientists, Protestant evangelists, and some orthodox Jewish sects, practice faith healing.

What is the evidence?

Although it is known that a small percentage of people with cancer experience remissions of their disease which cannot be explained, there is no scientific evidence that faith healing can actually cure physical ailments. When a person has a strong belief that a healer can create a cure, a "placebo effect" can occur which makes the person feel better. The placebo effect is an improvement that occurs because of a powerful belief in the treatment. The patient usually credits the improvement to the healer. Taking part in faith healing can evoke the power of suggestion, which promotes peace of mind. This can help people cope more effectively with their illness.

One review published in 1998 looked at 172 cases of fatalities among children treated by faith healing instead of conventional methods. These researchers found that if conventional treatment had been given, the survival rate for these children could have exceeded 90%, with the remainder of the children also having a good chance of survival.

Are there any possible problems or complications?

People who seek help through faith healing and are not cured can develop feelings of hopelessness, failure, guilt, worthlessness, and depression. Relying on this type of treatment alone, and avoiding conventional medical care, may have serious health consequences. There are some organizations working towards creating laws to protect children from inappropriate treatment by faith healers.

References

Alternative Medicine: Expanding Medical Horizons. A Report to the National Institutes of Health on Alternative Medical Systems and Practices in the United States. Washington, DC: US Government Printing Office; 1994. NIH publication 94-066.

Asser SM, Swan R. Child fatalities from religion-motivated medical neglect. Pediatrics. 1998;101:625-629.

Barrett S. Some thoughts about faith healing. Quackwatch Web site. Available at: http://www.quackwatch.com. Accessed October 21, 1999.

Complementary and Alternative Methods. Faith Healing. American Cancer Society Web site. Available at: http://www.cancer.org. Accessed January 26, 2000.

US Congress, Office of Technology Assessment. Unconventional Cancer Treatments. Washington, DC: US Government Printing Office; 1990. Publication OTA-H-405.

Feng Shui

Other common name(s)	Scientific/medical name(s)
None	None

DESCRIPTION

Feng shui is the ancient Chinese philosophy and art of placing objects, ornaments, furniture, rooms, buildings, and even towns in position so they promote the beneficial flow of vital energy or life force called qi (or chi). The words feng shui literally mean wind and water.

OVERVIEW

The ancient Chinese art of feng shui rests on placement of things so they are in harmony with one another and with the environment. There is no scientific evidence to support the claim that feng shui can influence health.

How is it promoted for use?

Chinese adherents to feng shui hold that the same natural elements that form the earth, such as wind and water, can bring healthy energy into homes, buildings, and cities if the placement of these man-made elements permits energy to flow through the environment.

By extension, some believe that living and work environments that are out of balance may promote disease, including cancer, and prevent those who live in the environment from responding to treatment. Changes in the environment, proponents claim, may help prevent disease and promote healing. For example, simply placing the bed of a person with cancer, or at risk of cancer, in a new position is thought to prevent the development or progression of the disease.

What does it involve?

The idea behind feng shui is to orient physical objects to allow humankind to live in harmony with the environment and the universe. In order to accomplish this goal, a feng shui practitioner will first study the physical environment outside a person's home to make sure the house is positioned in a way that will promote a positive flow of energy. Next, the inside of the house is examined. Furniture may be moved or set at angles until rooms are more open and free of clutter or obstacles which may hinder energy from flowing around the house. A feng shui practitioner will also analyze the electromagnetic energy in a person's home sometimes using a specialized compass and surrounding property to make sure the energy is balanced in order to promote good health and well being.

What is the history behind it?

Feng shui has been practiced in China since the Qin Dynasty beginning in about 221 BC. In ancient China, feng shui began as an oral tradition and was only taught to a select few by a master. The techniques were a well-guarded secret.

In 1929, a German baron, Gustave von Pohl, reportedly linked an unusually high cancer rate in the German village of Vilsbiburg to "radiation" coming from geological faults below the city. In 1932, von Pohl published a book called *Earth Currents: Causative Factors of Cancer and Other Diseases*. Currently, some alternative medical practitioners have cited von Pohl's theories as proof that imbalances in the natural energy or magnetic force of a physical area can cause illness. They claim that feng shui can be used to rebalance a physical environment and restore well being. The philosophy of feng shui has spread to the Western world where it has become popular for interior and building design.

What is the evidence?
There is no scientific evidence that feng shui has any effect on cancer or any other disease.

Are there any possible problems or complications?

No adverse effects have been reported with the use of feng shui. However, consultants in feng shui are not licensed, and relying on this type of treatment and avoiding conventional medical care may have serious health consequences.

References
Rossbach S. Feng shui explores relationship between design and health—ancient Chinese art of placement. *Calif Hosp.* 1991;5:29-31.

Von Pohl GF. *Earth Currents: Causative Factor of Cancer and Other Diseases.* Stuttgart, Germany: Frech-Verlag, 1983.

Holistic Medicine

Other common name(s)	Scientific/medical name(s)
Holistic Health, Holism	None

DESCRIPTION
Holistic medicine focuses on how the physical, mental, emotional, and spiritual elements of the body are interconnected to maintain wellness (holistic health). When one part of the body is not working properly, it is believed to affect the whole person. The treatment concentrates on the whole body rather than focusing narrowly on the illness or part of the body that is not healthy.

OVERVIEW
There is no scientific evidence that holistic medicine alone is effective in treating cancer or any other disease. However, many health professionals promote healthy lifestyle habits such as exercising, eating a nutritious diet, and not smoking as important in maintaining good health. Holistic methods can be used as complementary therapy.

How is it promoted for use?
Holistic medicine approaches health and disease from several angles and suggests that a person should not only treat the illness, but his or her whole self to reach a higher level of wellness. For example, practitioners treat cancer by changing diet and behavior, taking botanical supplements, and undergoing complementary therapies (see Acupuncture, Aromatherapy, Art Therapy, Hypnosis, Psychotherapy, Spirituality and Prayer, and Yoga). These approaches can be used along with conventional medicine such as

chemotherapy, surgery, radiation therapy, and hormone therapy. By combining these different techniques, a person can take control of the disease and obtain a feeling of total wellness—spiritually, physically, and mentally.

Some proponents claim, however, that conventional medicine does not work and that only the holistic approach to cancer and other diseases is effective. They offer not just a treatment but a "cure" based on anecdotal reports, or personal experience. Some of the different kinds of cancer which proponents claim can be cured by holistic approaches include bone, breast, tongue, liver, lung, throat, skin, testicle, prostate, ovarian, uterus, stomach, intestinal, colon, brain, pancreatic, spleen, kidney, and bladder, as well as leukemia, lymphoma, and melanoma. There is no scientific evidence to support these claims.

What does it involve?

The field of holistic medicine is very diverse and covers a broad continuum. Some providers define holistic oncology as care that doesn't ignore emotional and spiritual aspects, while others focus on these aspects to the exclusion of the physical. There are many different techniques and approaches in holistic medicine, depending on the person and the illness. All, however, stress the use of treatments that encourage the body's natural healing system and take into consideration the person as a whole.

Holistic medicine can involve the use of conventional and alternative therapies but focuses mostly on lifestyle changes. A holistic approach to stomach cancer might include reducing sodium intake, increasing intake of antioxidants through food or vitamins, eliminating *Helicobacter pylori* (a bacteria that exists in the stomach), quitting smoking, improving oral hygiene, avoiding foods that contain genotoxic agents, and increasing the amount of vegetables and fruits consumed.

Holistic medicine can also include natural supplements that cause the same changes as conventional drugs. For instance, synthetic interferon is currently used to treat people with cancer. A holistic approach might be to take high doses of intravenous vitamin C instead, in an attempt to stimulate the body's production of its own interferon.

The American Holistic Association says that healthy lifestyle habits will improve a person's energy and vitality. Those habits might include exercising, eating a nutritious diet, getting enough sleep, learning how to breath properly, taking antioxidants and supplements, acupuncture, acupressure, healing touch, craniosacral therapy, qigong, and other methods.

What is the history behind it?

Holistic medicine has its roots in several ancient healing traditions that stress healthy living and being in harmony with nature. Socrates promoted a holistic approach. Plato was another advocate of holism, advising physicians to respect the relationship between mind and body. Hippocrates, emphasized the body's ability to heal itself and cautioned physicians not to interfere with that process.

It was not until 1926, however, that Jan Christiaan Smuts coined the term "holism," which has given us the more integrated concept of psychosomatic medicine now known as holistic medicine. In the 1970s, "holistic" became a more common term. Today, holistic medicine is known as an approach to life and health which brings together the physical, mental, and spiritual aspects of a person in order to create a total sense of well being.

What is the evidence?

Although there has been research on various complementary methods, that may be considered part of a holistic approach, there is no research focusing on holistic medicine by itself as a cure for cancer or any other disease. The president of the American Holistic Association said, "there is no published evidence that alternative practitioners are more effective than conventional physicians in persuading their patients to improve their lifestyle. Nor have any vitalistic approaches been proven effective or cost-effective against any disease."

Some health care professionals suggest that cancer pain and some side effects of treatment can be managed by incorporating different aspects of holistic medicine that include the physical, psychological, and spiritual factors involved with each individual. Increasingly, the health care team is playing an important role in the treatment provided by many research centers and hospitals. Members of this team are drawn from the specialties of medicine, nursing, surgery, radiation therapy, oncology, psychiatry, psychology, and social work. In addition, the team may call on dietitians, physical therapists, and the clergy for support. Health professionals realize that a person's health depends on the balance of physical, psychological, social, and cultural forces.

Are there any possible problems or complications?

Adopting healthy habits related to diet, exercise, emotional, and spiritual well being are considered important to maintaining good health. Relying on this type of treatment alone, and avoiding conventional medical care, may have serious health consequences.

References

Barrett S. Be wary of alternative health methods. Quackwatch Web site. Available at: http://www.quackwatch.com. Accessed October 14, 1999.

Hassed C. Cancer and chronic pain. *Aust Fam Physician*. 1999;28:17-21, 23-24.

National Center for Complementary and Alternative Medicine. March 23-24, 1998: AMPAC Meeting Minutes: IX. Public Comments. National Institutes of Health Web site. Available at: http://nccam.nih.gov/nccam/news-events/ampac/1998/mar/9.html. Accessed January 3, 2000.

Sitzia J, Huggins L. Side effects of cyclophosphamide, methotrexate, and 5-fluorouracil (CMF) chemotherapy for breast cancer. *Cancer Pract*. 1998;6:13-21.

Sugimura T. Cancer prevention: past, present, future. *Mutat Res*. 1998;402:7-14.

Humor Therapy

Other common name(s)	Scientific/medical name(s)
Laugh Therapy	None

DESCRIPTION

Humor therapy is the use of humor for the relief of physical and emotional difficulties. It is used as a complementary tool to promote health and cope with illness.

OVERVIEW

Although there is no scientific evidence that laughter can cure cancer or any other disease, it can reduce stress, promote health, and enhance the quality of life. Humor has physiological effects that can stimulate the circulatory system, immune system, and other systems in the body.

How is it promoted for use?

Humor therapy is generally used to improve quality of life, provide some pain relief, encourage relaxation, and reduce stress. Researchers have described different types of humor. Passive humor is created by observing a comic film, or reading a book, for example. Humor production is a type of humor that involves creating or finding humor in stressful situations. It is thought that being able to find humor in everyday events can be helpful.

What does it involve?

The physical effects of laughter on the body involve increased breathing, oxygen use, and heart rate, which stimulate the circulatory system. Many hospitals and ambulatory care centers have incorporated special rooms where humorous materials, and sometimes people, are there to help make people laugh. Materials commonly used include movies, audio and videotapes, books, games, and puzzles. Many hospitals use volunteer groups who visit patients for the purpose of providing opportunities for laughter.

What is the history behind it?

Humor has been used in medicine throughout recorded history. One of the earliest mentions of the health benefits of humor is in the book of Proverbs in the Bible. As early as the 13th century, some surgeons used humor to distract patients from the pain of surgery. Humor was also widely used and studied by the medical community in the early 20th century. In more modern times, the most famous story of humor therapy involved Norman Cousins, then editor of the *Saturday Review*. According to the story, Mr. Cousins "cured" himself from an unknown illness with a self-invented regimen of laughter and vitamins.

What is the evidence?

There is no scientific evidence that humor is effective in treating cancer or any other disease, however, laughter has many clinical benefits that include positive physiological changes and an overall sense of well being. One study found the use of humor lead to an increase in pain tolerance. It is thought laughter stimulates the release of special neurotransmitter substances in the brain (endorphins) that help control pain. Another study demonstrated neuroendocrine and stress-related hormones decreased during episodes of laughter, which provides support for the claim that humor can relieve stress. More studies are needed to clarify the impact of laughter on health.

Are there any possible problems or complications?

Humor therapy is considered safe when used as a complementary therapy.

References

Berk LS, Tan SA, Fry WF, et al. Neuroendocrine and stress hormone changes during mirthful laughter. *Am J Med Sci*. 1989;298:390-396.

Complementary and Alternative Methods. Humor therapy. American Cancer Society Web site. Available at: http://www.cancer.org. Accessed January 31, 2000.

Seaward BL. Humor's healing potential. *Health Prog*. 1992;73:66-70.

Weisenberg M, Tepper I, Schwarzwald, J. Humor as a cognitive technique for increasing pain tolerance. *Pain*. 1995;63:207-212.

Ziegler J. Immune system may benefit from the ability to laugh. *J Natl Cancer Inst*. 1995;87:342-343.

Hypnosis

Other common name(s)	**Scientific/medical name(s)**
Hypnotherapy, Hypnotic Suggestion	None

DESCRIPTION

Hypnosis is a state of restful alertness during which a person can be relatively unaware of, but not completely blind to, their surroundings.

OVERVIEW

Hypnosis is one of several relaxation methods that has been approved by an independent panel, convened by the National Institutes of Health (NIH), as a useful complementary therapy for treating chronic pain. The technique may also be effective in reducing fear and anxiety, treating pain during labor and delivery, reducing labor time, and controlling bleeding and pain during dental procedures. There is no scientific evidence that hypnosis can influence the development or progression of cancer, however, it can help to improve the quality of life for some people with cancer.

How is it promoted for use?

Practitioners say that hypnosis creates a state of deep relaxation, quiets the conscious mind, and leaves the unconscious part of the mind open to suggestions that can help to improve health and lifestyle. People who are hypnotized have selective attention and are able to concentrate intensely on a specific thought, memory, feeling, or sensation while blocking out distractions.

Hypnosis is commonly used to reduce stress and anxiety, and create a sense of well being. It can also be used to change undesirable behaviors, such as smoking, alcohol dependency, and bedwetting, and to overcome common fears, such as the fear of flying or meeting people. Some claim that hypnosis can be used to reduce chronic and acute pain. Hypnosis is sometimes used to relieve pain caused by cancer. Proponents do not claim that hypnosis can cure cancer or any other disease, or that it always results in the desired effects. However, they say that it can be a useful addition to conventional therapy for some conditions.

Hypnosis is occasionally substituted for anesthetic drugs during minor surgical and dental procedures, and during childbirth. Some supporters also believe hypnosis not only accelerates recovery after an operation, but also reduces the amount of surgical bleeding and enhances the body's immune system.

What does it involve?

There are many different hypnotic techniques. One method involves leading patients into a state of hypnosis by talking in gentle, soothing tones, and describing images meant to create a sense of relaxation, security, and well being. People under hypnosis may appear to be asleep but they are actually in an altered state of concentration and can focus intently when asked to do so by the hypnotherapist. While a patient is under hypnosis, the hypnotherapist may suggest particular goals, such as pain control, stabilizing emotions, and reducing stress, fear, or anxiety.

Contrary to what many believe, people under hypnosis are not under the control of the hypnotherapist nor can they be made to do something they do not want. Quite the opposite is true. Hypnosis is used to help patients gain more control over their behavior, emotions, and even physiological processes that cause undesired consequences. People cannot be hypnotized involuntarily, and not everyone can be put into a hypnotic trance. Success depends upon the patient's willingness and receptivity to the idea of undergoing hypnosis. Some people can learn to hypnotize themselves.

What is the history behind it?

Hypnosis and hypnotic suggestion have been a part of healing practices for thousands of years. The word comes from the Greek, "hypnos," which means sleep. The induction of trance-like states and the use of therapeutic suggestion were important features of the early Greek healing temples. Variations of those techniques were practiced throughout the ancient world.

Modern hypnosis can be credited to the Viennese physician, Franz Anton Mesmer, who believed that imbalances in magnetic forces in the human body were responsible for illness. Mesmer applied a therapy, which he called mesmerism, involving the use of tranquil gestures and soothing words to relax patients and restore the balance to their magnetic forces. Sigmund Freud, the father of psychotherapy, found hypnosis useful for treating hysteria, but later abandoned the practice after observing that his technique stirred up powerful emotions within his patients.

Eventually, the notion of using a state of altered awareness gained greater acceptance in conventional Western medicine. Today, hypnosis is used widely in the United States and other Western countries. People who practice hypnosis are licensed and are often trained in a variety of psychological techniques.

What is the evidence?

Numerous reports demonstrate that hypnosis can help patients reduce blood pressure, stress, anxiety, and pain; create relaxing brain wave patterns, modify negative behaviors such as smoking, alcohol consumption, and overeating; and eliminate or decrease the intensity of phobias. Some research has also demonstrated that hypnosis can be used to control nausea and vomiting caused by chemotherapy. According to a report from the NIH, there is strong evidence that hypnosis can relieve some pain associated with cancer.

Another NIH report, which reviewed several scientific studies, showed some interesting research findings about the therapeutic potential of hypnosis including the finding that women under hypnosis prior to childbirth experienced shorter labors and more comfortable deliveries. According to the report, hypnosis may also enhance the immune system. One study listed found that hypnosis raised the levels of immunoglobulin (an important component of the immune system) in healthy children. Another study reported that self-hypnosis led to an increase in white blood cell activity. The NIH report also looked at twelve different controlled studies, which showed that hypnosis is an excellent way to reduce the intensity or frequency of migraine headaches in children and teenagers. Another study on chronically ill patients found a 113% increase in pain tolerance among highly hypnotizable subjects versus those who were not hypnotized. According to the NIH report, the reasons why hypnosis causes these changes are not well understood.

Are there any possible problems or complications?

Hypnosis conducted under the care of a trained hypnotherapist is considered safe as a complementary method.

References

Alternative Medicine: Expanding Medical Horizons. *A Report to the National Institutes of Health on Alternative Medical Systems and Practices in the United States.* Washington, DC: US Government Printing Office; 1994. NIH publication 94-066.

Cassileth B. *The Alternative Medicine Handbook.* New York, NY: W. W. Norton & Co; 1998.

Levitan AA. The use of hypnosis with cancer patients. *Psychiatr Med.* 1992;10:119-131.

Morrow GR, Hickok JT. Behavioral treatment of chemotherapy-induced nausea and vomiting. *Oncology (Huntingt).* 1993;7:83-89.

NIH Technology Assessment Panel. Integration of behavioral and relaxation approaches into the treatment of chronic pain and insomnia. *JAMA.* 1996;276:313-318.

Imagery

Other common name(s)	Scientific/medical name(s)
Guided Imagery, Visualization	None

DESCRIPTION

Imagery involves mental exercises designed to enable the mind to influence the health and well being of the body.

OVERVIEW

Imagery involves the use of visualization techniques that are used as complementary therapies in people with cancer and other diseases. The techniques can help to reduce stress, anxiety, and depression, manage pain, lower blood pressure, ease some of the side effects of chemotherapy, and create feelings of being in control. There is no scientific evidence that imagery can influence the development or progression of cancer.

How is it promoted for use?

Imagery is said to be a relaxation technique, similar to meditation that has physical and psychological effects (see Meditation). Promoters claim it can relax the mind and body by decreasing heart rate, lowering blood pressure, and altering brain waves. Some proponents also claim imagery can relieve physical pain and emotional anxiety, improve the effectiveness of drug therapies, and provide emotional insights.

Practitioners use imagery to treat people with phobias and depression, reduce stress, increase motivation, promote relaxation, increase control over one's life, improve communication, and even to stop smoking. Imagery is also used in biofeedback, hypnosis, and neuro-linguistic programming (see Biofeedback, Hypnosis, and Neuro-Linguistic Programming).

For people with cancer, some supporters of imagery have found the techniques can alleviate nausea and vomiting associated with chemotherapy, relieve stress associated with having cancer, enhance the immune system, facilitate weight gain, combat depression, and lessen pain.

What does it involve?

There are many different imagery techniques. One popular method is called palming, which involves placing the palms of your hands over your eyes and imagining a color you associate with anxiety or stress (such as red), and then a color you associate with relaxation or calmness (such as blue). Visualizing a calming color is supposed to make you feel relaxed and improve your health and sense of well being.

Another common technique is known as guided imagery, which involves visualizing a specific image or goal to be achieved and then imagining achieving that goal. Athletes use this technique to improve their game. One type of guided therapy used for cancer patients is called the Simonton method, which was developed in the 1970s by O. Carl Simonton, a radiation oncologist, and Stephanie Matthews-Simonton, a psychotherapist. In the Simonton method, people with cancer are asked to imagine their bodies fighting cancer cells and winning the battle.

One popular exercise is modeled on the old Pac Man video game. Patients are to picture tiny Pac Men eating and destroying tumor cells, just like Pac Man destroyed his enemies in the game. The Simontons used their method as complementary therapy with conventional cancer treatments.

The techniques can be done as self-taught therapy with the help of one of a number of books or learning tapes published on the subject or they can be practiced under the guidance of a trained therapist. Imagery sessions with a health professional may last 20 to 30 minutes.

What is the history behind it?

Imagery is believed to have been used as a medical therapy for centuries. There is recorded evidence that Tibetan monks in the 13th and 14th centuries began meditating to Buddha and imagining that Buddha would cure diseases. Some say the techniques even go back to the ancient Babylonians, Greeks, and Romans. The Simontons popularized these therapies in a best-selling 1978 book titled Getting Well Again. The book described their experiences in treating cancer patients with their imagery method and other therapies.

Currently, imagery is used in clinics at medical centers and local hospitals. It is often combined with other behavioral treatments.

What is the evidence?

A review of 46 studies conducted from 1966 to 1998 found that guided imagery was effective in managing stress, anxiety, and depression, and lowering blood pressure, pain, and the side effects of chemotherapy. The authors suggested a need for systematic, well-designed research to determine the specifics of how guided imagery can be most effectively used.

A recent randomized clinical trial involving women with early stage breast cancer found guided imagery was also useful for easing anxiety related to radiation therapy, including fears about the equipment, surgical pain, and recurrence of cancer.

According to some studies, guided imagery may help reduce some of the side effects of conventional cancer treatment. Some studies also suggest that imagery can directly effect the immune system. Although one uncontrolled, exploratory study suggested that guided imagery can increase survival rates for people with cancer, there is no scientific evidence these techniques can cure cancer or any other disease.

Are there any possible problems or complications?

Imagery techniques are considered safe, especially under the guidance of a trained health professional. They are best used as complementary therapy along with conventional treatment.

References

Alternative Medicine: Expanding Medical Horizons. *A Report to the National Institutes of Health on Alternative Medical Systems and Practices in the United States.* Washington, DC: US Government Printing Office; 1994. NIH publication 94-066.

Barrett S, Herbert V. Questionable cancer therapies. Quackwatch Web site. Available at: http//:www.quackwatch.com. Accessed October 8, 1999.

Cassileth B. *The Alternative Medicine Handbook.* New York, NY: W. W. Norton & Co; 1998.

Eller LS. Guided imagery interventions for symptom management. *Annu Rev Nurs Res.* 1999;17:57-84.

Kolcaba K, Fox C. The effects of guided imagery on comfort of women with early stage breast cancer undergoing radiation therapy. *Oncol Nurs Forum.* 1999;26:67-72.

Richardson MA, Post-White J, Grimm EA, Moye LA, Singletary SE, Justice B. Coping, life attitudes, and immune responses to imagery and group support after breast cancer treatment. *Altern Ther Health Med.* 1997;3:62-70.

Spencer JW, Jacobs JJ. *Complementary/Alternative Medicine: An Evidence-Based Approach.* St. Louis, MO: Mosby, Inc; 1999.

Walker LG, Walker MB, Ogston K, et al. Psychological, clinical and pathological effects of relaxation training and guided imagery during primary chemotherapy. *Br J Cancer.* 1999;80:262-268.

Kirlian Photography

Other common name(s)	Scientific/medical name(s)
None	None

DESCRIPTION

Kirlian photography involves recording the responses of high voltage electricity, passed through a metal plate, onto a piece of photographic paper.

OVERVIEW

There is no evidence that Kirlian photography is useful in diagnosing cancer or any other disease.

How is it promoted for use?

Kirlian photography advocates believe that all objects, including humans, emit auras that represent the body's energy fields or life forces. These auras are invisible, believers say, but Kirlian photography captures them on film. Proponents claim Kirlian photographs of the human body carry information about the subject's physiological, psychological, and psychic state. The various colors of the photographs are said to reflect the subject's mood, energy level, and health. For example, they say that predominantly red auras indicate repressed anger; green auras suggest drug or alcohol addiction; gray or brown auras are signs of emotional or physical deficiency. The photographs are used to diagnose problems with specific organs such as kidney disorders, nutritional deficiencies, substance abuse, mental illness, anxiety, confusion, and even cancer. There is no scientific evidence to support these claims.

What does it involve?

Kirlian photography does not actually involve a photographic lens or camera. The apparatus to produce a Kirlian photograph consists of a high-voltage electrical source that is attached to a metal plate. A glass plate sits on top of the metal plate, and a piece of photographic paper is laid on top of the glass plate. The object being photographed, such as a hand or foot, is placed directly on the photographic paper. A Kirlian photograph emerges consisting of jagged, colored lines that outline the shape of the photographed object. The resulting image is said to represent an aura, or outline of the body's life force.

What is the history behind it?

Kirlian photography was invented by a Russian electrician, Semyon Kirlian, and his wife Valentina in the 1950s. In 1978, researchers in Romania claimed that the technique could detect malignant tumors; however, these claims have not been proven.

What is the evidence?

There is no scientific evidence demonstrating that Kirlian photographs can be used to diagnose physical or psychological problems. Research has shown that the images are caused by a variety of factors, none of which are an indication of health problems.

Scientists explain that Kirlian film images reflect differences in skin temperature, position and pressure of the finger or object on the plate, air temperature, moisture levels, and other physiologic changes, rather than auras. Changes in voltage and length of exposure can also affect images captured in the films.

Are there any possible problems or complications?

Kirlian photography is generally considered safe. However, relying on this method alone for diagnosis, and avoiding conventional medical care, may have serious health consequences.

References

Complementary and Alternative Methods. Kirlian photography. American Cancer Society Web site. Available at: http://www.cancer.org. Accessed January 24, 2000.

Stanwick M. Aura photography: mundane physics or diagnostic tool? *Nurs Times.* 1996;92:39-41.

Labyrinth Walking

Other common name(s)	Scientific/medical name(s)
Labyrinths	None

DESCRIPTION

Labyrinth walking is a form of meditation that involves walking on labyrinths (winding pathways drawn or laid on the ground). These labyrinths have only one path from start to finish and can be found indoors and outdoors.

OVERVIEW

Labyrinth walking should not be used to prevent or treat cancer or other serious diseases. However, it may be helpful as a complementary method to decrease stress and create a state of relaxation.

How is it promoted for use?

Labyrinth walking is used as a form of meditation. In fact, it is described by many as walking meditation. People walk through labyrinths to reach any number of goals, such as inner peace, heightened spirituality, personal insight, prayer, relaxation, stress relief, or just "letting go" (see Meditation).

What does it involve?

Labyrinth walkers follow the labyrinth path from a specified beginning, through a well-defined central area and continue on to the exit. They might pray, reflect on life, consider a particular problem, let the mind wander or seek spiritual awakening and unity as they move along the twisting trail. Their aim is not to reach the finish, but to become immersed in all aspects of the labyrinth walking process, and potentially to experience some degree of personal transformation.

What is the history behind it?

Labyrinths may date back 4,000 years, though their origins are shrouded in mystery. During the middle ages, labyrinths were built in a number of large European churches so worshippers could make a symbolic "pilgrimage" to the Holy Land. The labyrinth on the floor of the famous Chartres cathedral in France was built in the year 1220.

Many religious traditions incorporate labyrinths. In Judaism, the Tree of Life, called the Kaballah, takes the form of an elongated labyrinth. The Hopi medicine wheel is another example of a labyrinth. Labyrinths are undergoing a rediscovery of sorts and can now be found not only in places of worship, but also in retreat centers, hospitals, prisons, parks, airports and community centers. By one estimate, there are more than 1,000 labyrinths in the United States alone. One of the most common labyrinth designs is the eleven-circle labyrinth, which is named for the eleven paths that lead to the center.

What is the evidence?

There is no scientific evidence that labyrinth walking can be used to treat cancer or any other disease. However, many health care practitioners consider any activity that promotes relaxation and relieves stress beneficial to overall health.

Are there any possible problems or complications?

Labyrinth walking is generally considered safe as a complementary therapy.

References

Condren D. Labyrinth walking explores spiritual path to inner peace. *The Buffalo News.* July 11, 1999:1C.

Spilner, M. Treading ancient paths. *Prevention.* 1997;49:143.

Meditation

Other common name(s)	Scientific/medical name(s)
Transcendental Meditation®	None

DESCRIPTION

Meditation is a mind-body process that uses concentration or reflection to relax the body and calm the mind in order to create a sense of well being.

OVERVIEW

Meditation is one of several relaxation methods approved by an independent panel, convened by the National Institutes of Health (NIH), as a useful complementary therapy for treating chronic pain and insomnia. There is no scientific evidence that meditation is effective in treating cancer or any other disease, however, it can help to improve the quality of life for people with cancer.

How is it promoted for use?

The NIH National Center for Complementary and Alternative Medicine reports that regular meditation can increase longevity and quality of life; and reduce chronic pain, anxiety, high blood pressure, cholesterol, health care use, substance abuse, post-traumatic stress syndrome in Vietnam veterans, and blood cortisol levels initially brought on by stress.

Practitioners also claim meditation improves mood, improves immune functioning, and enhances fertility. Proponents further claim meditation increases mental efficiency and alertness, and raises self-awareness which contributes to relaxation.

What does it involve?

There are different forms of meditation. Meditation is usually done while sitting, but there are also moving forms of meditation, like tai chi, walking in Zen Buddhism, and the Japanese martial art aikido (see Tai Chi). Meditation can be self-directed, or guided by doctors, psychiatrists, other mental health professionals, and yoga masters.

Self-directed meditation is done by selecting a quiet place free from noise and distraction, sitting or resting quietly with eyes closed (usually on a floor), and trying to achieve a feeling of peace. The person achieves a relaxed yet alert state by concentrating on a pleasant idea or thought, chanting a phrase or special sound, or by focusing on the sound of his or her own breathing. The ultimate goal of meditation is to separate oneself mentally from the outside world. Some practitioners recommend two 15 to 20 minute sessions a day.

What is the history behind it?

Meditation is an important part of ancient Eastern religious practices, particularly in India, China, and Japan, but can be found in all cultures of the world. Meditation began to attract attention in the West in the 1960s when the Indian leader Maharishi Mahesh Yogi brought his method called Transcendental Meditation (TM) to the United States. In 1968, a Harvard cardiologist named Herbert Benson was asked by TM practitioners to test them on their ability to lower their own blood pressures. Benson later developed a popular relaxation technique called the relaxation response. Interest in the use of meditation in the treatment of people with cancer began in the 1970s and early 1980s, when Ainslie Meares, MD, an Australian psychiatrist, studied the use of meditation for enhancing the immune system in order to reduce the size of tumors.

Today, universities and continuing education programs provide training in behavioral medicine, including meditation. Some clinics at major medical centers and local hospitals practice meditation as a form of behavioral medicine.

What is the evidence?

In the last 15 years, meditation has been studied in clinical trials as a way of reducing stress on both the mind and body. Research shows that meditation can reduce anxiety, stress, blood pressure, chronic pain, and insomnia. An NIH panel found evidence that regular meditation can also reduce cholesterol, post-traumatic stress syndrome in Vietnam veterans, substance abuse, health care use, and increase longevity and quality of life.

A cross-sectional study of 16 women found that meditation increased levels of melatonin. Melatonin is thought to help different functions in the body that maintain health and prevent disease, such as breast and prostate cancer. More research is needed to determine the role of melatonin in the treatment of cancer (see Melatonin).

Are there any possible problems or complications?

Most experts agree that the positive effects of meditation outweigh any negative reactions. Complications are rare, however, a small number of people who meditate have become disoriented and experienced some negative feelings.

References

Alternative Medicine: Expanding Medical Horizons. *A Report to the National Institutes of Health on Alternative Medical*

Systems and Practices in the United States. Washington, DC: US Government Printing Office; 1994. NIH publication 94-066.

Benson H. *Timeless Healing: The Power of Biology and Belief.* New York, NY: Scribner; 1996.

Coker KH. Meditation and prostate cancer: integrating a mind/body intervention with traditional therapies. *Semin Urol Oncol.* 1999;17:111-118.

Massion AO, Teas J, Hebert JR, Wertheimer MD, Kabat-Zinn J. Meditation, melatonin and breast/prostate cancer: hypothesis and preliminary data. *Med Hypotheses.* 1995;44:39-46.

National Center for Complementary and Alternative Medicine. Mind-Body Control - Fields of Practice. National Institutes of Health Web site. Accessed October 12, 1999. Available at: http://nccam.nih.gov/nccam/what-is-cam/fields/mind.shtml#meditation. Accessed November 4, 1999.

NIH Consensus Development Program. Integration of behavioral and relaxation approaches into the treatment of chronic pain and insomnia. National Institutes of Health Web site. Available at: http://mantis.cit.nih.gov/temp/CDC/consensus/ta/017/017_statement.htm. Accessed November 4, 1999.

Spencer JW, Jacobs JJ. *Complementary/Alternative Medicine: An Evidence-Based Approach.* St. Louis, MO: Mosby, Inc; 1999.

US Congress, Office of Technology Assessment. *Unconventional Cancer Treatments.* Washington, DC: US Government Printing Office; 1990. Publication OTA-H-405.

Music Therapy

Other common name(s)	Scientific/medical name(s)
Sound Therapy	None

DESCRIPTION
Music therapy is a method that consists of the active or passive use of music in order to promote healing and enhance quality of life.

OVERVIEW
There is some evidence that when used along with conventional treatment, music therapy can help to reduce pain and relieve chemotherapy-induced nausea and vomiting. It may also relieve stress and provide an overall sense of well being. Some studies have found that music therapy can lower heart rate, blood pressure, and breathing rate.

How is it promoted for use?
Because of its soothing quality, proponents use music therapy for a variety of physical, emotional, and psychological symptoms. Music therapy is often used in cancer treatment to help reduce pain, anxiety, and nausea caused by chemotherapy. Some proponents believe music therapy may enhance the health care of pediatric oncology patients by promoting social interaction and cooperation.

There is some evidence that music therapy reduces high blood pressure, rapid heart beat, depression, and sleeplessness. There are no claims music therapy can cure cancer or other diseases, but medical experts do believe it can reduce some symptoms, aid healing, improve physical movement, and enrich a patient's quality of life.

What does it involve?

Music therapists design music sessions for individuals and groups based on individual needs and tastes. Some aspects of music therapy include music improvisation, receptive music listening, song writing, lyric discussion, imagery, music performance, and learning through music. Individuals can also perform their own music therapy at home by listening to music or sounds that help relieve their symptoms. Music therapy can be conducted in a variety of places including hospitals, cancer centers, hospices, at home, or anywhere people can benefit from its calming or stimulating effects.

A related practice called music thanatology is sometimes used at the end of a patient's life to ease the person's passing. It is practiced at home and in hospices or nursing homes.

What is the history behind it?

Music has been used in medicine for thousands of years. Ancient Greek philosophers believed that music could heal both the body and the soul. Native Americans have included singing as part of their healing rituals for centuries. The more formalized approach to music therapy began in World War II when US Veterans Administration hospitals began to use music to help treat soldiers suffering from shell shock. In 1944, Michigan State University established the first music therapy degree program in the world.

Today, about 70 colleges and universities have degree programs that are approved by the American Music Therapy Association. There are over 5,000 professional music therapists working in health care settings in the United States today. They serve as part of cancer-management teams in many hospitals and cancer centers, helping to plan and evaluate treatment.

What is the evidence?

Scientific studies have shown the positive value of music therapy on the body, mind, and spirit of children and adults. Researchers have found that music therapy used along with antiemetic drugs (drugs that relieve nausea and vomiting) for patients receiving high-dose chemotherapy can be effective in easing the physical symptoms of nausea and vomiting.

A number of clinical trials have shown the benefit of music therapy for acute pain, including pain from cancer. When used in combination with pain-relieving drugs, music has been found to decrease the overall intensity of the patient's experience of pain. Music therapy can sometimes result in a decreased use of pain medication.

Other clinical trials have revealed a reduction in heart rate, blood pressure, breathing rate, insomnia, depression, and anxiety with music therapy. No one knows exactly how music benefits the body, but one theory holds that our muscles, including the heart muscle, learn to synchronize to the beat of the music. Another suggests that music and sound distract the mind from focusing on pain and anxiety.

Are there any possible problems or complications?

In general, music therapy has a positive effect on people and is considered safe when used as a complementary therapy.

References

Ezzone S, Baker C, Rosselet R, Terepka E. Music as an adjunct to antiemetic therapy. *Oncol Nurs Forum.* 1998; 25:1551-1556.

Johnston K, Rohaly-Davis J. An introduction to music therapy: helping the oncology patient in the ICU. *Crit Care Nurs Q.* 1996;18:54-60.

Lane D. Music therapy: a gift beyond measure. *Oncol Nurs Forum.* 1992;19:863-867.

Lane D. Music therapy: gaining an edge in oncology management. *J Oncol Manag.* 1993;Jan/Feb:42-46.

Watkins GR. Music therapy: proposed physiological mechanisms and clinical implications. *Clin Nurse Spec.* 1997;11:43-50.

Native American Healing

Other common name(s)	Scientific/medical name(s)
None	None

DESCRIPTION

Native American healing combines religion, spirituality, herbal medicine, and rituals to treat medical and emotional problems.

OVERVIEW

There is no scientific evidence that Native American healing can cure cancer or any other disease. However, the communal support provided by this approach to health care can have some worthwhile physical, emotional, and spiritual benefits.

How is it promoted for use?

Native American healing is based on the belief that health is interconnected with morality, spirituality, and harmonious relationships with community and nature. Proponents claim it can help cure physical diseases, injuries, and emotional problems. Native American healers claim to have cured conditions such as heart disease, diabetes, thyroid problems, skin rashes, asthma, and cancer. There is no scientific evidence to support these claims.

Practitioners of Native American healing presume illness stems from spiritual problems. They believe a person under psychological distress cannot be healed. They also claim that diseases are more likely to invade the body of a person who is imbalanced, has negative thinking, and lives an unhealthy lifestyle. Many Native American healers believe that inherited conditions, such as birth defects, are caused by the parents' immoral lifestyles and are not easily treated. Native American healing practices are claimed to find balance and wholeness in an individual to restore one to a healthy and spiritually pure state.

Native American healing is promoted in many different ways. Some of the most com-mon aspects of Native American healing include the use of herbal remedies, purifying rituals, shamanism, and spiritual healing to treat illnesses of both the body and spirit. Herbal remedies are used to treat many physical conditions (see Chapter on Herb, Vitamin, and Mineral Methods). Practitioners use purifying rituals to cleanse the body, which they claim makes the person more susceptible to other Native American healing techniques. One kind of Native American healer, a shaman, focuses on using spiritual healing powers to treat people with illness based on the idea that spirits have caused the illness (see Shamanism). Symbolic healing rituals, which can involve family and friends of the sick person, are used to invoke the spirits to help heal the sick person.

What does it involve?

Native American healing practices vary greatly because there are about 500 Native American Nations (commonly called tribes). However, they do have some basic rituals and healing practices in common. Because of their extensive knowledge of herbs, one of the most common forms of Native American healing involves the use of herbal remedies which can include teas, tinctures, and salves. For example, one remedy for joint pain uses bark from a willow tree.

Purifying and purging the body is also an important technique used in Native American healing. Sweat lodges (similar to a steam bath) and special teas which induce vomiting, are used for this purpose. Smudging (cleansing a place or person with the smoke of sacred plants) is also used to bring about an altered state of consciousness and sensitivity, making a person more open to the healing techniques. Because some illnesses are believed to come from angry spirits, shamans are sometimes used to invoke the healing powers of spirits or to help appease the angered spirits (see Shamanism).

Another practice of Native American healing, symbolic healing rituals, can involve a shaman and even entire communities. These rituals use ceremonies which can include chanting, singing, painting bodies, dancing, exorcisms, sand paintings, and even the use of mind altering substances (like peyote) to persuade the spirits to heal the sick person. Rituals can last minutes or weeks. Prayer is also an essential part of all Native American healing techniques (see Spirituality and Prayer).

What is the history behind it?

Native American healing has been practiced in North America for up to 40,000 years. It has roots in different cultures, such as ancient Ayurvedic (Indian) and Chinese traditions, but has also been influenced by what they learned about nature, plants, and animals (see Ayurveda). Other healing practices were influenced over time by the migration of tribes and contact with other tribes along trade routes. The tribes gathered many herbs from the surrounding environment and sometimes traded over long distances.

Today, Native American Indian community-based medical systems still practice some Native American healing practices and rituals.

What is the evidence?

One recent clinical trial examined 116 people with a variety of ailments (such as infertility, chest and back pain, asthma, depression, diabetes, and cancer) who were treated with traditional Native American healing. More than 80% showed some benefit after a 7 to 28 day intensive healing experience. Five years later, 50 of the original participants said they were cured of their diseases while another 41 said they felt better. Another 9 showed no change, 5 were worse, and 2 had died. However, the comparison group who received different treatments also showed benefits. More clinical studies are needed to confirm the benefits of the specific healing methods.

Although Native American healing has not been shown to cure disease, anecdotal reports suggest that it can reduce pain and stress, and improve quality of life. The communal support provided by this type of healing could have beneficial effects. Prayers, introspection, and meditation can be calming and can help to reduce stress.

Because Native American healing is based on spirituality and mysticism, there are very few scientific studies to support the validity of the practices. It is difficult to study Native American healing under accepted scientific standards because practices differ between various Nations, shamans, and illnesses. Many Native Americans do not want their practices studied because they believe sharing such information exploits their culture and weakens their power to heal.

Are there any possible problems or complications?

Like other complementary therapies, Native American healing practices may be used in relieving certain symptoms of cancer and side effects of cancer treatment. People with cancer and other chronic conditions should consult their physician before pursuing purification rituals or herbal remedies. Relying on this type of treatment alone, and avoiding conventional medical care, may have serious health consequences.

References

Alternative Medicine: Expanding Medical Horizons. *A Report to the National Institutes of Health on Alternative Medical Systems and Practices in the United States.* Washington, DC: US Government Printing Office; 1994. NIH publication 94-066.

Cohen K. Native American medicine. *Altern Ther Health Med.* 1998;4:45-57.

Complementary and Alternative Methods. Native American healing. American Cancer Society Web site. Available at: http://www.cancer.org. Accessed January 24, 2000.

Mehl-Madrona LE. Native American medicine in the treatment of chronic illness: developing an integrated program and evaluating its effectiveness. *Altern Ther Health Med.* 1999;5:36-44.

Naturopathic Medicine

Other common name(s)	Scientific/medical name(s)
Naturopathy, Natural Medicine	None

DESCRIPTION

Naturopathic medicine integrates a wide range of complementary approaches such as nutrition, herbal medicine, physical manipulation, exercise, stress reduction, and acupuncture with conventional medicine. It is a holistic approach (designed to treat the whole person) that enlists the healing power of the body and nature to fight disease (see Holistic Medicine).

OVERVIEW

There is no scientific evidence that naturopathic medicine can cure cancer or any other disease. Specific methods within naturopathic medicine vary in terms of effectiveness. Some methods, such as homeopathy, may be of little value (see Homeopathy). Others, however, have shown some evidence of effectiveness in prevention and symptom management. Examples include the importance of diet in lowering the risk of severe illnesses such as heart disease and cancer, and the usefulness of acupuncture to reduce pain.

How is it promoted for use?

Proponents claim naturopathic medicine uses the healing power of nature to maintain and restore health. The whole person is supported to create a healthy environment inside and outside the body. Supporters claim naturopathic medicine prevents illness because people are taught to incorporate healthy diets and lifestyles to avoid disease. Diagnosis and treatment is focused on the cause of the disease, rather than on the symptoms. Naturopaths diagnose illness with many of the same methods used in conventional medicine. They use x-rays, lab tests, and physical exams. However, naturopathic treatment does not involve the use of drugs, modern medical technology, or major surgery.

Naturopathic medicine is promoted for the treatment of migraine headaches, chronic lower back pain, enlarged prostate, menopause, AIDS, and cancer. Practitioners claim they use "natural methods" to strengthen the body's inner ability to heal itself. They claim that this type of care causes fewer side effects and costs less than conventional treatment. However, practitioners often refer complicated cases or people needing major treatment to conventional medical professionals.

What does it involve?

Naturopathic medicine uses many different techniques and methods. Practitioners act mostly as teachers. They decide how to treat a particular patient based on case history, observation, medical records, clinical nutrition information, and previous experience. Naturopathic treatment can include nutritional medicine and therapeutic fasting; herbs, minerals, and vitamins; homeopathy; Chinese medicine; manipulation of muscles, bones and the spine; natural childbirth including pre- and post-natal care; acupuncture; counseling and hypnotherapy; massage, colonic enemas; hydrotherapy, heat, and cold applications; therapeutic exercise; and some minor surgery. For more information about some of the treatments involved in naturopathic medicine, see Acupuncture, Homeopathy, Hypnosis, Colon Therapy, and Chapters on Herb, Vitamin, and Mineral Methods, and Diet and Nutrition Methods.

Counseling or behavioral medicine is an important part of naturopathic medicine. Practitioners are trained in counseling, biofeedback, stress reduction, and other means to improve mental health (see Biofeedback and Psychotherapy). They may also use other unproven techniques, such as ozone therapy, for people with cancer and AIDS.

Chiropractors, massage therapists, holistic nurses, and nutritionists offer naturopathic remedies, but may not have educational training in naturopathic medicine. Treatment by naturopathic doctors is not covered by Medicare or most insurance policies.

What is the history behind it?

Naturopathic medicine began with Sebastian Kneipp in the 1800s. Kneipp, a German priest, opened a water cure center and developed herbal treatments. Later, a student of Kneipp's, Benedict Lust opened a water cure institute in New York which used Kneipp's drugless therapies. Lust went on to acquire degrees in osteopathy, and chiropractic, homeopathic, and eclectic medicine. In 1902, Lust purchased the rights to naturopathic medicine from another Kneipp student and opened the American Institute of Naturopathy.

By the early 1900s, there were more than 20 schools of naturopathic medicine. With the advances in medicine after World War II, however, interest in naturopathic medicine began to decline until the mid-1950s when the National College of Naturopathic Medicine was founded in Portland, Oregon. In 1968, the US Department of Health, Education, and Welfare issued a report stating that the educational programs for practitioners of naturopathic medicine did not adequately prepare them to make accurate diagnoses or treatment decisions. The report also concluded that naturopathic medicine was not based on widely accepted scientific principles of health, disease, and health care.

The American Naturopathic Medical Association was founded in 1981 and has approximately 2,000 members. The Council on Naturopathic Medical Education was approved by the US Secretary of Education in 1987 as an accrediting body for full-time schools. Doctor of naturopathic medicine (ND) degrees are offered by four-year graduate-level programs. Naturopathic doctors take some of the same basic science courses as conventional doctors (MDs), however, the ND curriculum includes courses on disease prevention, wellness, clinical nutrition, acupuncture, homeopathic medicine, botanical medicine, psychology, and counseling. Naturopathic doctors do not receive residency training. There are currently three schools that offer accredited ND programs in the United States, and eleven states license naturopathic doctors. Some ND degrees are currently available through non-accredited correspondence schools.

What is the evidence?

There have been no randomized clinical studies showing the effectiveness of naturopathic medicine. Most of the documentation of treatment includes case history observations, medical records, and summaries of practitioners' clinical experiences. Naturopathic medicine uses several methods that have been shown to vary in how effective they are.

It involves the use of several unproven methods such as homeopathy and colonic irrigation, which have not shown any positive effects for cancer or any other disease. Other aspects of naturopathic medicine, like proper diet and nutrition are believed to lower the risk of severe illnesses such as heart disease and cancer. Another component, acupuncture, may reduce pain. Some aspects of naturopathic medicine may be useful as complementary methods to conventional medical treatment.

Are there any possible problems or complications?

Most naturopathic methods are not harmful. However, some herbal preparations can be toxic (see specific herbs for more information). Excessive fasting, dietary restrictions, or use of enemas may be dangerous. Relying on this type of treatment alone, and avoiding conventional medical care, may have serious health consequences.

References

Alternative Medicine: Expanding Medical Horizons. *A Report to the National Institutes of Health on Alternative Medical Systems and Practices in the United States.* Washington, DC: US Government Printing Office; 1994. NIH publication 94-066.

Barrett S. A close look at naturopathy. Quackwatch Web site. Available at: http://www.quackwatch.com. Accessed October 3, 1999.

Complementary and Alternative Methods. Naturopathic medicine. American Cancer Society Web site. Available at: http://www.cancer.org. Accessed January 24, 2000.

Spencer JW, Jacobs JJ. *Complementary/Alternative Medicine: An Evidence-Based Approach.* St. Louis, MO: Mosby, Inc; 1999.

Neuro-linguistic Programming

Other common name(s)	Scientific/medical name(s)
NLP	None

DESCRIPTION

Neuro-linguistic programming (NLP) uses a number of techniques or tools to teach people to identify personal goals, change unhelpful beliefs, reach a higher level of achievement, and communicate better with others. Special attention is paid to the relationship between language, thoughts, and behavior.

OVERVIEW

Some smaller studies have reported positive effects of NLP in such areas as increasing relaxation and treating phobias. There is no scientific evidence, however, that NLP is effective in treating cancer or any other disease.

How is it promoted for use?

Practitioners of NLP claim it is used to identify and change unconscious patterns of thinking and behavior to help treat a wide range of physical conditions. They also claim NLP can be used to help people with phobias, allergies, arthritis, migraines, Parkinson's disease, AIDS, and cancer. There is no scientific evidence to support these claims.

NLP is based on the belief that the brain (ie, neuro) controls how the body functions, language (ie, linguistic) determines how people communicate, and programming is used to develop models for interaction. NLP involves studying the relationship between all three parts. They claim thinking is closely tied to the five senses, that experiences are recreated in memories through the senses, and that is what controls people's abilities and beliefs. NLP proponents claim that once people understand that they create their own internal world, they realize they have the power to change their health and behavior. Practitioners claim people who have problems healing from physical conditions often have negative beliefs about their health.

What does it involve?

NLP practitioners may ask a person questions about his or her life or physical condition then analyze eye movements, body posture, voice tone, muscle tension, gestures, and language to understand and correct problems. This observational information is used to show how people are consciously and unconsciously relating to their life and condition, and what limiting beliefs may exist. Practitioners claim some illnesses or other problems can be cured with one NLP session although some conditions may require a few repeated sessions.

What is the history behind it?

In the early 1970s, John Grinder, PhD and Richard Bandler, PhD studied the thinking processes, and language and behavioral patterns of several successful people, including Fritz Perls, the father of Gestalt therapy Virginia Satir,

an accomplished family therapist; Milton Erickson, a prominent hypnotherapist; and Gregory Bateson, a well-known anthropologist and author in the field of communication theory. Grinder and Bandler believed that by studying and learning the internal processes of these successful people, they could learn to teach anyone the skills necessary to increase their level of success. Grinder and Bandler made connections between the body language and speaking patterns of these people and related this information to the internal thinking process of each person studied.

They applied the information they learned to help people who were experiencing emotional difficulties by asking people questions about their problems while observing their body language. Once the unconscious patterns were known, they found the person could be helped to learn new, more useful patterns. This process was called neuro-linguistic programming.

Today, NLP practitioners can receive training in the process from affiliated organizations such as The Society for Neuro-Linguistic Programming.

What is the evidence?

Although there have been anecdotal and case reports of the effectiveness of NLP, there have been no large-scale randomized clinical trials of the method. One small-scale study found that NLP might be effective in treating phobias. However, a National Research Council committee did not find the theories or practices of NLP to be well founded. Several reviews of the literature have reported there is little or no evidence to support the effectiveness of NLP. A recent survey of 139 psychologists listed in the National Register of Health Service Providers in Psychology found that the soundness of NLP was questionable. More scientific research is needed to determine if NLP holds any benefit for any medical condition.

Are there any possible problems or complications?

Not all NLP practitioners will have a background in medical settings and some may not even be properly trained. Someone without training or experience in the field may not be skilled or sensitive to the needs and issues important to someone living with cancer and could cause psychological harm if they are not careful.

References

Barrett S. Mental help: procedures to avoid. Quackwatch Web site. Available at: http://www.quackwatch.com. Accessed September 4, 1999.

Beyerstein BL. Brainscams: neuromythologies of the new age. *Intern J Mental Health.* 1990;19:27-36.

Einspruch EL, Forman BD. Neuro-linguistic programming in the treatment of phobias. *Psych Priv Prac.* 1988;6:91-100.

Sharpley CF. Research findings on neurolinguistic programming: nonsupportive data or an untestable theory? *J Counsel Psych.* 1987;34:103-107.

Starker S, Pankratz L. Soundness of treatment: a survey of psychologists' opinions. *Psychol Rep.* 1996;78:288-290.

Swets JA, Bjork RA. Enhancing human performance: an evaluation of "New Age" techniques considered by the U.S. Army. *Psychol Sci.* 1990;1:85-86.

Psychotherapy

Other common name(s)	Scientific/medical name(s)
Therapy, Counseling, Psychological Intervention, Psychotherapeutic Treatment	None

DESCRIPTION

Psychotherapy covers a wide range of approaches designed to help people change their ways of thinking, feeling, or behaving.

OVERVIEW

Research has shown that psychotherapy may improve a patient's quality of life. It can help reduce anxiety and depression that sometimes occurs in people with cancer. Psychotherapy has not, however, been demonstrated to increase survival in people with cancer.

How is it promoted for use?

The idea of the existence of a mind-body connection has been around for a very long time, and has received more support and attention in recent years. Psychotherapists believe that what a person experiences mentally and emotionally affects his or her body. They also believe psychotherapy can help people, including those with cancer, find the inner strength they need to improve their coping skills, allowing them to more fully enjoy their lives. Psychotherapy can be used to help people deal with the diagnosis and treatment of cancer. It can also be useful in overcoming depression and anxiety, which many people with cancer experience.

Psychotherapy is available in many forms. People may seek individual therapy, where there is a one-on-one relationship with a therapist. There are also therapists who work with couples and/or entire families, in order to deal with the impact of the cancer and its diagnosis on those most closely affected. Psychotherapy is also practiced in a group format, where a number of people meet together to discuss common experiences and issues and to learn specific coping techniques (see Support Groups).

What does it involve?

There are many different kinds of therapy, from discussion of emotional experiences to active participation in homework assignments. People can get referrals by asking members of their health care team, or by contacting professional organizations for names of psychotherapists who specialize in the area. Oncology units of hospitals sometimes have departments that staff therapists. Most individual psychotherapy is held in the therapist's office, but there are situations when different arrangements can be made (eg, the hospital or person's home). Sessions typically last 50 minutes, and occur at a frequency determined by the client and therapist, although most are weekly and only short-term (3-4 months). There are a wide range of psychotherapeutic approaches and techniques. These include the following:

Behavioral Therapy (Behavior Modification)

This therapy focuses on replacing problematic behavior patterns (eg, obsessive-compulsive behavior) with more healthy responses. A behavioral therapist may use techniques such as biofeedback and muscle relaxation (see Biofeedback). This kind of therapy deals only with the symptoms of a problem.

Client-Centered Therapy

This form of therapy focuses on the feelings and current experiences of the individual. The therapist encourages the patient to direct the sessions while providing empathy and support. The goal is to help patients help themselves. The length of this therapy varies.

Body-Oriented Therapy

This kind of therapy is based on the belief that emotions become stored in the body and may be expressed in the form of physical tension and restriction. Breathing techniques, movement, manual pressure, and probing are used to help people release emotions that have built up in the body (see Bioenergetics).

Cognitive Therapy

Cognitive therapy is directed at changing behavior by addressing the repeated, faulty, negative thoughts that affect behavior. Cognitive therapists help people learn to re-program harmful internal messages and create positive self-talk (internal dialogue/thoughts). This kind of therapy can include homework assignments for the patient such as making a list of ten things he or she likes about himself or herself.

Family/Couples Therapy

Family therapy focuses on relationship patterns and all family members may be involved in therapy sessions. A therapist involved in this type of therapy acts as a facilitator to help the family/couple communicate their feelings more effectively. Although usually short-term, this therapy can last longer depending on the needs of the family or couple.

Group Therapy

Group therapy varies widely in size and format, as well as duration. Some groups are small, and meet weekly without a scheduled agenda, while others meet monthly and offer information, teach coping skills, help reduce anxiety, and provide a place to share common concerns and emotional support.

Psychodynamic Therapy

Rooted in traditional psychoanalysis (eg, Freud), the goal of this form of therapy is to change life-long personality patterns by uncovering the connections between current emotional reactions and early childhood experiences. This form of therapy is long-term (several years) and focuses on the underlying causes of a problem.

Whatever approach is used, when a person has a serious physical illness such as cancer, the therapy is likely to focus on the emotional stress resulting from the illness. It will also focus on depression and anxiety if present, as well as exploring past or present issues that may affect the person's adjustment to the illness. Attention may be paid to the person's previous experiences with loss, in general, as well as with the specific illness now being faced.

What is the history behind it?

The influence of personality characteristics on health has been examined for many years. Research by Lawrence LeShan, PhD during the early 1950s on the relationship between personality characteristics and cancer found that many patients experienced a loss of hope in finding true meaning in their lives well before they were diagnosed with cancer. He also found that for men, the rate of occurrence of cancer was highest in the period shortly following their job retirement. Dr. LeShan developed a specific approach to psychotherapy designed to treat people living with cancer. This approach focuses on helping patients use their own inner self-healing abilities and live more fulfilled, enjoyable, and personally meaningful lives.

Over the past 20 years, several books on the role of emotions and behavior in recovery from serious illness have become popular. Books by Norman Cousins, Bernie Siegel, MD, and Carl Simonton, MD, have focused on developing effective coping strategies to manage feelings of hopelessness, passivity, and depression that can occur with life-threatening illness. Psychological and behavioral methods are now becoming a regular part of cancer treatment.

Psychotherapy is practiced by licensed mental health professionals, including psychologists, psychiatrists, social workers, nurses, counselors, and marriage and family therapists. Specialized training and experience in the issues involved in treating people with cancer is necessary, and some professionals specifically work as psycho-oncologists.

What is the evidence?

Research has consistently shown that psychotherapy can be beneficial to people with cancer in a variety of ways. A psychologist at the University of California School of Medicine in Los Angeles reported in 1999 that behavior therapy is most useful in managing anxiety related to specific treatment concerns such as phobic reactions to needles, fears related to surgery or chemotherapy, and claustrophobic feelings during MRIs (magnetic resonance imaging). A 1996 study reported weekly individual cognitive therapy and bi-monthly family counseling improved both depression and quality of life of women diagnosed with non-metastatic breast cancer. Research has generally shown that, for people with cancer, psychotherapy can help them reduce anxiety and depression, make better use of their time, and help them return to work. Psychotherapy can also help people learn to communicate better with their doctors, and be more compliant with medical instructions because they feel their own needs are being recognized.

Research has not clearly shown, however, that individual psychotherapy can prolong the life of cancer patients. Few controlled studies of this nature have been conducted. In 1982, researchers studied 120 end-stage male cancer patients. Approximately half were randomly assigned to a control group and the other half received individual counseling. While those receiving psychotherapy showed improvement on quality of life measures, no difference was found between groups in survival rate after one year.

In a 1997 study, 5 out of 35 patients with cancer that was no longer responsive to medical treatment showed an arrest in tumor growth during and immediately after a 12-session course of individual counseling that focused on present concerns coupled with bi-weekly group therapy. Four of these five maintained this state for 3 to 9 months and one maintained it for 2 years. This was a small, non-controlled study, however, so it cannot be concluded that the effects were the result of the counseling program. It is not clear whether support groups or group counseling actually lead to a longer life. Research has revealed contradictory results about the ability of support groups or group therapy to extend life (see Support Groups).

Are there any possible problems or complications?

Psychotherapists vary in the amount of their training and experience in dealing with issues relevant to the treatment of people with cancer. Difficult personal issues that arise from psychotherapy can also be emotionally upsetting or uncomfortable. Some physicians have raised a concern that an "alternative" method such as psychotherapy may lead to a delay of conventional treatment, although most now view psychotherapy as complementary to standard medical intervention.

References

Cassileth BR. The aim of psychotherapeutic intervention in cancer patients. *Support Care Cancer.* 1995;3:267-269.

de Vries MJ, Schilder JN, Mulder CL, Vrancken AM, Remie M, Garssen B. Phase II study of psychotherapeutic intervention in advanced cancer. *Psychooncology.* 1997;6:129-137.

Fox BH. The role of psychological factors in cancer incidence and prognosis. *Oncology (Huntingt).* 1995;9:245-253.

Linn MW, Linn BS, Harris R. Effects of counseling for late stage cancer patients. *Cancer.* 1982;49:1048-1055.

Marchioro G, Azzarello G, Checchin F, et al. The impact of a psychological intervention on quality of life in non-metastatic breast cancer. *Eur J Cancer.* 1996;9:1612-1615.

Sourkes BM, Massie MJ, Holland JC. *Psychotherapeutic issues.* In Holland JC, ed. *Psycho-oncology.* New York: Oxford University Press; 1998.

Spiegel D. Essentials of psychotherapeutic intervention for cancer patients. *Support Care Cancer.* 1995;3:252-256.

US Congress, Office of Technology Assessment. *Unconventional Cancer Treatments.* Washington, DC: US Government Printing Office; 1990. Publication OTA-H-405.

Wellisch DK. Treating cancer patients: a growing area for psychologists. *The National Psychologist.* May/June;1999:26-27.

Qigong

Other common name(s)	Scientific/medical name(s)
Chi-kung	None

DESCRIPTION

Qigong is a Chinese system of self-care designed to enhance the natural flow of vital energy called qi (or chi) in the body. The process of working toward a regulated, smooth flow of qi is called "gong."

OVERVIEW

There is no scientific evidence showing that qigong is effective in treating cancer or any other disease; however, it may be useful to enhance quality of life. According to limited scientific literature, qigong may reduce chronic pain for a short period of time and relieve anxiety.

How is it promoted for use?

Proponents of qigong believe disease, injury, and stress can disrupt the vital energy or life force of the body (qi). By correcting these disruptions, individuals can lead healthier, less stressful lives (see Electromagnetic Therapy). Qigong is promoted to strengthen the body or to enhance other conventional health care treatments, not to cure existing disease. Practitioners claim it may be helpful in managing pain and reducing anxiety. There is some limited evidence for these claims.

Some promoters also claim that qigong can help to prevent cancer by improving the oxygen supply to the body and regulating the autonomic nervous system. They further claim qigong can be used to treat hypertension, stroke, heart and other circulatory diseases, abnormal sex hormone levels, low bone density, and senility. Some qigong masters even claim they can cure a person with the energy released from their fingertips. There is no scientific evidence to support any of these claims.

What does it involve?

The goal of qigong is to facilitate the flow of energy through the body. Qigong consists primarily of meditation, physical movements, and breathing exercises (see Meditation). Internal qigong involves exercises that individuals can do on their own. External qigong involves skilled masters who claim to use their own qi to help heal other people. The qigong master does not have to touch a person in order to promote healing.

A typical qigong session might require a person to sit or stand quietly while thinking about the qi flowing through his or her body and performing breathing and movement exercises at the same time. The breathing and movement used in qigong is slow, deliberate, and controlled. Qigong can also be used to target specific areas of the body where problems may exist.

Hospitals in China include qigong as part of their health care programs. Only in rural China is qigong practiced without complementary forms of conventional health care. Qigong classes are offered for various fees at health clubs, schools, hospitals, YMCAs, and community-fitness facilities as part of continuing adult-education programs in the United States. There are also a number of "qigong institutes" that charge a small fee to present classes about qigong. Qigong is also taught through videotapes and printed materials.

What is the history behind it?

Qigong is a form of traditional Chinese medicine based on the theory of yin-yang (interaction of opposite forces). People in China have been practicing qigong for at least 7,000 years to maintain health and achieve long life. Initially, the ancient Chinese realized that certain body movements and mental concentration could adjust and enhance body functions. Qigong techniques even became part of religious rituals.

Over the past few centuries, qigong slowly separated from religious beliefs and a more conventional form of qigong was developed in the 1970s. In the early 1980s, Chinese scientists began scientific investigations of qigong. Hundreds of medical applications were subsequently published in Chinese literature, but many studies only involved a few patients and did not use well-controlled, randomized methods. By the 1990s, the Chinese government began to manage qigong and made it an official part of the Chinese health plan.

Today, qigong is widely practiced and studied in China. In the United States, qigong is used as a form of relaxation and meditation in some health clubs and fitness centers.

What is the evidence?

While some scientists believe that qigong may be useful as a form of exercise to help to alleviate stress, improve coordination, and generally improve a person's quality of life, there is no scientific evidence that qigong can cure cancer or any other disease.

One study recently published in the United States found that for people with chronic pain, qigong training resulted in a short-term reduction of pain and a long-term reduction in anxiety. However, this was a small study involving only 26 patients. More well-controlled clinical research, using larger groups of patients, is needed to determine what effect qigong may have in treating various medical conditions.

A review of animal research studies in China reported that external qigong slowed the growth of tumors in mice. Animal studies may show that a certain therapy holds promise as a beneficial treatment, but further studies are necessary to determine if the results apply to humans. It was also reported that one clinical study found patients who practiced qigong (2 hours each day for 3 to 6 months) showed improvement in strength and immune system functioning, appetite, freedom from diarrhea, and weight gain. These findings, however, were reported in proceedings from a scientific meeting in Shanghai with no publications appearing in scientific journals. Results were not provided in English.

Are there any possible problems or complications?

Qigong is generally considered safe because of the slow, deliberate exercises involved. Those with a history of muscle aches and joint pain should realize that the deliberate, slow movement of qigong may cause muscle fatigue and joint pain if overdone. People with cancer and chronic conditions such as arthritis and heart disease should consult with their physician before undergoing any type of therapy that involves manipulation of joints and muscles.

References

Cassileth B. *The Alternative Medicine Handbook*. New York, NY: W. W. Norton & Co; 1998.

Eisenberg DM, Kessler RC, Foster C, Norlock FE, Calkins DR, Delbanco TL. Unconventional medicine in the United States. *NEngl J Med*. 1993;328:246-252.

Sancier KM. Medical applications of qigong. *Altern Ther Health Med*. 1996;2:40-46.

Wu WH, Bandilla E, Ciccone DS, et al. Effects of qigong on late-stage complex regional pain syndrome. *Altern Ther Health Med*. 1999;5:45-54.

Shamanism

Other common name(s)	Scientific/medical name(s)
Shaman	None

DESCRIPTION
Shamanism is a form of folk medicine which uses spiritual healing and is performed by a shaman, an individual recognized by a people or a tribe who is believed to have special religious and/or magical powers of healing (see Native American Healing).

OVERVIEW
Although anecdotal stories have existed for centuries and many people around the world continue to practice shamanism today, there is no scientific evidence that it can cure cancer or any other disease. Some key elements of shamanism, such as the use of imagery, have been shown to reduce stress and anxiety (see Imagery).

How is it promoted for use?

Shamanism is based on the belief that healing has a spiritual dimension that must be addressed before healing can begin. The goal of shamanism is to help people discover meaning within themselves as well as in society and nature. Proponents claim that shamanism can heal both the body and soul, as well as restore harmony to the community and nature. Shamans claim they communicate with the spirits in order to help heal. Some shamans claim they can heal spiritual, psychic, and physical wounds as well as communities and global conditions.

Not all shamans claim the ability to cure every disease. Many shamans are very selective in choosing which people they will treat because if they fail to cure someone, they may be punished by the tribe. For example, shamans who believe that their brand of healing will not influence the course of cancer are not likely to work with a person who has been diagnosed with cancer.

What does it involve?

The shaman enters a trance, either self-induced or through the aid of hallucinogens or fasting, and then prays, sings, chants, dances, and/or drums around the patient. Storytelling and other art forms may also be used. During the trance, the shaman's soul is believed to travel in the quest to help the sick individual. The soul is said to leave the body and ascend to the spiritual world. This is where the shaman communicates with the evil spirits thought to be responsible for the illness. Although the shaman is in a state of trance, he is still conscious, which enables him to bargain with the spirits that are responsible for the patient's illness. Successful bargaining results in a cure. Today, some shamans also use herbal medicine or even conventional medicine in an effort to heal.

Each shaman must complete rigorous training, especially in the ability to achieve the trance required for communication with the spirits. Shamans work both with individual patients and with groups. It is common practice for Native American shamans to conduct healing sessions at night, most often in places with some religious connection or significance.

What is the history behind it?

Shamanism may be the oldest of all healing practices, dating back as far as 40,000 years. It is believed to have originated in the Altai and Ural Mountains of western China and Russia, probably in the form of a religion. In the Tungusu-Manchurian language, the word shaman means, "to know."

Many early cultures had their own forms of shamanism. These included people on the North American and South American continents, Asia, India, Africa, the South Pacific and Australia. Each early culture throughout the world had its own shamans. The shaman was thought to be the only person in the tribe able to communicate with the spirits of ancestors and with the gods and demons.

Today, shamanism is still practiced as folk medicine in some parts of Europe, Africa, and Asia. In the United States, many Native American tribes also practice shamanism.

What is the evidence?

There are many stories about the success of shamans throughout history. Most of these stories are not unlike the reports of religious "miracles" at shrines such as Lourdes. There is no scientific evidence that demons exist, that a shaman can communicate with and influence them, or that illness is caused by spirits.

Those who accept shamanism believe it works in a spiritual dimension of life that must be cleansed of all evil spirits. There is no proof of shamanic ability to cure disease, any results are most likely due to the placebo effect, in which believing that something can or will happen generates a positive result. Pain may subside because the patient believes the shaman made it subside.

Some key elements of shamanism, such as the use of imagery, have been shown to reduce stress and anxiety. One researcher at Stanford University reported that some aspects of shamanism might be helpful in changing destructive thought patterns in people with cancer. However, there is no scientific evidence that shamanism is effective in treating cancer or any other disease.

Are there any possible problems or complications?

Shamanism is generally considered safe and may be useful as a complementary therapy to help people with cancer deal with their emotions and certain symptoms of cancer and side effects of cancer treatment. Relying on this type of treatment alone, and avoiding conventional medical care, may have serious health consequences.

References

Alternative Medicine: Expanding Medical Horizons. *A Report to the National Institutes of Health on Alternative Medical Systems and Practices in the United States.* Washington, DC: US Government Printing Office; 1994. NIH publication 94-066.

Cassileth B. *The Alternative Medicine Handbook.* New York, NY: W.W. Norton & Co; 1998.

Money M. Shamanism and complementary therapy. *Complement Ther Nurs Midwifery.* 1997;3:131-135.

Spirituality and Prayer

Other common name(s)	Scientific/medical name(s)
Religion	None

DESCRIPTION
Spirituality is generally described as an awareness of something greater than the individual self and is usually expressed through religion and/or prayer.

OVERVIEW
Studies have found spirituality and religion are very important to the quality of life for some people with cancer. Although research has not shown that spirituality can cure cancer or any other disease, some studies have found intercessory prayer (praying for others) may be an effective addition to conventional medical care. The psychological benefits of prayer may include reduction of stress and anxiety, promotion of a more positive outlook, and the strengthening of the will to live.

How is it promoted for use?
Proponents of spirituality claim that prayer can decrease the negative effects of disease, speed recovery, and increase the effectiveness of medical treatments. Many people believe the spiritual dimension in healing is important, especially for coping with serious illness. Religious attendance has been associated with improvement of various health conditions such as heart disease, hypertension, stroke, colitis, uterine and other cancers, and overall health status, however the scientific evidence is mixed.

Some religious groups, such as Christian Scientists, claim prayer can cure any disease.

These groups often rely entirely on prayer in place of conventional medicine. This belief is based on a spiritual, rather than a biological explanation of how disease develops. There have been some reported cases that prayer has lead to tumor regression. There is no scientific evidence to support these claims.

What does it involve?

Spirituality has many forms and can be practiced in several ways. Prayer, for example, may be silent or spoken out loud and can be done alone in any setting or in groups (as in a church or temple). Another form of spirituality, regular attendance at a church or temple, may involve prayer which focuses on one's self (supplication) or on others (intercessory prayer). In this type of setting, the entire congregation of a church may be asked to pray for a sick person or the person's family.

Some religions set aside certain times of the day and special days of the week for praying. Standard prayers written by religious leaders are often memorized and repeated during private sessions and in groups. Prayers often ask a higher being for help, understanding, wisdom, or strength in dealing with life's problems.

Many medical institutions and practitioners include spirituality and prayer as important components of healing. In addition, hospitals have chapels, and contracts with ministers, rabbis, and voluntary organizations to serve their patients' spiritual needs.

What is the history behind it?

Since the beginning of recorded history all cultures throughout the world have developed systems of religion and spirituality. Earlier religions of ancient Egypt and Greece have given way to more modern religions such as Christianity, Judaism, Hinduism, Islam, Buddhism.

Within each culture, some form of spirituality and prayer have served as the institutionalized means of seeking assistance from the supreme being or beings perceived as powerful enough to alter nature, health, and disease. Different religions hold different beliefs about a supreme being. Today, spirituality, especially in the form of prayer, is practiced by billions of people throughout the world.

What is the evidence?

Studies done on the impact of prayer and spirituality generally focus on the effect of religious beliefs and behavior on health, survival, and quality of life and the effects of intercessory prayer. The results of many of these studies have been mixed. Although some research has found that religious groups with orthodox beliefs and behavior have lower cancer death rates, other studies have not found any health benefits related to religion and health.

The US Office of Technology Assessment (OTA) reported that a survey spanning 10 years of issues of the *Journal of Family Practice* found that 83% of studies on religiosity found a positive effect on physical health. Another study on 12 years of issues of two major psychiatric journals found that for the studies that measured religiosity, 92% showed a benefit for mental health, 4% were neutral, and 4% showed harm. Religiosity was measured by participation in religious ceremony, social support, prayer, and belief in a higher being.

There also has been research done on the effects of intercessory prayer (praying for others) in coronary care patients. A randomized clinical trial conducted in 1988 at a San Francisco hospital coronary care (heart attack) unit found that those seriously ill patients who were prayed for were less likely to need antibiotics and had fewer complications, although length of hospital stay and death rates did not differ between groups. A larger randomized clinical trial conducted at a Kansas City hospital coronary care unit found similar findings. Overall length of hospital stay and time in critical care unit did not differ between groups. However, the group that had been prayed for had 11% fewer complications. The researchers concluded that these results suggest that prayer may be an effective complementary therapy to conventional medical treatment.

Are there any possible problems or complications?

Patient consent is important before conducting any activity that may impact health. Those who do not believe in prayer and those who do not wish to be healed are among those who may object to being the object of intercessory prayer. Relying on this type of treatment alone, and avoiding conventional medical care, may have serious health consequences.

References

Alternative Medicine: Expanding Medical Horizons. *A Report to the National Institutes of Health on Alternative Medical Systems and Practices in the United States.* Washington, DC: US Government Printing Office; 1994. NIH publication 94-066.

Byrd RC. Positive therapeutic effects of intercessory prayer in a coronary care unit population. *South Med J.* 1988;81:826-829.

Complementary and Alternative Methods. Prayer and spirituality. American Cancer Society Web site. Available at: http://www.cancer.org. Accessed January 24, 2000.

Dwyer JW, Clarke LL, Miller MK. The effect of religious concentration and affiliation on county cancer mortality rates. *J Health Soc Behav.* 1990;31:185-202.

Harris WS, Gowda M, Kolb JW, et al. A randomized, controlled trial of the effects of remote, intercessory prayer on outcomes in patients admitted to the coronary care unit. *Arch Intern Med.* 1999;159:2273-2278.

Marcus A. Lord, please heal whatshisname: anonymous prayer helps heart patients, study finds. HealthScout Web site. Available at: http://www.healthscout.com. Accessed October 15, 1999.

Mytko JJ, Knight SJ. Body, mind and spirit: towards the integration of religiosity and spirituality in cancer quality of life research. *Psychooncology.* 1999;8:439-450.

Spencer JW, Jacobs JJ. *Complementary/Alternative Medicine: An Evidence-Based Approach.* St. Louis, MO: Mosby, Inc; 1999.

US Congress, Office of Technology Assessment. *Unconventional Cancer Treatments.* Washington, DC: US Government Printing Office; 1990. Publication OTA-H-405.

Support Groups

Other common name(s)	Scientific/medical name(s)
Group Therapy, Group Psychotherapy, Psychosocial Interventions, Psychosocial Treatment	None

DESCRIPTION

Support groups present information, provide comfort, teach coping skills, help reduce anxiety, and provide a place to share common concerns and emotional support.

OVERVIEW

Preliminary research has shown that many groups can enhance quality of life. There is no scientific evidence, however, that support groups can actually extend the survival time of people with cancer.

How is it promoted for use?

Support group participants believe that people can live healthier, happier lives in the company of others. They believe that when relatives and friends lend support, it is easier for people to deal with their health and social problems. Some proponents claim the bonds formed between members of support groups help them feel stronger. They further claim that sharing feelings and experiences within support groups can reduce stress, fear, and anxiety, and help to promote healing. Evidence suggests that support groups can improve quality of life for people with cancer.

What does it involve?

Support groups are composed of education, behavioral training, and group interaction. Behavioral training can involve muscle relaxation or meditation to reduce stress or the effects of chemotherapy or radiation therapy (see Meditation). People with cancer are often encouraged by health care professionals to seek support from groups of individuals that have direct or indirect experiences with the same type of cancer.

Many different kinds of support groups are available and they vary in their structure and activities. Some are time-limited, while others are ongoing. There are also support groups composed of people with the same type of cancer, while others are composed of people who are undergoing the same kind of treatment. Support groups are available for patients, family members, and other caregivers of people with cancer. The format of different groups varies from lectures and discussions to exploration and expression of feelings. Topics discussed by support groups are those of concern among the members and those considered of value by a therapist who may lead the group.

Support groups are different from group therapy. Support groups may be lead by survivors, group members, or trained professionals, while therapy groups are always facilitated by licensed counselors such as marriage and family therapists, nurses, psychologists, psychiatrists, and social workers. Group therapy is generally longer, more involved, and focuses on in-depth personal growth (see Psychotherapy). Support groups focus on learning to manage current concerns and situations. Most support groups involve little or no cost to the participants, while there is usually a fee for group therapy.

Support group meetings can be held in hospitals, school classrooms, community centers, office buildings, or one of the group member's homes. Some support groups also exist through the Internet, which usually involves interacting with people by sending and receiving messages through the computer. These groups vary widely in quality, and some are lead by moderators in chat-rooms, while others are not.

What is the history behind it?

In the late 1970s, encounter groups became popular, and group-intervention studies began appearing in a variety of science journals. An influential study by David Spiegel, PhD in 1989 reported that group therapy helped women with breast cancer to cope and possibly live longer. The demand for support groups from people with cancer has grown in the last ten years. Today, there are many hospital-based, independent, and national networks of support groups for people with various forms of cancer and other diseases, as well as their families.

What is the evidence?

The scientific community believes that support groups can enhance the quality of life for people with cancer by providing information and support to overcome the feelings of helplessness that sometimes accompany a diagnosis of cancer. Research has shown that people with cancer are better able to deal with their disease when supported by others in similar situations.

One clinical trial found that support groups helped in reducing tension, anxiety, fatigue, and confusion. Some research has shown that there is a link between group support and greater toleration of cancer treatment and treatment compliance. One psychologist found that an educational, supportive intervention improved patient compliance with oral medication, which lead to an increase in survival rates.

Research has shown contradictory results about the ability of groups to extend life. A randomized clinical trial by Dr. Spiegel found that women with metastatic breast cancer lived 18 months longer if they had participated in supportive group therapy. However, another clinical trial found no significant difference in survival between breast cancer patients who participated in group therapy and those who did not. Another clinical trial found that patients with malignant melanoma lived longer if they had participated in a group psycho-educational course. It is not clear whether support groups or group therapy actually lead to a longer life.

One study at the Ontario Cancer Institute found that women with breast cancer who lacked support from families and friends were helped the most from support groups. Researchers at Carnegie Mellon University recently found that educational groups helped women adjust to a diagnosis of early stage breast cancer. However, they also found there were some negative effects from group discussion. Some of the women in the group that were already receiving support at home gained no benefit from the group and became depressed and lethargic.

Although more research is needed to determine what types of groups are most effective with what type of people, support groups may be useful as a complementary therapy for people with cancer and other diseases.

Are there any possible problems or complications?

Support groups vary in quality. People with cancer may find that the support group they have joined does not discuss topics relevant to their personal situation. Some people may find a support group upsetting because it stirs up too many uncomfortable feelings or because the leader is not skilled. Support groups that exist through the Internet should be used with caution. This method cannot always assure confidentiality, and the people involved may have no special training or qualifications, especially if found in unmonitored chat rooms.

References

Alternative Medicine: Expanding Medical Horizons. *A Report to the National Institutes of Health on Alternative Medical Systems and Practices in the United States.* Washington, DC: US Government Printing Office; 1994. NIH publication 94-066.

Azar B. Does group therapy mean longer life? *APA Monitor.* 1999;30:13-14.

Cunningham AJ, Edmonds CV, Jenkins GP, Pollack H, Lockwood GA, Warr D. A randomized controlled trial of the effects of group psychological therapy on survival in women with metastatic breast cancer. *Psychooncology.* 1998;7:508-517.

Edmonds CV, Lockwood GA, Cunningham AJ. Psychological response to long-term group therapy: a randomized trial with metastatic breast cancer patients. *Psychooncology.* 1999;8:74-91.

Fawzy FI, Fawzy NW, Arndt LA, Pasnau RO. Critical review of psychosocial interventions in cancer care. *Arch Gen Psychiatry.* 1995;52:100-113.

Helgeson VS, Cohen S, Schulz R, Yasko J. Education and peer discussion group interventions and adjustment to breast cancer. *Arch Gen Psychiatry.* 1999;56:340-347.

Kogon MM, Biswas A, Pearl D, Carlson RW, Spiegel D. Effects of medical and psychotherapeutic treatment on the survival of women with metastatic breast carcinoma. *Cancer.* 1997;80:225-230.

Richardson JL, Shelton DR, Krailo M, Levine AM. The effect of compliance with treatment on survival among patients with hematologic malignancies. *J Clin Oncol.* 1990;8:356-364.

Spiegel D, Bloom JR, Kraemer HC, Gottheil E. Effect of psychosocial treatment on survival of patients with metastatic breast cancer. *Lancet.* 1989;2:888-891.

US Congress, Office of Technology Assessment. *Unconventional Cancer Treatments.* Washington, DC: US Government Printing Office; 1990. Publication OTA-H-405.

Tai Chi

Other common name(s)	Scientific/medical name(s)
T'ai Chi, Tai Chi Chuan, Tai Chi Chih, Tai Ji Juan, Tai Ji Quan, Tai Ji, Shadow Boxing	None

DESCRIPTION

Tai chi is an ancient Chinese form of martial arts. It is a mind-body, self-healing system that uses movement, meditation, and breathing to improve health and well being.

OVERVIEW

Research has shown tai chi is useful as a form of exercise that may improve posture, balance, muscle mass and tone, flexibility, stamina, and strength in older adults. Tai chi is also recognized as a method to reduce stress that can provide the same cardiovascular benefits as moderate exercise, such as lowered heart rate and blood pressure.

How is it promoted for use?

People who practice the deep breathing and physical movements of tai chi report it makes them feel more relaxed, younger, agile, and helps their circulation. Its slow, graceful movements, accompanied by rhythmic breathing, relax the body as well as the mind. Research has found that tai chi can reduce stress, lower blood pressure and reduce the risk of heart disease. See Qigong and Yoga for other Eastern methods of exercise. There is also evidence that tai chi is particularly suited for older adults, or for others who are not physically strong or healthy.

Proponents claim tai chi balances the flow of vital energy or life force called qi (or chi), which serves to prevent illness, improve general health, and extend life. It is also based on the theory of yin and yang (interaction of opposite forces). Practitioners claim tai chi is designed to balance yin and yang forces to achieve inner harmony.

What does it involve?

Tai chi students begin by learning a series of gentle, deliberate movements called forms. Each form contains between 20 to 100 moves, and requires up to 20 minutes to complete. Each form derives its name from nature, for example, "Wave Hands Like Clouds," or "Grasping the Bird's Tail." In order to balance the yin and yang, the movements are practiced in pairs of opposites. For example, a turn to the right follows one to the left. While performing these exercises, the individual is urged to pay close attention to his or her breathing, which is centered in the diaphragm. Tai chi relies entirely on technique rather than strength or power. Meditative concentration is focused on a point just below the navel, from which it is believed qi radiates throughout the body.

Tai chi is taught in many health clubs, schools, and recreational facilities. Practitioners believe that daily practice is necessary in order to get the most benefit. Once an individual has mastered a form, it can be practiced at home.

What is the history behind it?

Tai chi is based on the philosophy of Taoism, a Chinese belief system first developed in the 6th century BC that also includes qigong and acupuncture (see Qigong and Acupunture). Taoism includes beliefs in the existence of qi and the yin and yang. Tai chi originated as a martial art and has been practiced as an exercise in China for many centuries.

Tai chi became a sports event in the 1990 XI Asian Games. Tai chi has recently gained popularity in the United States and other Western countries as a general exercise technique, especially for older adults. Today, there are classes, videotapes, and books available on tai chi.

What is the evidence?

Researchers have focused on studying the benefits of relaxation and exercise that result from practicing tai chi. Clinical trials found that tai chi improves posture, balance, flexibility, muscle mass and tone, stamina, and strength in older adults and may help prevent falls and fractures.

One randomized clinical trial found that tai chi lead to a sense of improvement in overall well being in older adults and increased motivation to continue exercising. As an exercise, the benefits have also been noted for older individuals with chronic diseases such as arthritis, osteoporosis, chronic obstructive pulmonary disease, and peripheral artery disease. Research has found that tai chi can reduce stress and provide the same cardiovascular benefits as moderate exercise, such as reduced heart rate and blood pressure. There is no scientific evidence that tai chi cures cancer or any other disease, however, it may be useful as a complementary therapy to conventional treatment.

Are there any possible problems or complications?

Tai chi is considered to be a relatively safe, moderate physical activity. As with any form of exercise, it is important to be aware of physical limitations. People with cancer and chronic conditions such as arthritis and heart disease should consult with their physician before undergoing any type of therapy that involves manipulation of joints and muscles.

References

Channer KS, Barrow D, Barrow R, Osborne M, Ives G. Changes in haemodynamic parameters following Tai Chi Chuan and aerobic exercise in patients recovering from acute myocardial infarction. *Postgrad Med J.* 1996;72:349-351.

Complementary and Alternative Methods. Tai Chi. American Cancer Society Web site. Available at: http://www.cancer.org. Accessed January 24, 2000.

Kutner NG, Barnhart H, Wolf SL, McNeely E, Xu T. Self-report benefits of Tai Chi practice by older adults. *J Gerontol B Psychol Sci Soc Sci.* 1997;52:242-246.

Lan C, Lai JS, Wong MK, Yu ML. Cardiorespiratory function, flexibility, and body composition among geriatric Tai Chi Chuan practitioners. *Arch Phy Med Rehabil.* 1996;77:612-616.

Province MA, Hadley EC, Hornbrook MC, et al. The effects of exercise on falls in elderly patients. A preplanned meta-analysis of the FICSIT trials. Frailty and injuries: cooperative studies of intervention techniques. *JAMA.* 1995;273:1341-1347.

Ross MC, Presswalla JL. The therapeutic effects of Tai Chi for the elderly. *J Gerontol Nurs.* 1998;24:45-47.

Schaller KJ. Tai Chi Chih: an exercise option for older adults. *J Gerontol Nurs.* 1996;22:12-17.

Wolf SL, Barnhart HX, Kutner NG, McNeely E, Coogler C, Xu T. Reducing frailty and falls in older persons: an investigation of Tai Chi and computerized balance training. Atlanta FICSIT Group. Frailty and Injuries: Cooperative Studies of Intervention Techniques. *J Am Geriatr Soc.* 1996; 44:489-497.

Wolfson L, Whipple R, Derby C, et al. Balance and strength training in older adults: intervention gains and Tai Chi maintenance. *J Am Geriatr Soc.* 1996;44:498-506.

Yoga

Other common name(s)	Scientific/medical name(s)
Hatha Yoga	None

DESCRIPTION

Yoga is a form of nonaerobic exercise that involves a program of precise posture and breathing activities. In ancient Sanskrit, the word yoga means "union."

OVERVIEW

Yoga can be a useful method to help relieve some symptoms associated with chronic diseases such as cancer, arthritis, and heart disease, and can lead to increased relaxation and physical fitness. There is no scientific evidence that yoga is effective in treating cancer or any other disease; however, it may enhance quality of life.

How is it promoted for use?

Yoga is promoted as a system of personal development. It is a way of life based on the Hindu philosophy that combines ethical standards, dietary guidelines, physical exercise, and meditation to create a union of mind, body, and spirit. Yoga is said to cultivate prana, which is similar to qi (or chi) in traditional Chinese medicine meaning vital energy or life force. People who practice yoga claim it leads to a state of physical health, relaxation, happiness, peace, and tranquility. There is some evidence which shows that yoga can lower stress, increase strength, and provide a good form of exercise.

Proponents also claim yoga can be used to stop smoking, eliminate insomnia, and increase stamina. They further claim that the mastery of yoga can give people supernormal mental and physical powers. Yogis, who are masters and teachers of yoga, claim they can obtain heightened senses, overcome hunger and thirst, and develop almost total control over physiological processes such as heartbeat and respiration.

What does it involve?

There are different variations and aspects of yoga. There are many different types of yoga, including mantra, hatha, shiva, dissha, and bhakti. The most common form of yoga involves the use of movement, breathing exercises, and meditation to achieve a connection with the mind, body, and spirit. The goal of yoga is perfect concentration to attain the ancient Hindu ideal of samadhi—separation of pure consciousness from the outside world through the development of intuitive insight. Hatha yoga uses forbearance, religious observances, breath control, withdrawal of senses, attention, concentration, and meditation to attain samadhi. The three most commonly used aspects of yoga today include the postures of hatha yoga, the breathing techniques of pranayama yoga, and meditation (see Meditation).

Practitioners say yoga should be done either at the beginning or the end of the day. A typical session can last between 20 minutes and 1 hour. A yoga session starts with the person sitting in an upright position and performing gentle movements, all of which are executed very slowly, while taking slow, deep breaths from the abdomen. A session may also include guided relaxation, meditation, and sometimes visualization (see Imagery). It often ends with the chanting of a mantra (a meaningful word or phrase) to achieve a deeper state of relaxation. Yoga requires several sessions a week in order to become proficient. Yoga can be practiced at home without an instructor, or in adult education classes, or classes usually offered at health clubs and community centers. There are also numerous books and videotapes available on yoga.

What is the history behind it?

Yoga is one of the oldest mind-body health systems in existence and was first practiced in India over 5,000 years ago. In the United States, yoga was first practiced by the Concord transcendentalists in the 1840s but it did not become well known until the 1880s when the English translation of Yoga Sutras was published. This ancient book gave a detailed description of yoga techniques and the Hindu quest for samadhi, which is central to yoga beliefs. Over the past 80 years, the therapeutic potential of yoga has been researched. Today, some health plans offer members access to yoga instructors as a form of exercise and relaxation.

What is the evidence?

Research has shown that yoga can be used to control physiological functions such as blood pressure, heart rate, respiration, metabolism, body temperature, brain waves, skin resistance, and other bodily functions. This can result in improved physical fitness, lower levels of stress, and increased feelings of relaxation and well being.

According to a report to the National Institutes of Health, there is also some evidence to suggest yoga may be useful as a complementary therapy to conventional medical treatment to help relieve symptoms associated with cancer, asthma, diabetes, drug addiction, high blood pressure, heart disease, and migraine headaches. Yoga may also help to reduce cholesterol levels when used with diet and exercise. Randomized clinical trials have shown that yoga helps relieve the pain of arthritis, and is more effective than wrist splinting in relieving some symptoms and signs of carpal tunnel syndrome.

Are there any possible problems or complications?

Some yoga postures are difficult to achieve. People with cancer and chronic conditions, such as arthritis and heart disease, should consult their physician before undergoing any type of therapy that involves manipulation of joints and muscles.

References

Alternative Medicine: Expanding Medical Horizons. *A Report to the National Institutes of Health on Alternative Medical Systems and Practices in the United States.* Washington, DC: US Government Printing Office; 1994. NIH publication 94-066.

Complementary and Alternative Methods. Yoga. American Cancer Society Web site. Available at: http://www.cancer.org. Accessed January 24, 2000.

Garfinkel MS, Schumacher HR Jr, Husain A, Levy M, Reshetar RA. Evaluation of a yoga-based regimen for treatment of osteoarthritis of the hands. *J Rheumatol.* 1994;21:2341-2343.

Garfinkel MS, Singhai A, Katz WA, Allan DA, Reshetar R, Schumacher HR Jr. Yoga-based intervention for carpal tunnel syndrome: a randomized trial. *JAMA.* 1998;280:1601-1603.

Taylor E. Yoga and meditation. *Altern Ther Health Med.* 1995;1:77-78.

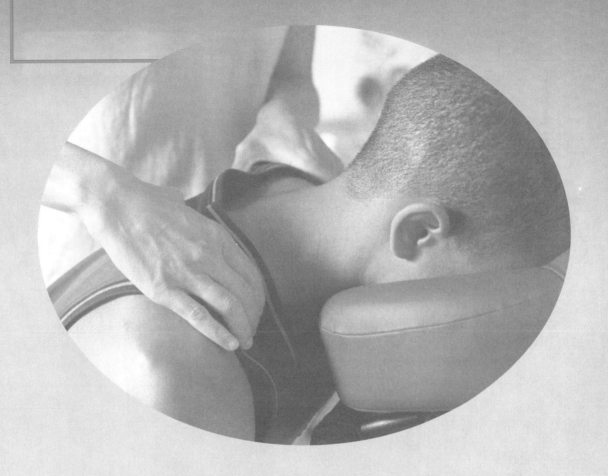

Chapter 6

Manual Healing and Physical Touch Methods

Treatment methods in this category involve

touching, manipulation, or movement of the

body. These techniques are based on the idea

that problems in one part of the body

often affect other parts of the body.

Acupuncture

Other common name(s)	**Scientific/medical name(s)**
Acupuncture Therapy, Zhenjiu	None

DESCRIPTION

Acupuncture is a technique in which very thin needles of varying lengths are inserted through the skin to treat a variety of conditions.

OVERVIEW

Although there is no evidence that acupuncture is effective as a treatment for cancer, clinical studies have found it to be effective in treating nausea caused by chemotherapy drugs and surgical anesthesia, and in relieving pain following dental surgery. The technique may also assist people who are trying to stop addictive behaviors, such as smoking or alcoholism, and may be useful for treating headaches, helping in rehabilitation from strokes, and treating a number of musculoskeletal conditions.

How is it promoted for use?

There is evidence that acupuncture eases nausea caused by chemotherapy and surgical anesthesia, and relieves postoperative dental pain. It may also assist withdrawal from addiction to drugs and alcohol, and help relieve headaches, menstrual cramps, tennis elbow, low back pain, carpal tunnel syndrome, and asthma.

In China, acupuncture is used as an anesthetic during surgery and is believed to have the power to cure diseases and relieve symptoms of illness. The teachings of traditional Chinese medicine explain that acupoints lie along invisible meridians, which are channels for the flow of vital energy or life force called qi (or chi) that is present in all living things. Meridians also represent an internal system of communication that is said to connect specific organs or networks of organs. There are 12 major meridians in the human body, one for each month of the year. Illness is claimed to occur when the energy flow along one or more meridians is blocked or out of balance. Some practitioners in the West reject the traditional philosophies of Chinese medicine and claim that acupuncture relieves pain by stimulating the production of natural substances in the body responsible for relieving pain called endorphins.

What does it involve?

In traditional acupuncture, needles are inserted at specific locations, called acupoints. In order to restore balance and a healthy energy flow to the body, needles are inserted at acupoints just deep enough into the skin to keep them from falling out. They are usually left in place for less than half an hour. Skilled acupuncturists cause virtually no pain. The acupuncturist may twirl the needles, and apply heat or a weak electrical current to enhance the effects of the therapy. Acupuncture is sometimes accompanied by less well-known traditional healing techniques (see Moxibustion and Cupping).

In acupressure, a popular variation of acupuncture, therapists press on acupoints with their fingers instead of using needles. This technique is used by itself or as part of an entire system of manual healing such as in shiatsu (see Bodywork). In other variations of acupuncture, heat, laser beams, sound waves, friction, suction, magnets, and electrical impulses are directed to acupoints (see Electromagnetic Therapy).

What is the history behind it?

Acupuncture originated 2,000 to 3,000 years ago and is an important component of current traditional Chinese medicine. Originally, 365 acupoints were identified, corresponding to the number of days in a year, but gradually, the number of acupoints grew to more than 2,000. Traditional acupuncture needles were made of bone, stone, or metal, including silver and gold. Modern acupuncture needles are made of very thin stainless steel and are disposable. In 1996, the FDA approved the use of acupuncture needles by licensed practitioners. By law, needles must be labeled for one-time use only.

In China, acupuncture is commonly accepted as a treatment for many diseases. Acupuncture has also become quite popular in the United States and Europe, where the technique is used primarily to control pain and relieve symptoms of disease such as nausea caused by chemotherapy drugs, but not to cure the disease itself. It is estimated that there are over 10,000 acupuncturists in the United States, and about 32 states have established training standards for licensing the practice of acupuncture. Medicare does not cover acupuncture, but it is covered by some private health insurance plans and HMOs. The American Academy of Medical Acupuncture maintains a current referral list of doctors who practice acupuncture.

What is the evidence?

There is no scientific evidence that acupuncture is effective as a treatment for cancer, but it appears to be useful as a complementary method for relieving some symptoms related to cancer and other conditions. Acupuncture has been the subject of numerous clinical studies. According to a National Institutes of Health (NIH) expert panel consisting of scientists, researchers, and health care providers, acupuncture is an effective treatment for nausea caused by chemotherapy drugs and surgical anesthesia, and the treatment of dental pain following surgery. Acupuncture *may* also be useful by itself or combined with conventional therapies to treat addiction, headache, menstrual cramps, tennis elbow, fibromyalgia, myofascial pain, osteoarthritis, lower back pain, carpal tunnel syndrome and asthma, and to assist in the rehabilitation of stroke patients. There is also some evidence that acupuncture may lessen the need for conventional pain-relieving drugs. A small clinical trial recently found acupuncture was effective in reducing the number of hot flashes men experienced after prostate cancer hormonal therapy.

Are there any possible problems or complications?

When conducted by a trained professional, acupuncture is generally considered safe. The number of complications reported have been relatively few, but there is a risk that a patient may be harmed if the acupuncturist is not well trained. When performed improperly, acupuncture can cause fainting, local internal bleeding, convulsions, hepatitis B, dermatitis, and nerve damage. Acupuncture also poses risks such as infection from contaminated needles or improper delivery of treatment. Relying on this type of treatment alone, and avoiding conventional medical care, may have serious health consequences.

References

Barrett S. Acupuncture, qigong, and "chinese medicine." Quackwatch Web site. Available at: http://www.quackwatch.com. Accessed October 12, 1999.

Cassileth B. The Alternative Medicine Handbook. New York, NY: W.W. Norton & Co; 1998.

Hammar M, Frisk J, Grimas O, Hook M, Spetz AC, Wyon Y. Acupuncture treatment of vasomotor symptoms in men with prostatic carcinoma: a pilot study. *J Urol.* 1999;161:853-856.

He JP, Friedrich M, Ertan AK, Muller K, Schmidt W. Pain-relief and movement improvement by acupuncture after ablation and axillary lymphadenectomy in patients with mammary cancer. *Clin Exp Obstet Gynecol.* 1999;26:81-84.

National Institutes of Health National Center for Complementary and Alternative Medicine Clearing House. Acupuncture Information Package. National Institutes of Health Web site. Available at: http://nccam.nih.gov. Accessed October 12, 1999.

Applied Kinesiology

Other common name(s)	Scientific/medical name(s)
Muscle Testing, AK	None

DESCRIPTION

Applied kinesiology is a technique used to diagnose illness by testing muscles for strengths and weaknesses.

OVERVIEW

There is no scientific evidence that applied kinesiology can diagnose or treat cancer. Muscle-testing methods appear to have no health benefits.

How is it promoted for use?

The fundamental notion of applied kinesiology is that every problem with an organ is accompanied by weakness in a corresponding muscle. For instance, a weak muscle in the chest might indicate liver disease, while weakness of the lower back or leg muscles may be the result of lung problems. Practitioners claim by discovering the weak muscle, they can identify the underlying illness and make decisions about subsequent treatment. They claim strengthening the weak muscles will restore the health of internal organs. Applied kinesiology is usually used for evaluation purposes, but claims have been made that after undergoing an AK session, it is possible to observe the "spontaneous remission" of cancer. There is no scientific evidence to support these claims.

Kinesiologists claim muscle weakness may be caused by a number of internal energy disruptions, such as nerve damage, drainage impairment of the lymph system, reduced blood supply, chemical imbalances, or organ and gland dysfunction. Practitioners usually recommend people confirm the diagnosis with conventional diagnostic techniques, such as laboratory testing and x-rays.

What does it involve?

Applied kinesiologists assess their patients by observing posture, gait, muscle strength, range of motion, and by palpation (touching). These observations may be combined with more conventional methods of diagnosis, such as a clinical history, a routine physical examination, and laboratory tests. They may also test for environmental or food sensitivities.

During the therapy, the patient might be asked to hold his or her arm parallel to the floor and resist the downward push of the practitioner, then repeat the exercise with the other arm. The relative strength differences supposedly help the kinesiologist diagnose internal imbalances. The practitioner might also press on key "trigger points" to detect muscle weakness.

To restore muscle strength, the applied kinesiologist may apply manual stimulation and relaxation techniques to key muscles. The therapy can include joint manipulation or mobilization, dietary management, reflex procedures, and cranial manipulation.

What is the history behind it?

Applied kinesiology was developed by Michigan chiropractor George J. Goodheart, Jr in 1964. Dr. Goodheart reported that a patient with an immobile shoulder visited his office. An examination revealed no abnormalities, even though the patient had complained of the problem for more than 15 years. When Dr. Goodheart pressed on small nodules near the origin of the pain, the muscle strength returned to normal and the shoulder's motion was restored. By "tugging" on particular trigger points, Goodheart claimed he could stimulate muscles to regain lost strength and function. He later incorporated disease diagnosis into his kinesiology system.

Today, practitioners who use applied kinesiology include chiropractors, naturopaths, physicians, dentists, nutritionists, physical therapists, massage therapists, and nurse practitioners. In order to practice as an applied kinesiologist, certification is available from the International College of Applied Kinesiology. To reach the highest level of certification, over 300 hours of instruction, several proficiency exams, and submission of original research papers are required. However, this college is not recognized by the Council on Chiropractic Education (see Chiropractic).

What is the evidence?

A few researchers have investigated kinesiology muscle-testing procedures in controlled clinical studies. The results showed that applied kinesiology was not an accurate diagnostic tool, and that muscle response was not any more useful than random guessing. In fact, one study found that applied kinesiologists made very different assessments regarding nutrient status for the same patients.

Some anecdotal accounts of successful applied kinesiology treatments do exist. However, there is no scientific evidence that kinesiology cures cancer or any other disease. A review of research papers published by the International College of Applied Kinesiology from 1981 to 1987 found that none of the studies used adequate statistical analyses.

Are there any possible problems or complications?

Applied kinesiology is considered relatively safe. However, relying on this diagnostic method alone, and avoiding or delaying conventional medical diagnosis and treatment, may have serious health consequences.

References

Barrett S. Applied kinesiology: muscle-testing for allergies and nutrient deficiencies. Quackwatch Web site. Available at: http://www.quackwatch.com. Accessed May 8, 2000.

Haas M, Peterson D, Hoyer D, Ross G. Muscle testing response to provocative vertebral challenge and spinal manipulation: a randomized controlled trial of construct validity. *J Manipulative Physiol Ther.* 1994;17:141-148.

Kenney JJ, Clemens R, Forsythe KD. Applied kinesiology unreliable for assessing nutrient status. *J Am Diet Assoc.* 1988;88:698-704.

Klinkoski B, Leboeuf C. A review of the research papers published by the International College of Applied Kinesiology from 1981 to 1987. *J Manipulative Physiol Ther.* 1990;13:190-194.

Biological Dentistry

Other common name(s)	Scientific/medical name(s)
None	None

DESCRIPTION

Biological dentistry is the removal of dental fillings or teeth claimed to contain toxins, which may cause systemic diseases or pain.

OVERVIEW

There is no scientific evidence that removing teeth or fillings can prevent cancer or any other disease. In 1987, the American Dental Association (ADA) declared that the unnecessary removal of silver amalgam is improper and unethical.

How is it promoted for use?

Practitioners of biological dentistry claim the mercury in ordinary fillings can escape, travel to distant organs, and contribute to the development of diseases, including cancer. They claim replacing metal fillings with synthetic, nontoxic compounds will eliminate toxins from the body and increase resistance to disease. Proponents of biological dentistry claim dental health has an impact on the health of the entire body.

Some practitioners also claim decaying teeth produce a chemical called dimethyl sulfide, which can cause cancer and other illnesses. They further claim there are infected cavities within jawbones that are not detectable by x-ray which must be scraped out. They call this condition "cavitational osteopathosis."

Practitioners claim that because each tooth is related to a corresponding organ in the body, an unhealthy, misaligned, or filled tooth (which may contain a "toxic" material such as mercury) disturbs the flow of vital energy or life force called qi (or chi) that flows freely through a healthy person. By removing the tooth or filling, or realigning the jaw, practitioners claim they can stop the production of dental toxins and restore the proper flow of energy (qi), resulting in improved health. Some biological dentists also claim that root canal procedures increase the risk of disease in other parts of the body.

One biological dentist has claimed patients with conditions such as chronic fatigue syndrome, allergies, and thyroid problems all improved after their mercury-containing fillings were removed. A Swiss physician claimed that 90% of the women with breast cancer he treated had dental problems that may have contributed to formation of the disease. There is no scientific evidence to support these claims.

What does it involve?

Biological dentistry involves the replacement of mercury-containing dental fillings with synthetic substitutes. Practitioners approach their patients holistically, meaning they consider the entire body rather than just the diseased area (see Holistic Medicine). A biological dentist may also prescribe other remedies or diets that claim to detoxify the body and strengthen the immune system. Biological dentistry can also involve oral acupuncture, surgical scraping, chelation therapy, neural therapy, laser therapy, and "mouth balancing," which is the attempt to improve structural deformities in the mouth and jaw (see Chelation Therapy and Neural Therapy).

What is the history behind it?

Dentists have used silver amalgam, which contains about 50% mercury, to fill cavities for over 160 years. A German physician, Dr. Josef Issels, was among the first to state that toxins from dental fillings could harm a person's overall health, and that root canal procedures posed the threat of infection to various organ systems. Dr. Issels also claimed there was a connection between the growth of tumors and the presence of dental toxins. He stated that 98% of his adult patients with cancer had from 2 to 10 teeth that had undergone root canal procedures. Such teeth, he believed, must be removed in order to decrease the level of toxicity in the body.

In 1999, a practitioner who removed fillings containing mercury was placed on probation by his state's Board of Dental Examiners for 5 years. They ruled on the basis of extensive complaints from patients who claimed their health and safety had been compromised. A few years earlier, a group of patients filed a lawsuit against several practitioners of biological dentistry, claiming that perfectly healthy teeth had been removed without any improvement in health. About 2,000 to 3,000 dentists practice biological dentistry in the United States today.

What is the evidence?

The few clinical studies that have been published in peer-reviewed medical journals found no association between teeth fillings and the development of cancer. The amount of mercury absorbed by the body from amalgams is so small it is considered harmless.

Typical dental fillings do contain materials such as mercury, copper, and silver, but there is no solid evidence showing the presence of these metals in teeth fillings causes disease in other parts of the body. A 1998 study concluded "there was no clear evidence that dental radiography (x-rays) or amalgam fillings is related to the development of tumors of the central nervous system." Another study found there was no connection between amalgam fillings, cardiovascular disease, diabetes, cancer, or early death.

In 1987, the ADA declared that removing perfectly good fillings (even if they contained mercury) is unethical. They stated dental amalgam was reviewed and found to be safe. At a 1991 conference, NIH experts concluded there was no evidence to support the idea that dental fillings caused health problems.

Are there any possible problems or complications?

Many dentists and other health experts believe the removal of healthy teeth or fillings is improper and unethical and should be avoided. Relying on this treatment alone, and avoiding conventional medical care, may have serious health consequences.

References

ADA Council on Scientific Affairs. Dental amalgam: update on safety concerns. *J Am Dent Assoc*. 1998;129:494-503.

ADA Daily News. England health department's amalgam report 'may cause unnecessary anxiety.' American Dental Association Web site. Available at: http://www.ada.org/adapco/daily/archives/9805/0501amal.html. Accessed May 8, 2000.

Ahlqwist M, Bengtsson C, Lapidus L. Number of amalgam fillings in relation to cardiovascular disease, diabetes, cancer and early death in Swedish women. *Community Dent Oral Epidemiol*. 1993;21:40-44.

Barrett S. Be wary of 'fad diagnoses.' Quackwatch Web site. Available at: http://www.quackwatch.com. Accessed May 8, 2000.

Barrett S. The mercury amalgam scam. Quackwatch Web site. Available at: http://www.quackwatch.com. Accessed May 8, 2000.

Dodes JE, Schissel M. Cavitational osteopathosis, NICO, and 'biological dentistry.' Quackwatch Web site. Available at: http://www.quackwatch.com. Accessed May 8,2000.

National Institutes of Health *Technology Assessment Conference. Effects and Side Effects of Dental Restorative Materials.* Bethesda, Md: National Library of Medicine;1991.

Rodvall Y, Ahlbom A, Pershagen G, Nylander M, Spannare B. Dental radiography after 25 years, amalgam fillings and tumours of the central nervous system. *Oral Oncol*. 1998;34:265-269.

Bodywork

Other common name(s)	**Scientific/medical name(s)**
Movement Therapy, Rolfing®, Alexander Technique®, Feldenkrais Method, Trager Approach, Shiatsu Massage	None

DESCRIPTION

Bodywork refers to a variety of physically-oriented techniques. Some forms of bodywork involve hands-on manipulation of joints or soft tissue, realigning the body, and correcting posture imbalances. Others focus on increasing a person's awareness of their own body through gentle, deliberate movement and breathing exercises.

OVERVIEW

There is no scientific evidence that bodywork is effective in treating cancer, but it can be used to enhance quality of life. Many forms of bodywork have the potential to bring pain relief and stress reduction although the effectiveness of these techniques has not yet been proven scientifically.

How is it promoted for use?

Various forms of bodywork are generally promoted to relieve pain, reduce stress, soothe injured muscles, stimulate blood and lymphatic circulation, and promote relaxation. Practitioners also claim that through bodywork, their patients become more comfortable with their bodies by learning how to move more freely, gracefully, and efficiently.

Some practitioners claim bodywork and movement therapy are effective treatments for many conditions, including cancer, circulation problems, colic, depression, headaches, heart problems, high blood pressure, hyperactivity, insomnia, sinus infections, and tension. There is no scientific evidence to support these claims.

What does it involve?

Many of the most commonly used bodywork therapies resemble traditional massage, but each differs from massage in one or more notable ways.

Rolfing

Rolfing is a form of myofascial massage guided by the contours of the body (see Myotherapy). Rolfers use their fingers, hands, elbows, and knees to place deep pressure and shift bones into proper alignment. Their goal is to increase range of motion and make movement easier by correcting posture misalignments. Rolfing can sometimes be quite painful.

Shiatsu

Shiatsu consists of pressing with the fingers on acupuncture points (see Acupuncture). Shiatsu practitioners use their fingers to press on vital points or holes to stretch and open pathways for the body's flow of vital energy or life force called qi (or chi).

The Feldenkrais Method

This technique involves a slow and gentle sequence of movements to help people develop a heightened awareness of their bodies, improve mobility, and break habits of poor posture and inefficient motion that can cause pain and discomfort. No attempt is made to alter the structure or alignment of the body.

The Alexander Technique

The Alexander Technique involves gently mobilizing parts of a patient's body that appear to be strained. Therapists also explain how to relax and move the body properly. The technique is designed to improve the mechanical relationships among body parts, and to align the head, neck, torso, and spine.

The Trager Approach

The Trager Approach uses gentle, rhythmical touch combined with movement exercises. The therapist feels how the client is holding his or her body, then applies various rocking, pulling, and rotational movements to the head, neck, torso, arms, and legs. Practitioners ask their clients to focus not on the effort of movement, but on the pleasure of it, so that the body can become an instrument of self-expression.

What is the history behind it?

Rolfing was developed in the 1930s by Ida Rolf, PhD, who believed that humans function most efficiently and comfortably when key parts of the body, such as the head, torso, pelvis, and legs, are properly aligned. There are different versions of Rolfing, such as Aston Patterning® and Hellerwork.

Shiatsu is a Japanese word that literally means, "finger-pressure." It is a system that evolved from acupressure and traditional Chinese practices. The goal is to improve the body's ability to heal itself and to promote overall health. Therapies similar to Shiatsu include reflexology, which focuses on massage and pressure points of the feet, and traditional Chinese massage (see Reflexology).

The Feldenkrais Method was developed during the first half of the 20th century by physicist Moshe Feldenkrais. A sports injury early in his life caused chronic pain and led Feldenkrais to explore unconventional methods of healing. He "reeducated" himself to walk again without pain using this method.

The Alexander Technique was developed by Frederick Matthias Alexander in the late 1800s. Alexander was an actor who kept losing his voice. He determined that he habitually moved his head back and down when he spoke, which caused him to suck in his breath and tense up his throat. He developed a method of breathing to alter this old habit and recovered his voice.

The Trager Approach was developed in 1927 by Milton Trager, MD. Dr. Trager was born with a spinal deformity. He overcame his handicap and became a dancer and gymnast. The physical movements of his therapy are intended not only to improve mobility and promote relaxation, but also to alter deep-seated thought patterns, which Dr. Trager believed were responsible for many physical problems.

There are many other variations of bodywork practiced today (see Myofascial Release, Myotherapy, Ohashiatsu®, Rosen Method, Rubenfeld Synergy® Method, Watsu®, and Tui-Na).

What is the evidence?

Many people who undergo one or more of these techniques enthusiastically report they feel more relaxed or can move with greater ease or less pain. However, very little scientific research has been done to find out what positive effects these treatments can offer.

Some people with cancer may find that these therapies help to relieve certain symptoms of cancer and side effects of treatments, but the evidence is anecdotal or based on very small research studies. There is no scientific evidence that any of these techniques are effective in treating cancer or any other disease.

Are there any possible problems or complications?

Rolfing can sometimes be quite painful. One concern for people with cancer is that therapies involving bodywork might increase the risk that tissue manipulation will cause cancer cells to travel to other parts of the body, however, there is no research to indicate that this will happen. People with rheumatoid arthritis, cancer that has spread to the bone, spine injuries, or bone diseases that could be aggravated by physical manipulation should avoid therapies that involve body manipulation because these conditions could worsen.

Manipulation of a bone where cancer metastasis is present could result in a bone fracture. People with cancer and chronic conditions, such as arthritis and heart disease, should consult their physician before undergoing any type of therapy that involves manipulation of joints and muscles.

References

Bernau-Eigen M. Rolfing: a somatic approach to the integration of human structures. *Nurse Pract Forum.* 1998;9:235-242.

Bower PJ, Rubik B, Weiss SJ, Starr C. Manual therapy: hands-on healing; use of hands in alternative medicine. *Patient Care.* 1997;31:69.

Burke C, Macnish S, Saunders J, Gallini A, Warne I, Downing J. The development of a massage service for cancer patients. *Clin Oncol.* 1994;6:381-384.

Gam AN, Warming S, Larsen LH, et al. Treatment of myofascial trigger-points with ultrasound combined with massage and exerciseña randomized controlled trial. *Pain.* 1998;77:73-79.

Cancer Salves

Other common name(s)	Scientific/medical name(s)
Black Salve, Escharotics, Escharotic Therapy, Botanical Salve, Curaderm	None

DESCRIPTION

Cancer salves are pastes, salves or poultices applied to external tumors or on the skin above internal tumor sites. There are many variations in the formulas, which can contain up to 10 ingredients or more in bases of olive oil, beeswax, and pine tar. Ingredients may include chaparral (Larrea tridentata), DMSO (dimethyl sulfoxide), chickweed (Stellaria media), Indian tobacco (Lobelia inflata), comfrey (Symphytum officinale), myrrh (Commiphora myrrha), marshmallow (Althaea officinalis), mullein (Verbascum thapsus) and other herbs, oils, and chemicals.

OVERVIEW

There is no scientific evidence that salves are effective in treating cancer or tumors. In fact, some ingredients may cause great harm to the body. There have been numerous reports of severe burns and permanent scarring.

How is it promoted for use?

Practitioners claim cancer salves have the power to kill cancer cells or draw them out of the body and that salves can cure any type of cancer. Some of the companies that sell cancer salves claim their products can heal cancer without the need for conventional treatments, such as surgery, chemotherapy, or radiation. One manufacturer has claimed the company's salves are successful at curing from 75% to 80% of cancer cases, and even 99% of one type of skin cancer. Other proponents claim their cancer salves have anti-tumor properties which cause no damage to healthy skin. There is no scientific evidence to support these claims.

One salve called curaderm is being promoted as a cure for three types of skin lesions—solar keratosis, basal cell carcinoma and squamous cell carcinoma—without leaving scars or harming normal skin. The cream contains chemicals called solasodine glycosides, derived from Sodom's apple *(Solanum sodomaeum),* also called devil's apple and kangaroo apple. Supporters do not claim the salve is effective against melanoma, the most deadly form of skin cancer. Curaderm is not approved by the FDA. There is no scientific evidence that curaderm is effective in treating any type of skin cancer.

What does it involve?

For skin cancers, the salves are rubbed directly onto the tumor. For other types of cancers, the salves are rubbed on the skin above the internal location of the tumor. Because the salves are widely available, some people apply them at home, while others receive salve treatments from naturopaths (see Naturopathic Medicine).

What is the history behind it?

The use of cancer salves to cure disease dates back centuries, perhaps even to ancient Egypt. The use of salves to cure cancer became relatively common in the 18th and 19th centuries. One 18th century English cancer surgeon, Dr. Richard Guy, used a black salve to treat dozens of cancer patients, particularly those with breast cancer. His claims of a high success rate were never verified. Another physician, Dr. Eli G. Jones, claimed he had miraculous results curing cancer patients using a salve made of figwort syrup. Many home grown salve formulations have been handed down through families for generations.

Cancer salves fall into a category of naturopathic medicine called "escharotics." An escharotic is a corrosive substance that creates an eschar (a thick, crusty scar) on the skin. Eschars often form after a person has been burned by heat or caustic chemicals.

What is the evidence?

All claims that cancer salves cure cancer are based on anecdotal reports and testimonials. There have been no clinical studies of cancer salves and there is no scientific evidence that cancer salves cure cancer or any other disease.

Are there any possible problems or complications?

There have been numerous reports of severe scarring and burns associated with the use of cancer salves. The FDA does not regulate cancer salves. The contents of different cancer salves vary and can contain potentially dangerous substances. Women who are pregnant or breast-feeding should not use cancer salves.

References

Jarvis WT. How quackery harms. Quackwatch Web site. Available at: http://www.quackwatch.com. Accessed May 8, 2000.

Moss R. *Herbs Against Cancer*. New York, NY: Equinox Press; 1998.

Castor Oil

Other common name(s)	Scientific/medical name(s)
Castor, Castor Bean, Palma Christi	*Ricinus communis*

DESCRIPTION

Castor oil is extracted from the seeds of Ricinus communis, an herb considered native to Africa and India.

OVERVIEW

There is no scientific evidence that castor oil is effective in preventing or treating cancer. However, researchers are currently studying castor oil as a vehicle for delivering chemotherapy drugs to cancerous tumors.

How is it promoted for use?

Castor oil is used as a laxative in conventional medicine. It may also be used to treat some eye irritations and skin conditions.

Alternative practitioners claim castor oil boosts the immune system by increasing lymphocytes (white blood cells that help the body fight infection) and other immune cells. They also claim castor oil helps dissolve cysts, warts, and tumors, as well as soften bunions and corns. Other claims for castor oil include treating lymphoma, bacterial and viral diseases (including HIV), arthritis, skin and hair conditions, eye irritations, diseases of the colon and gallbladder, bursitis, multiple sclerosis, and Parkinson's disease. There is no scientific evidence to support these claims.

What does it involve?

Treatment involves massaging castor oil into the body or using a warm or hot castor oil pack or compress. The castor oil is massaged along the problem region, spine, abdomen, and lymph drainage pattern. Promoters say application of castor oil is supposed to continue until the problem is healed.

What is the history behind it?

Ancient Egyptians were the first to record the use of castor oil for medicinal purposes, and since then it has been used by many cultures as a folk medicine. Castor oil was reportedly used as a medicine during the early Middle Ages in Europe. In his Encyclopedia of Healing, Edgar Cayce claimed that castor oil helped to heal the lymphatic tissue in the small intestines, thus increasing absorption of fatty acids and allowing for tissue growth and repair. Most of the plants used in producing castor oil are now grown in India and Brazil.

What is the evidence?

Castor oil is used in conventional medicine as a laxative and to treat some eye irritations. It is also an ingredient in some hair conditioners and skin products. There have been no scientific studies to support any other claims.

Researchers are currently studying the possibility of using castor oil as a vehicle for delivering chemotherapy drugs to cancerous tumors. Castor oil shows promise as a carrier of Taxol®, a drug used to treat metastatic breast cancer and other tumors. However, a study on high-intensity focused ultrasound therapy for liver cancer found castor oil did not work as well as iodized oil in producing a higher and faster temperature rise in the area of the tumor.

Researchers at Texas Tech University, Harvard University, the National Cancer Institute, and other institutions are studying ricin, a strong poison produced by the castor bean. Early clinical trials indicate that when combined with a monoclonal antibody (antibodies made in the laboratory designed to target specific substances), ricin may shrink tumors in lymphoma patients. There is no scientific evidence that castor oil cures cancer or any other disease.

Are there any possible problems or complications?

Castor oil is considered safe in proper doses for conventional uses as a laxative. However, side effects can include abdominal pain or cramping, colic, nausea, vomiting, and diarrhea. Long-term use of castor oil can lead to fluid and electrolyte loss. Women who are pregnant or breast-feeding should not use castor oil, as well as people with intestinal obstruction, acute inflammatory intestinal disease, appendicitis, or abdominal pain.

Castor beans are extremely poisonous and can lead to death if chewed or swallowed. Also, handling the seeds over a period of time can lead to allergic reactions.

References

Bown D. *Encyclopedia of Herbs & Their Uses.* New York, NY: DK Publishing Inc; 1995.

Cheng SQ, Zhou XD, Tang ZY, Yu Y, Bao SS, Qian DC. Iodized oil enhances the thermal effect of high-intensity focused ultrasound on ablating experimental liver cancer. *J Cancer Res Clin Oncol.* 1997;123:639-644.

Fetrow CW, Avila JR. *Professional's Handbook of Complementary and Alternative Medicines.* Springhouse, Pa: Springhouse Corp; 1999.

Fjallskog ML, Frii L, Bergh J. Paclitaxel-induced cytotoxicityóthe effects of cremophor EL (castor oil) on two human breast cancer cell lines with acquired multidrug resistant phenotype and induced expression of the permeability glycoprotein. *Eur J Cancer.* 1994;30A:687-690.

Henderson CW. Researchers know beans about cancer research. Cancer Weekly Plus. November 2, 1998. Accessed in the Information Access Company's Newsletter Database.

Medical Economics. *PDR for Herbal Medicines.* Montvale, NJ: Medical Economics Company; 1998.

Rischin D, Webster LK, Millward MJ, et al. Cremophor pharmacokinetics in patients receiving 3-, 6-, and 24-hour infusions of paclitaxel. *J Natl Cancer Inst.* 1996;88:1297-1301.

Chiropractic

Other common name(s)	Scientific/medical name(s)
Chiropractic Techniques, Spinal Manipulation	None

DESCRIPTION

Chiropractic is a treatment involving manipulation (moving) of the spine to correct medical problems.

OVERVIEW

There is no scientific evidence that chiropractic treatment cures cancer or any other disease. However, it has been shown to be effective in treating lower back pain and other pain due to muscle or bone problems. It can also promote relaxation and stress reduction. Complications may occur in a small number of cases.

How is it promoted for use?

Chiropractic is most commonly used to treat lower back pain and other pain due to muscle or bone problems. While there is evidence that it is effective for this use, there is no scientific evidence for other health claims. For example, some chiropractors claim to be able to treat health problems such as heart disease, epilepsy, impotence, and allergies, among other conditions. They claim the spine plays a vital role in nearly all health problems.

The basic concept of chiropractic is that illness stems from underlying "subluxations," or blockages, along the nerve bundles inside the spinal cord. Chiropractors do not treat the illness directly. Instead, they seek to correct the spine-related cause. Chiropractic is based on the idea that the human body has the ability to heal itself, and that the body always seeks to maintain a balance among its systems and organs. Practitioners claim this is achieved through the nervous system. Illness is thought to result from a blockage of the nerve impulses. Chiropractors claim manipulating the spine is designed to correct these blockages or other unnatural relationships between bones and nerves.

What does it involve?

The chiropractor first diagnoses the person's ailment through a personal interview, visual and touch examination, and x-rays of the spine. The person's flexibility and posture also may be examined. Electrical activity of the nerves and muscles may be measured. The examination is designed to pinpoint the source of the symptoms. For example, if a person complains of a pain in the shoulder, the chiropractor will search for the cause of the pain in the spinal column. Then the chiropractor will try to restore proper realignment and nerve function through manipulation of the vertebrae.

To receive treatment, a person lies face down on a specially designed treatment table. The chiropractor stands at the side and uses hands, elbows, and specially designed equipment to manipulate the spine, working to correct misalignments or other irregularities. Some chiropractors may also prescribe exercises to correct health problems, especially those that involve the skeletal and nervous systems.

What is the history behind it?

Chiropractic comes from the Greek words cheir (hands) and praktikos (efficient). It was practiced by priest healers in ancient Egypt, and for centuries, by Asian healers. Modern chiropractic was founded by Daniel D. Palmer, a grocer and mystic healer, who applied his knowledge of the nervous system to a man who had lost his hearing in the 1890s. He thrusted on a thoracic vertebra and the man's hearing was restored. Although Palmer wasn't the first to use this thrusting technique, he was the first to use the vertebrae as levers for manual contact. Palmer founded the first chiropractic school. In the three decades that followed, many other chiropractic colleges were opened and a variety of concepts developed regarding how to approach the practice of chiropractic.

Chiropractic colleges require at least four years of academic and professional training. The Council on Chiropractic Education establishes accreditation criteria for education. More than 55,000 licensed chiropractors are currently practicing in the United States.

What is the evidence?

Chiropractic has been shown to be effective in treating lower back pain and other pain due to muscle or bone problems. Chiropractors have also treated headaches, sports injuries, and carpal tunnel syndrome with some success.

There were two major reviews of the literature in 1992. One examined 22 randomized clinical trials involving spinal manipulation. The authors concluded that manipulation offers some positive short-term results for the treatment of people with low back pain. Other researchers evaluated 51 reviews and concluded spinal manipulation is of short-term benefit in some patients, especially for those who have uncomplicated, acute low back pain. Both reviews concluded there is not enough information to determine if chiropractic has any long-term benefits for low back pain.

Are there any possible problems or complications?

Chiropractic is considered relatively safe. However, there have been some reported cases of complications and even death following chiropractic care as well as misdiagnoses of patients' conditions. Several people with cancer developed paraplegia (paralysis of the legs) and quadriplegia (full-body paralysis) after manipulation of the spine when cancer had spread to the bones. People with cancer and chronic conditions, such as arthritis and heart disease, should consult their physician before undergoing any type of therapy that involves manipulation of joints and muscles.

References

Abenhaim L, Bergeron AM. Twenty years of randomized clinical trials of manipulative therapy for back pain: a review. *Clin Invest Med.* 1992;15:527-535.

Agency for Health Care Policy and Research. Acute pain management: Operative or medical procedures and trauma. Rockville, Md; 1992. Publication AHCPR 92-0032.

Alternative Medicine: Expanding Medical Horizons. A Report to the National Institutes of Health on Alternative Medical Systems and Practices in the United States. Washington, DC: US Government Printing Office; 1994. NIH publication 94-066.

Assendelft WJ, Koes BW, Knipschild PG, Bouter LM. The relationship between methodological quality and conclusions in reviews of spinal manipulation. *JAMA.* 1995;274:1942-1948.

Cassileth B. *The Alternative Medicine Handbook.* New York, NY: W. W. Norton & Co; 1998.

Shekelle PG, Adams AH, Chassin MR, Hurwitz EL, Brook RH. Spinal manipulation for low-back pain. *Ann Intern Med.* 1992;117:590-598.

Spencer JW, Jacobs JJ. *Complementary/Alternative Medicine: An Evidence-Based Approach.* St. Louis, MO: Mosby, Inc; 1999.

Manual Healing / Physical Touch

Cold Laser Therapy

Other common name(s)	Scientific/medical name(s)
None	None

DESCRIPTION / OVERVIEW

Cold laser therapy is similar to acupuncture, but it involves the use of laser beams to stimulate the body's acupoints rather than needles (see Acupuncture). The term cold laser refers to the use of low-intensity or low levels of laser light. This treatment regimen appeals to those who fear the pain of needles. Proponents claim that cold laser therapy can reduce pain and inflammation. There is no scientific evidence to support these claims. This method should not be confused with conventional laser surgery, used as a valid treatment for some cancers, which involves vaporizing tissue with hot lasers.

Colon Therapy

Other common name(s)	Scientific/medical name(s)
Colonic Irrigation, High Colonic, Detoxification Therapy, Colon Hydrotherapy, Coffee Enemas, Enema Irrigation, Hydro-Colon Therapy, High Enema	None

DESCRIPTION

Colon therapy is the cleansing of the large intestine (colon) through the administration of water, herbal solutions, or other substances, such as coffee.

OVERVIEW

There is no scientific evidence that colon therapy is effective in treating cancer or any other disease. Colon therapy can be dangerous, and can cause infection or death.

How is it promoted for use?

Proponents of colon therapy consider it to be a method of detoxifying the body through the removal of accumulated waste from the colon. Because they claim detoxification increases the efficiency of the body's natural healing abilities, it is sometimes promoted as a treatment for illness. It is often promoted as a general preventive health measure, or as part of a routine internal hygiene regimen by practitioners.

Coffee enemas have been promoted as part of several controversial cancer treatment regimens. People who promote the use of coffee enemas to detoxify the body claim that an "unpoisoned" body or a "clean" colon has the ability to recognize and destroy cancer cells. Practitioners claim coffee enemas can stimulate the liver and gallbladder into releasing toxins and flushing them from the body, allowing the body's immune system to battle malignant cells (see Gerson Therapy and Metabolic Therapy). There is no scientific evidence to support these claims.

What does it involve?

A high colonic is administered by a colonic hygienist or colon therapist, and is accomplished through the use of plastic tubes inserted through the rectum and into the colon. A machine or gravity driven pump sends large quantities of liquid (up to 20 gallons) into the large intestine. In contrast, regular enemas only flush out the rectum, and generally use about a quart of fluid. After filling the colon with water, the therapist massages the abdomen to facilitate the removal of waste material from the colon wall, fluid and waste are carried out of the body through another tube. The procedure is generally repeated several times, and the average session lasts from 45 to 60 minutes. Coffee enemas vary in frequency and may be incorporated into the entire treatment program.

What is the history behind it?

As far back as the ancient Egyptians, enemas and other "cleansing rituals" were commonly used to rid the body of toxic waste products believed to cause disease and death. In the 19th century, proponents described the large intestine as a sewage system, and claimed stagnation caused toxins to form and be absorbed by the body, which led to the theory of "autointoxication." Laxatives, purges, and enemas were routinely recommended to prevent the accumulation of waste.

Colon therapy became very popular in the United States in the 1920s and 1930s, when irrigation machines were commonly found in hos-

pitals and physicians' offices. Although the procedure became less popular when advances in science and medicine did not support its founding theory, colon therapy has recently experienced an increase in popularity.

In 1985, the California Department of Health Services issued a statement which listed some of the potential hazards of colon therapy as infection and death from contaminated equipment, death from electrolyte depletion, and perforation of the intestinal wall leading to life-threatening infection or death. The FDA classifies colonic irrigation machines as Class III devices that cannot be legally marketed except for medically indicated colon cleansing (such as before a radiologic or endoscopic examination). No colonic irrigation machine or system has been approved for routine use.

What is the evidence?

There is no scientific evidence supporting the claims on which colon therapy is based. It is known that most digestive processes take place in the small intestine, where nutrients are absorbed into the body. What remains enters the large intestine, where it passes to the rectum for elimination after water and minerals are extracted. There is no scientific evidence that toxins accumulate on intestinal walls, or that toxicity results from poor elimination of waste from the colon.

Are there any possible problems or complications?

The machines used for colon therapy are illegal unless used during conventional medical treatment. Colon therapy can be dangerous, leading to death from contaminated equipment, electrolyte (salt and mineral) depletion, or perforation of intestinal walls. Relying on this type of treatment alone, and avoiding conventional medical care, may have serious health consequences.

References

Barrett S. Gastrointestinal quackery: colonics, laxatives, and more. Quackwatch Web site. Available at: http://www.quackwatch.com. Accessed May 8, 2000.

Brown BT. Treating cancer with coffee enemas and diet. *JAMA*. 1993;269:1635-1636.

Cassileth B. *The Alternative Medicine Handbook*. New York, NY: W. W. Norton & Co; 1998.

Green S. A critique of the rationale for cancer treatment with coffee enemas and diet. *JAMA*. 1992;268:3224-3227.

Craniosacral Therapy

Other common name(s)	Scientific/medical name(s)
Cranial Balancing, Cranial Osteopathy, Cranial Sacral Manipulation, Craniopathy	None

DESCRIPTION

Craniosacral therapy involves the gentle massage of bones in the skull (including the face and mouth), vertebral column (spine), and pelvis to ease stress in the body and improve physical movement.

OVERVIEW

There is no scientific evidence that craniosacral therapy is effective in treating cancer or any other disease. However, it may help people with cancer feel more relaxed. The gentle, hands-on method is non-invasive and may offer some relief for symptoms of stress, headaches, and muscle tension.

How is it promoted for use?

Craniosacral therapy is a variation of chiropractic and osteopathic medicine (see Chiropractic and Osteopathic Medicine). Proponents claim gentle massage of the bones of the head, spine, and pelvis increases the flow of cerebrospinal fluid, which can cure any number of ailments. They say it normalizes, balances, and eliminates obstructions in various systems throughout the body. By removing obstructions, they claim the body can function in a healthy manner.

Promoters claim this therapy can be used to help relieve headaches, neck and back pain, temporomandibular joint dysfunction, chronic fatigue, motor coordination difficulties, eye problems, depression, hyperactivity, attention deficit disorder, problems with the central nervous system, the immune system, the endocrine system, and many other conditions.

Practitioners also claim the birthing process can have a negative effect on growth of the cartilage and membranes surrounding an infant's skull and offer this treatment to fix this problem. There is no scientific evidence to support these claims.

What does it involve?

Craniosacral therapy is usually performed by osteopaths, chiropractors, and massage therapists. The treatment involves either gentle massage or manipulation to the bones of the skull. Sessions last from 30 minutes to 1 hour.

What is the history behind it?

Dr. William G. Sutherland developed cranial osteopathy in the early 1930s. John E. Upledger, DO, developed craniosacral therapy, a derivative of Sutherland's work, in the 1970s. Upledger opened the Upledger Institute of Florida, where thousands of health care professionals attend his program every year to learn about releasing stresses in the skull and the membranes surrounding the brain.

What is the evidence?

There are only anecdotal reports of successful treatment with craniosacral therapy. Some patients report that it helps to reduce stress, tension, and headaches. However, there have been no controlled clinical studies of this method. In a report to the National Institutes of Health Office of Alternative Medicine, it was stated that successes have not been documented in formal studies. The US Air Force Academy Physical Therapy Clinic conducted a study to determine the reliability of measurements obtained during craniosacral therapy. They found no evidence to support the claims made about the therapy.

Are there any possible problems or complications?

Craniosacral therapy should not be used in children under age two because the bones of the skull are not fully developed. People with cancer and chronic conditions, such as arthritis and heart disease, should consult their physician before undergoing any type of therapy that involves manipulation of joints and muscles.

References

Alternative Medicine: Expanding Medical Horizons. A Report to the National Institutes of Health on Alternative Medical Systems and Practices in the United States. Washington, DC: US Government Printing Office; 1994. NIH publication 94-066.

Barrett S. Jarvis W. Holistic dentistry: a brief overview. Quackwatch Web site. Available at: http://www.quackwatch.com. Accessed May 8, 2000.

Barrett S. Dubious aspects of osteopathy. Quackwatch Web site. Available at: http://www.quackwatch.com. Accessed May 8, 2000.

Cassileth B. *The Alternative Medicine Handbook.* New York, NY: W. W. Norton & Co; 1998.

Rogers JS, Witt PL, Gross MT, Hacke JD, Genova PA. Simultaneous palpation of the craniosacral rate at the head and feet: intrarater and interrater reliability and rate comparisons. *Phys Ther.* 1998;78:1175-1185.

Manual Healing / Physical Touch

Cupping

Other common name(s)	Scientific/medical name(s)
Cupping, Fire Cupping, Body Vacuuming, The Horn Method	None

DESCRIPTION

Cupping involves warming the air inside a glass, metal, or wooden cup and inverting it over a part of the body to treat various health conditions.

OVERVIEW

There is no scientific evidence that cupping leads to any health benefits.

How is it promoted for use?

Cupping is a practice of Chinese medicine recommended primarily for treating bronchial congestion, arthritis, and pain. It is also promoted to ease depression and reduce swelling. There is no evidence to support these claims.

Cupping is supposed to realign and balance the flow of vital energy or life force called qi (or chi). In the presence of illness or injury proponents say, the qi is disturbed and may become excessive or deficient at certain points. The practitioner diagnoses any imbalances in the qi and attempts to restore them. Although not widely used as an alternative method of treatment for cancer, some practitioners may use it to rebalance energy in the body that has been blocked by certain tumors.

What does it involve?

A flammable substance, such as alcohol, herbs, or paper is placed in a cup made of glass, metal, wood, or bamboo. The material inside the cup is set on fire. As the fire goes out, the cup is placed upside down over qi pathways associated with the patient's illness, where it remains for 5 to 10 minutes.

As the air inside the jar cools, it creates a vacuum, which causes the skin to rise. This is supposed to open up the skin's pores and create a route for toxins to escape the body. The skin under the cup reddens as blood vessels expand. In a more modern version of cupping, a rubber pump attached to the jar is used to create the vacuum.

In "wet" cupping, the skin is punctured before treatment. When the cup is applied, blood flows out of the punctures, supposedly carrying along harmful substances and toxins. In "dry" cupping, the skin is left intact. Some practitioners sterilize the cups in an autoclave, which heats the cups to more than 250° F.

What is the history behind it?

Cupping is an ancient component of Chinese medicine. Besides "fire" cupping, other methods include acupuncture cupping, water cupping, and air-pump cupping.

What is the evidence?

No research or clinical studies have been done on cupping. Any reports of successful treatment with cupping are anectodal. There is no scientific evidence that cupping can cure cancer or any other disease.

Are there any possible problems or complications?

Cupping is considered relatively safe. However, the treatment may be uncomfortable and slightly painful. Cupping also leaves purplish marks on the skin that heal after several days and can cause swelling due to the accumulation of excess fluid around the cupped area.

References

Cassileth B. *The Alternative Medicine Handbook*. New York, NY: W. W. Norton & Co; 1998.

Raso J. Dictionary of metaphysical healthcare. Quackwatch Web site. Available at: http://www.quackwatch.com. Accessed February 22, 2000.

Electroacupuncture

Other common name(s)	Scientific/medical name(s)
None	None

DESCRIPTION / OVERVIEW

Electroacupuncture, considered an enhanced version of traditional acupuncture, involves applying electrical stimulation, with or without needles, to the acupoints that are targeted during traditional acupuncture. Controlled clinical studies have shown that this treatment method can benefit some people with postoperative pain, nausea associated with chemotherapy, and renal (kidney) colic (see Acupuncture).

Electrodermal Screening

Other common name(s)	Scientific/medical name(s)
None	None

DESCRIPTION / OVERVIEW

Electrodermal screening is used to diagnose disease by detecting energy imbalances along acupuncture meridians (see Acupuncture and Electronic Devices). It involves the use of devices to monitor energy signals from the skin. Proponents claim the devices can help select specific treatments, measure the progress of therapy, and even detect disease before it becomes apparent. There is no scientific evidence to support these claims.

Manual Healing / Physical Touch

Electromagnetic Therapy

Other common name(s)	**Scientific/medical name(s)**
Electromagnetism, Bioelectricity, Black Boxes, Energy Medicine, Electronic Devices, Electrical Devices, Zapping Machine, Rife Machine, Cell Com System, BioResonance Tumor Therapy	None

DESCRIPTION

Electromagnetic therapy involves the use of electrical and magnetic energy to diagnose or treat disease.

OVERVIEW

There is no scientific evidence that electromagnetic therapy is effective in diagnosing or treating cancer or any other disease. There are some medically approved uses for some electronic devices, such as the electroencephalogram (EEG), electrocardiogram (EKG), and transcutaneous electrical nerve stimulation units (TENS) which are used to diagnose nervous system and heart problems (see Transcutaneous Electrical Nerve Stimulation). However, many of the alternative electronic devices promoted to cure disease have not been scientifically proven to be effective.

How is it promoted for use?

Practitioners claim when electromagnetic frequencies or fields of energy within the body go out of balance, disease and illness occurs. They claim these imbalances disrupt the body's chemical makeup. By applying electrical energy from outside the body, usually with electronic devices, practitioners claim they can correct the imbalances in the body.

Practitioners claim these methods can treat ulcers, headaches, burns, chronic pain, nerve disorders, spinal cord injuries, diabetes, gum infections, asthma, bronchitis, arthritis, cerebral palsy, heart disease, and cancer. There is no scientific evidence to support any of the claims made for these devices.

Practitioners of BioResonance Tumor Therapy (a kind of electromagnetic therapy) use an electronic device they claim results in the self-destruction of tumor cells. They say it cures cancer in 80% of cases. However, there is no description of precisely how this is accomplished or reliable scientific data to substantiate the claim.

Another electronic device called the Cell Com System is promoted as a regulator of the chemical and electrical communication between cells. Proponents claim it can be used to relieve pain caused by cancer and for fighting recurrent infections, asthma, bronchitis, and arthritis. They further claim the device can stop the growth of cancer cells. There is no evidence to support this claim.

Practitioners claim the Rife Machine, another electronic device, can diagnose and eliminate diseases, including cancer, by tuning into electrical impulses emitted by diseased tissue. The Rife Machine then directs energy of the same frequency back at the diseased tissue. Promoters claim the device kills microorganisms that cause disease; however, there is no evidence for this.

Another electronic device that has been promoted to cure cancer is the Zapping Machine. Based on the claim that cancer is related to parasites, promoters say it kills the parasites that cause cancer; however, there is also no evidence for this claim.

What does it involve?

Electromagnetic therapy, which encompasses several different kinds of therapy, uses an energy field—electrical, magnetic, microwave, or infrared—to diagnose or treat an illness by detecting imbalances in the body's energy fields and then correcting them. Electronic devices, which emit some form of low-voltage electrical current or radio frequency, are often involved. Magnets and other unconventional treatments may also be a part of electromagnetic therapy (see Bioenergetics, Crystal Healing, Magnetic Therapy, Polarity Therapy, Qigong, Reiki, and Therapeutic Touch). The most commonly used electronic devices are listed below.

BioResonance Tumor Therapy

This therapy uses a small electronic device to generate oscillations that are supposed to "re-enliven" the p53 gene in order to cure cancer. Some reports estimate that the program can last up to six weeks.

Cell Com System

This device reportedly transmits low voltage electricity through electrodes that are placed on the hands and feet in order to regulate communication between cells in the body.

Rife Machine

(a.k.a. Frequency Therapy, Frequency Generator, Rife Frequency Generator)
This device is used to direct electrical impulses at the feet to break up the supposed accumulated deposits of toxins at nerve endings. During treatment, the patient places his or her feet in a plastic box attached to the Rife unit.

Zapping Machine

A zapping machine is a small, battery-powered device that produces a low-frequency electrical current. Wires connected to copper tubes transmit the electricity to patients.

What is the history behind it?

The effects of magnetism and energy forces have been examined since the time of the Greek and Roman empires. Chinese medicine uses one of the oldest energy based systems of healing. Traditional Chinese medicine is based on the concept of qi (or chi) which is considered to be the vital energy or life force that flows throughout the body. The concept of life force energy is also a central aspect of Indian medical beliefs.

In modern times, the discovery of electricity brought about the promotion of electromagnetic therapies. The use of various forms of electrical devices and frequency generators in medicine has intrigued practitioners and patients for generations. Since the mid 1800s, countless electronic machines have been applied to a long list of ailments. Most of these devices have never been proven effective. In some cases their use has resulted in serious injury or even death. However, some electromagnetic and electrical technologies have become mainstays of modern medical practice, such as diagnostic x-rays, radiation therapy, magnetic resonance imaging (MRI), and cardiac pacemakers.

The first known use of frequency therapy came in the late 1800s when Albert Abrams, MD, developed a number of devices he claimed could detect the frequencies of diseased tissue and heal the underlying imbalances. However, Dr. Abrams was never able to prove his devices were effective. Dozens of unconventional and unproven electronic devices have been marketed over the years. BioResonance Tumor Therapy, the Cell Com system, the Rife machine, and the Zapping machine are four popular systems on the market today.

BioResonance Tumor Therapy was developed by Martin Keymer, a German biophysicist, who claims the therapy is rooted in the age-old idea that it is possible to tap into the vital energy that flows throughout the body. A clinic offering the therapy, which opened in Tijuana, Mexico in 1998, has been the subject of a great deal of controversy. The Cell Com system which is said to increase communication between cells was invented by a Danish acupuncturist named Hugo Nielsen.

The Rife machine (or Rife frequency generator) was created by Royal Raymond Rife, an American who asserted that cancer was caused by bacteria. The machine supposedly emitted radio waves at the same frequency as those discharged by offending bacteria. According to Rife, the radio waves created vibrations that "shattered" the bacteria.

The most widely marketed zapping machine today is the Zapper designed by Hulda Clark, PhD, a physiologist with no formal clinical medical training. She currently uses her device to treat patients with cancer, AIDS, and other diseases in a Tijuana, Mexico medical clinic.

Electronic devices and other frequency generators are available through a number of companies. Treatment programs that incorporate the devices are offered in Mexican and Canadian clinics. Practitioners do not need a license to conduct frequency therapy in the United States.

The FDA has not approved any of the alternative machines or products connected to electrical sources (electronic devices) used to cure illness and does not recognize any frequency generator as a legitimate medical device. They have, however, launched an investigation into the industry.

What is the evidence?

Science has established the fact that electrical and magnetic energy exist in the human body. Electrical energy is used by physicians to re-start the heart after heart attacks and is even appled to promote bone growth. Some accepted electrical devices commonly used in hospitals include EEGs to measure electrical activity in the brain and EKGs to measure electrical patterns of heartbeats.

Low level electrical impulses or radio waves are not strong enough to produce a biological effect. There is no evidence radio waves destroy bacteria or any living cells.

There is no relationship between these conventional uses of electrical energy and the alternative devices or methods that use externally applied electrical forces. There is no scientific evidence that electromagnetic therapies are effective in diagnosing or treating cancer or any other disease.

Are there any possible problems or complications?

Untested, unproven electrical devices may pose some risk. There have been reports of injuries due to faulty electrical wiring, power surges during lightening storms, and misuse of equipment. Relying on this type of treatment alone, and avoiding conventional medical care, may have serious health consequences.

References

American Cancer Society. Questionable methods of cancer management: electronic devices. *CA Cancer J Clin*. 1994;44:115-127.

Alternative Medicine: Expanding Medical Horizons. A Report to the National Institutes of Health on Alternative Medical Systems and Practices in the United States. Washington, DC: US Government Printing Office; 1994. NIH publication 94-066.

Cassileth B. *The Alternative Medicine Handbook*. New York, NY: W.W. Norton & Co; 1998.

Rubik B. Energy medicine and the unifying concept of information. *Altern Ther Health Med*. 1995;1:34-39.

Heat Therapy

Other common name(s)	Scientific/medical name(s)
Hyperthermia, Heat Treatment	None

DESCRIPTION
Heat therapy involves exposing part or all of the body to high temperatures, usually to enhance other forms of therapy (eg, radiation and chemotherapy).

OVERVIEW
Although not part of routine cancer treatment, local and regional heat therapy is being studied as part of conventional treatment for some cancers. Whole-body heat therapy is currently investigational, and clinical trials are underway to study its use along with radiation and chemotherapy. The use of heat therapy outside clinical trials remains questionable and is an alternative treatment. There are some serious complications associated with whole-body heat therapy. More research is needed to determine the full benefits of heat therapy in cancer treatment.

How is it promoted for use?
There is some evidence that local and regional heat therapy may stop cancers from growing and increase the effectiveness of radiation and chemotherapy in some cases. It seems to work by increasing blood flow, which can make the cancer cells more responsive to conventional treatment.

Proponents of the alternative use of heat therapy claim it reduces or even eliminates the need for conventional treatment. They say it decreases the number of invading organisms so the immune system can handle them, acting much like a fever helping the body fight off disease. There is no scientific evidence for this theory.

What does it involve?
There are three major types of heat therapy: local, regional, and whole-body. Local heat therapy involves applying heat to a very small area, such as a tumor. The area may be heated externally, with high-frequency waves, or internally using one of several types of sterile probes (thin, heated wires or hollow tubes filled with warm implanted microwave antennae) and radiofre-quency electrodes. In regional heat therapy, an organ or limb is heated. One method, called perfusion, involves removing the patient's blood, heating it, and then pumping it into a region to be heated internally. Whole-body heat therapy is used to treat metastatic cancers (cancer that has spread). It involves the use of warm blankets, hot wax, inductive coils (similar to those in electric blankets), or thermal chambers (similar to large incubators).

What is the history behind it?
The first documented use of heat treatment dates back to 400 BC with Hippocrates. In 500 BC, the Greek physician Parmenides believed that if he could create fever, he could cure all illness. The early Romans used elaborate heat baths and Native Americans have used sweat lodges in cleansing practices for centuries (see Native American Healing).

The first scientific investigation of heat therapy began in 1866, when M. Busch, a German physician, described a patient with a neck sarcoma which disappeared after he experienced a high fever. Similar reports were made by others 20 years later. In 1893, F. Westermark, a Swedish gynecologist, administered bacterial toxins extracted from *Streptococcus* and *Serratia marcescens* to cause fever and used a coil containing hot water as a localized source of heat to treat uterine tumors. Reports followed of tumors responding to both localized and whole-body heat therapy treatments. However, the scientific evidence was weak and interest soon declined.

In the 1960s, a series of biochemical studies involving the effects of elevated temperature on normal and malignant cells were conducted using rodent cells. Based on their observations, researchers concluded that cancer cells were more sensitive to heat than normal cells. However, studies have since shown that there is little or no difference between cancer cells and normal cells in terms of their response to heat.

What is the evidence?
Numerous laboratory and clinical studies have demonstrated that heat therapy can enhance the effectiveness of radiation therapy in local and regional tumor control and the effectiveness of chemotherapy in some cancers.

Whole-body heat therapy is currently under investigation as a method to treat system-wide illnesses. A small, randomized clinical trial found that there were some positive effects of using the combination of whole-body heat therapy and melphalan (a chemotherapy drug), but more research is needed. The National Cancer Institute (NCI) is currently sponsoring three phase II clinical trials using whole-body heat therapy in combination with chemotherapy drugs in treating patients with advanced melanoma, advanced sarcoma, and metastatic and recurring lymphoma.

Are there any possible problems or complications?

Heat therapy can cause internal bleeding. The high death rate and labor-intensive methods associated with whole-body heat therapy have also caused concerns. Heat therapy should only be administered under careful supervision by qualified physicians. It should also be used with caution in people who have anemia, heart disease, diabetes, seizure disorders, and tuberculosis, as well as women who are pregnant, and people who are sensitive to the effects of heat. Relying on this type of treatment alone, and avoiding conventional medical care, may have serious health consequences.

References
Kapp DS, Hahn GM, Carlson RW. Principles of hyperthermia. In: Bast RC, Kufe DW, Pollock RE, Weichselbaum RR, Holland JF, Frei EF, eds. *Cancer Medicine*. 5th ed. Hamilton, Ontario: BC Decker; 2000:479-488.

Katschinski DM, Wiedemann GJ, Mentzel M, Mulkerin DL, Touhidi R, Robins HI. Optimization of chemotherapy administration for clinical 41.8°C whole body hyperthermia. *Cancer Lett.* 1997;115:195-199.

Murphy GP, Morris LB, Lange D. *Informed Decisions: The Complete Book of Cancer Diagnosis, Treatment, and Recovery.* New York, NY: Viking; 1997.

National Cancer Institute PDQ. NCI Fact Sheet: Hyperthermia in cancer treatment. National Cancer Institute Cancernet Web site. Available at: http://cancernet.nci.nih.gov. Accessed January 11, 2000.

Robins HI, Rushing D, Kutz M, et al. Phase I clinical trial of melphalan and 41.8°C whole-body hyperthermia in cancer patients. *J Clin Oncol.* 1997;15:158-164.

US Congress, Office of Technology Assessment. Unconventional Cancer Treatments. Washington, DC: US Government Printing Office; 1990. Publication OTA-H-405.

Hydrotherapy

Other common name(s)	Scientific/medical name(s)
Water Therapy	None

DESCRIPTION

Hydrotherapy is the use of water as a medical treatment, either internally or externally.

OVERVIEW

Hydrotherapy has been proven effective in various ways. It is used as a means of physical therapy, promoting relaxation, and relieving minor aches and pains. However, there is no evidence that any form of hydrotherapy is effective in preventing or treating cancer.

How is it promoted for use?

There are many medically accepted uses of hydrotherapy. Each involves water in the form of ice, liquid, or steam. Some of the more common examples of hydrotherapy include using water to clean wounds, warm water compresses, ice packs, whirlpool or steam baths, and drinking liquids to reduce dehydration.

Hydrotherapy includes the use of warm compresses, which expand blood vessels, increasing circulation to relax muscles and reduce pain, and speed rehabilitation. Warm water in the form of a bath, Jacuzzi, or hot tub also provides relaxation and stress relief. The steam used in a humidifier can reduce the discomfort of minor sore throats and colds. Steam, used in a sauna or "sweat lodge," causes perspiration, which helps rid the body of waste products. Hydrotherapy in the form ice packs is used to reduce inflammation and swelling. The coldness constricts blood vessels and reduces circulation to the applied area, thereby decreasing fluid and swelling.

Hydrotherapy is also used in physical rehabilitation, exercise, and child birthing. When performed in water, these activities can be more effective and cause less strain on the skeleton and joints. Dehydration, which can be a serious medical problem, is treated through the administration of water or liquids, either by drinking or intravenously (directly into a vein through a needle).

Some proponents claim one form of hydrotherapy, that involves frequent enemas, cleanses the bowels and helps cure cancer (see Colon Therapy). However, there is no scientific evidence to support this claim, and serious side effects may occur.

What does it involve?

In most types of hydrotherapy, water is either directly applied to the desired area (eg, an ice pack or a warm compress) or the body is immersed in water (eg, a hot tub or bath). Internal means of hydrotherapy range from drinking the recommended amount of water daily or receiving an intravenous (IV) infusion, to getting a large water enema.

What is the history behind it?

Hydrotherapy has been used throughout history by many diverse cultures. Even the Old Testament mentions the healing powers of mineral waters. By the time of the ancient Greeks, the use of water as a healing agent was well established. The early Roman and Turkish baths are still popular tourist attractions today.

The modern use of hydrotherapy is linked to Vincent Preissnitz who established the

"Graefenberg cure" for treating almost every ailment in the 1800s. This treatment involved the use of water in every conceivable way, often alternating between hot and cold water.

Today, Native Americans use sweat lodges as a remedy (see Native American Healing). They believe perspiration is a form of cleansing and purges poisons from the body. This belief is similar to the Scandinavians' use of saunas. Several of the springs first used by Native Americans have been converted into resorts and remain popular today. President Franklin D. Roosevelt's use of one such spring brought worldwide attention to the use of hydrotherapy.

What is the evidence?

Hydrotherapy is an accepted, useful form of symptom treatment for many conditions. The ability to promote relaxation in its many forms is well established. Certain types of hydrotherapy are good examples of conventional therapies that have been proven to be effective, such as ice packs for slight sprains and hot compresses for sore muscles. Water immersion is effectively used in physical therapy. Hydrotherapy is also useful for patients with severe burns, rheumatoid arthritis, spinal cord injuries, and bone injuries.

Hydrotherapy has not been proven effective in slowing the growth or spread of cancer. There is no scientific evidence that alternative uses of hydrotherapy, such as colon therapy, can cure cancer or any other disease.

Are there any possible problems or complications?

Most forms of hydrotherapy are safe. However, colon therapy can cause perforation of the colon, which can lead to death. Cases of bacterial infection due to improperly cleaned whirlpools and hot tubs have also been reported. Excessively hot or cold water applied directly to the skin for long periods of time may cause pain and tissue damage.

References

Burns SB, Burns JL. Hydrotherapy. *J Altern Complement Med.* 1997;3:105-107.

Cassileth B. *The Alternative Medicine Handbook.* New York, NY: W. W. Norton & Co; 1998.

Hyperbaric Oxygen Therapy

Other common name(s)	Scientific/medical name(s)
Hyperbaric Medicine, Hyperbarics, HBOT	None

DESCRIPTION

Hyperbaric oxygen therapy (HBOT) involves the breathing of pure oxygen that has been pressurized 1.5 to 3 times normal atmospheric pressure which is conducted in sealed chambers.

OVERVIEW

Research has shown HBOT is effective when used in addition to conventional therapy for the prevention and treatment of osteoradionecrosis (bone damage caused by radiation therapy). There is also some evidence suggesting HBOT may be helpful as an additional therapy for soft-

tissue injury caused by radiation. In the past, some head and neck cancers and cervical cancer were effectively treated using HBOT and radiation therapy; however, these treatments are no longer used in conventional medicine today. There is no evidence that HBOT cures cancer or any other disease.

How is it promoted for use?

HBOT is used in conventional treatment for decompression sickness and severe carbon monoxide poisoning. Decompression sickness, commonly known as "the bends," is an extremely painful and potentially dangerous condition that strikes scuba divers who surface too quickly and, occasionally, fighter pilots who ascend very quickly.

Claims about the alternative use of HBOT include that it destroys disease-causing microorganisms, cures cancer, alleviates chronic fatigue syndrome, and decreases allergy symptoms. A few proponents also claim HBOT helps patients with arthritis, multiple sclerosis, cyanide poisoning, autism, stroke, cerebral palsy, senility, cirrhosis, and gastrointestinal ulcers. There is no scientific evidence to support these claims.

What does it involve?

HBOT can be conducted in single person chambers or chambers which can contain more than a dozen people at a time. A single person chamber (monoplace) consists of a clear plastic tube about seven feet long. The patient lies on a padded table that slides into the tube. The chamber is gradually pressurized with pure oxygen. Patients are asked to relax and breathe normally during treatment. Chamber pressures typically rise to 2.5 times normal atmospheric pressure. Patients may experience ear popping or mild discomfort, which usually disappears if the pressure is lowered a bit. At the end of the session, which can last from 30 minutes to 2 hours, technicians slowly depressurize the chamber.

After an HBOT session, patients often feel light headed and tired. Monoplace chambers cost less to operate than multiplace chambers and are relatively portable. Some health insurance policies cover medically approved uses of HBOT.

What is the history behind it?

HBOT chambers were developed in the 1940s to treat deep-sea divers who suffered from decompression sickness. In the 1950s, HBOT was first used as a treatment, in addition to radiation, for head and neck cancers and cervical cancer. Clinical trials found that this treatment was most effective in less advanced tumors. This method is no longer used for these treatment purposes. HBOT has since been used for other health-related applications. It has been the subject of a great deal of controversy because there is a lack of scientific proof to support many of the other applications for which it is used.

What is the evidence?

There is strong scientific evidence showing HBOT is an effective treatment for decompression sickness, arterial gas embolism, and severe carbon monoxide poisoning. It may also be useful as an additional therapy for the prevention and treatment of osteoradionecrosis (bone damage caused by radiation therapy), clostridial myonecrosis (a life-threatening bacterial infection that invades the muscle), and for assisting skin grafts and flap healing. Other evidence suggests HBOT may be helpful for less severe carbon monoxide poisoning and as a complementary therapy for radiation-induced, soft-tissue injury; anemia due to severe blood loss (when transfusions are not an option); or crushing injuries, poor wound healing, and refractory osteomyelitis (chronic bone inflammation). There is conflicting evidence about whether HBOT is helpful in treating thermal burns and rapidly growing infections of the skin and underlying tissues.

The lack of randomized clinical studies makes it difficult to judge the value of HBOT for many of its claims. There is no scientific evidence that HBOT stops the growth of cancer cells, destroys disease-causing microorganisms, decreases allergy symptoms, or helps patients who have chronic fatigue syndrome, arthritis, multiple sclerosis, cyanide poisoning, autism, stroke, cerebral palsy, senility, cirrhosis, or gastrointestinal ulcers.

Are there any possible problems or complications?

HBOT is a relatively safe method for approved medical treatments. Complications can be minimized if pressures within the hyperbaric chamber remain below 3 times normal atmospheric pressure and sessions last no longer than two hours.

Milder problems associated with HBOT include claustrophobia (in monoplace chambers), fatigue, and headache. More serious complications include myopia (short sightedness) that can last for weeks or months, sinus damage, ruptured middle ear, and lung damage. A complication called oxygen toxicity can result in convulsions, fluid in the lungs, and even respiratory failure. Pregnant women should not be treated with HBOT. Hyperbaric chambers may also present a fire hazard. Fires or explosions in hyperbaric chambers have caused about 80 deaths worldwide.

References

Ashamalla HL, Thom SR, Goldwein JW. Hyperbaric oxygen therapy for the treatment of radiation-induced sequelae in children. The University of Pennsylvania experience. *Cancer.* 1996;77:2407-2412.

Brizel DM, Hage WD, Dodge RK, Munley MT, Piantadosi CA, Dewhirst MW. Hyperbaric oxygen improves tumor radiation response significantly more than carbogen/nicotinamide. *Radiat Res.* 1997;147:715-720.

Carl UM, Hartmann KA. Hyperbaric oxygen treatment for symptomatic breast edema after radiation therapy. *Undersea Hyperb Med.* 1998;25:233-234.

Coles C, Williams M, Burnet N. Hyperbaric oxygen therapy. Combination with radiotherapy in cancer is of proved benefit but rarely used. *BMJ.* 1999;318:1076-1077.

Grim PS, Gottlieb LJ, Boddie A, Batson E. Hyperbaric oxygen therapy. *JAMA.* 1990;263:2216-2220.

Kalns J, Krock L, Piepmeier E Jr. The effect of hyperbaric oxygen on growth and chemosensitivity of metastatic prostate cancer. *Anticancer Res.* 1998;18:363-367.

Kohshi K, Kinoshita Y, Imada H, et al. Effects of radiotherapy after hyperbaric oxygenation on malignant gliomas. *Br J Cancer.* 1999;80:236-241.

Leach RM, Rees PJ, Wilmshurst P. Hyperbaric Oxygen Therapy. *BMJ.* 1998;317:1140-1143.

London SD, Park SS, Gampper TJ, Hoard MA. Hyperbaric oxygen for the management of radionecrosis of bone and cartilage. *Laryngoscope.* 1998;108:1291-1296.

Mathews R, Rajan N, Josefson L, Camporesi E, Makhuli Z. Hyperbaric oxygen therapy for radiation induced hemorrhagic cystitis. *J Urol.* 1999;161:435-437.

Niezgoda JA, Cianci P, Folden BW, Ortega RL, Slate JB, Storrow AB. The effect of hyperbaric oxygen therapy on a burn wound model in human volunteers. *Plast Reconstr Surg.* 1997;99:1620-1625.

Tibbles PM, Edelsberg JS. Review Articles: Medical progress: Hyperbaric-Oxygen Therapy. *N Engl J Med.* 1996;334:1642-1648.

Woo TC, Joseph D, Oxer H. Hyperbaric oxygen treatment for radiation proctitis. *Int J Radiat Oncol Biol Phys.* 1997; 38:619-622.

Manual Healing / Physical Touch

Light Therapy

Other common name(s)	Scientific/medical name(s)
Light Boxes, Ultraviolet Light Therapy, Chromatotherapy, Colored Light Therapy, Ultraviolet Blood Irradiation	None

DESCRIPTION
Light therapy involves the use of visible or ultraviolet (UV) light to treat a variety of conditions.

OVERVIEW
There is no evidence that the alternative use of light therapy is effective in treating cancer or any other condition. However, some forms of light therapy are used in conventional medicine and can be helpful. For example, the use of light boxes is a proven medical treatment for seasonal affective disorder (SAD), and UV light therapy is currently used to treat psoriasis and cutaneous T-cell lymphoma (a type of cancer that first appears on the skin). A special form of UV blood irradiation, called photopheresis, may inhibit T-cell lymphoma.

How is it promoted for use?
Conventional medical professionals may recommend light boxes, photopheresis, or UV light therapy for the treatment of a few conditions for which studies have shown these methods to be safe and effective.

However, several forms of light therapy are currently being promoted for alternative use which include light boxes, UV light therapy, colored light therapy, and UV blood irradiation. There is no scientific evidence to support claims by proponents of any of the alternative methods described below.

Proponents claim light box therapy relieves high blood pressure, insomnia, premenstrual syndrome, migraines, carbohydrate cravings, hyperactivity in children, and improves sexual functioning. Proponents of UV light therapy claim that it neutralizes toxins in the body and cures or weakens disorders of the immune system, bacterial infections, and cancer.

Supporters of colored light therapy claim the therapy relieves a variety of conditions, including sleep disorders, shoulder pain, diabetes, impotence, and allergies. Practitioners of one system called chromatotherapy believe that shining colored lights on the body will harm cancer cells.

Proponents of UV blood irradiation claim that UV light exposure kills infectious organisms, such as viruses, bacteria, and fungi, and that it neutralizes toxins in the blood. They claim when the blood re-enters the circulatory system of the patient, it stimulates the immune system and increases attacks against invading organisms, including cancer cells.

What does it involve?
Light boxes contain lights that approximate the wavelength of light produced by the sun. Patients undergoing this kind of therapy sit in front of the light box for a prescribed amount of time each day. In ultraviolet light therapy, patients are exposed to UVA, UVB, and UVC light. Psoriasis treatment may involve the use of UVB and UVA light along with drugs, which make the skin sensitive to the light.

Colored light therapy involves the use of

colored lights such as blue, red, and violet that the practitioner shines directly on the patient. Sometimes the lights flash in patterns.

Ultraviolet blood irradiation (photopheresis) as used in conventional treatment involves 1) administering a phototoxic drug to sensitize a patient's cells to the light; 2) removing some of the patient's blood; 3) separating the white blood cells (WBCs) from the red blood cells; 4) exposing the WBCs to UVA radiation; and 5) returning the treated WBCs back into the patient. This treatment is FDA-approved for T-cell lymphoma involving the skin. It is also used in clinical trials for the treatment of immune system diseases, such as multiple sclerosis, rheumatoid arthritis, lupus, and graft-versus-host disease (a complication related to stem cell transplants).

What is the history behind it?

Interest in the relationship between light and health dates back centuries. All forms of light therapy now in use originated during the 20th century. The first reports of ultraviolet blood irradiation date back to the 1930s.

What is the evidence?

There is no scientific evidence that light box therapy can cure cancer, however, it does have some medically accepted uses. Light box therapy has been shown to be effective in treating SAD, a type of depression caused by insufficient exposure to bright light. UV light therapy is commonly used to treat psoriasis. There is also evidence that UVB light therapy inhibits the growth of cutaneous (skin) T-cell lymphoma. One group of researchers noted that it has resulted in many long-term remissions and cures among patients in the early-stage of the disease. However, the other claims for UV light therapy have not been scientifically proven.

While there is no evidence to support the use of colored light therapy, ultraviolet blood irradiation is currently under study at a number of institutions. According to some researchers, the treatment may also show promise for treating cutaneous T-cell lymphoma, even though it is still not well understood. None of the other claims made for this therapy have been proven.

Are there any possible problems or complications?

Light therapy that involves primarily visible light (light boxes and colored light therapy) is considered safe. Light box therapy should not be confused with a tanning bed, which is not a medical therapy and is dangerous due to high levels of ultraviolet radiation. Any treatment that exposes the patient to ultraviolet radiation presents some danger, including premature aging of the skin and an increased risk for skin cancer. Patients undergoing long-term UV light treatment for psoriasis may experience a greater-than-average number of skin-related problems.

References

American Cancer Society. Questionable methods of cancer management: electronic devices. *CA Cancer J Clin.* 1994;44:127-128.

Cassileth B. *The Alternative Medicine Handbook.* New York, NY: W. W. Norton & Co; 1998.

el-Ghorr AA, Norval M. Biological effects of narrow-band (311 nm TL01) UVB irradiation: a review. *J Photochem Photobiol B.* 1997;38:99-106.

Herrmann JJ, Roenigk HH Jr, Honigsmann H. Ultraviolet radiation for treatment of cutaneous T-cell lymphoma. Hematol *Oncol Clin North Am.* 1995;9:1077-1088.

Overview of ultraviolet light therapy. National Psoriasis Foundation Web site. Available at: http://www.psoriasis.org/overview.html. Accessed September 20, 1999.

Tanew A, Radakovic-Fijan S, Schemper M, Honigsmann H. Narrowband UV-B phototherapy vs photochemotherapy in the treatment of chronic plaque-type psoriasis: a paired comparison study. *Arch Dermatol.* 1999;135:519-524.

Taylor A, Gasparro FP. Extracorporeal photochemotherapy for cutaneous T-cell lymphoma and other diseases. *Semin Hematol.* 1992;29:132-141.

Magnetic Therapy

Other common name(s)	Scientific/medical name(s)
Magnetic Field Therapy, Magnet Therapy	None

DESCRIPTION
Magnetic therapy involves the use of magnets of varying sizes and strengths which are placed on the body in order to relieve pain and treat disease.

OVERVIEW
Although there are anecdotal reports of healing with magnetic therapy, there is no scientific evidence to support these claims. The FDA considers magnets harmless and of no use for medical purposes.

How is it promoted for use?
Many claims about magnetic therapy come from the fact that some cells and tissues in the human body generate electromagnetic impulses. Some practitioners think the presence of illness or injury disrupts these fields (see Electromagnetic Therapy). They claim strategically positioning magnets that are strong enough to penetrate the human body will correct disturbances and restore health to the afflicted systems, organs, and cells.

Proponents claim magnetic therapy can relieve pain caused by arthritis, headaches, migraines, and stress, and can also heal broken bones, improve circulatory problems, reverse degenerative diseases, and cure cancer. Practitioners also claim that placing magnets over areas of pain or disease intensifies the body's healing ability. They claim magnetic fields increase blood flow, alter nerve impulses, increase oxygen delivery to cells, decrease fatty deposits on artery walls, and realign thought patterns to improve emotional well being.

Proponents of magnetic therapy assert that magnetic fields produced from the negative pole of the magnet have healing powers. Negative magnetic fields presumably stimulate metabolism, increase the amount of oxygen available to cells, and create an alkaline environment within the body. Because they believe cancer cells cannot thrive when alkalinity is high, they claim the effects of negative magnetic fields can halt or reverse the spread of tumors. For the same reasons, it is thought negative magnetic fields hasten the healing of cuts, broken bones and infections, and counter the effects of toxic chemicals, addictive drugs, and other harmful substances. There is no scientific evidence to support these claims.

What does it involve?
Magnetic therapy involves the use of thin metallic wafer-like magnets attached to the body alone or in groups. They are sometimes mounted on bracelets and necklaces, or attached to adhesive patches that hold them in place. Some magnets are placed in bands or belts that can be wrapped around the wrist, elbow, knee, ankle, foot, waist, or lower back. There are even magnetic insoles, blankets, and slumber pads. These magnets may be worn for just a few minutes or for weeks, depending on the condition being treated and the practitioner.

What is the history behind it?
Interest in magnets as a source of healing dates

back many centuries. A 16th century physician, Paracelsus, hypothesized that because magnets attract iron they might attract and eliminate diseases from the body. The modern version of magnet therapy reportedly began in the 1970s when researcher Albert Roy Davis, PhD, noticed that positive and negative magnetic charges had different effects on human biological systems. He claimed that magnets could kill cancer cells in animals and could also cure arthritis pain, glaucoma, infertility, and other conditions.

Magnetic therapy has recently become a large industry in the United States and Europe and has been used widely in Japan and China for many years.

What is the evidence?

Magnetic therapy has undergone very little scientific investigation. Most of the success stories have come from a few isolated sources that have not provided proof that the treatment actually works. One well-publicized randomized clinical trial conducted at the Baylor College of Medicine concluded that the permanent placement of small magnets reduced pain in postpolio patients. However, the study has been criticized because two of the primary investigators had used magnets personally to relieve knee pain prior to the study, and the reports of pain relief are highly subjective.

One physician reported numerous cases involving the use of magnetic therapy to relieve pain but offered no documentation to verify his claims. There is no scientific evidence that magnetic therapy cures cancer or any other disease.

Are there any possible problems or complications?

According to the FDA, magnets used for magnetic therapy are generally considered safe. However, relying on this type of treatment alone, and avoiding conventional medical care, may have serious health consequences.

References

Alternative Medicine: Expanding Medical Horizons. A Report to the National Institutes of Health on Alternative Medical Systems and Practices in the United States. Washington, DC: US Government Printing Office; 1994. NIH publication 94-066.

Barrett S. Magnet therapy. Quackwatch Web site. Available at: http://www.quackwatch.com. Accessed May 8, 2000.

Livingston JD. Magnetic therapy: Plausible attraction? Committee for the Scientific Investigation of Claims of the Paranormal (Skeptical Inquirer Magazine) Web site. Available at: http://www.csicop.org. Accessed May 8, 2000.

Vallbona C, Hazlewood CF, Jurida G. Response to pain to static magnetic fields in postpolio patients: a double-blind pilot study. *Arch Phys Med Rehabil.* 1997;78:1200-1203.

Massage

Other common name(s)	Scientific/medical name(s)
Massage Therapy	None

DESCRIPTION

Massage involves manipulation, rubbing, and kneading of the body's muscle and soft tissue.

OVERVIEW

Some recent studies show massage can decrease stress, anxiety, depression, and pain, and increase alertness. Many health care professionals recognize massage as a useful addition to conventional medical treatment that is non-invasive and may offer some relief for these symptoms.

How is it promoted for use?

Massage is recommended by some health care professionals as a complementary therapy. They believe massage can help people with serious illnesses, such as cancer, reduce stress, anxiety, and pain. It is also known to relax muscles. Many people find that massage brings a temporary feeling of well being and relaxation. Massage is also used to relieve joint pain and stiffness, increase mobility, rehabilitate injured muscles, and reduce pain associated with headaches and backaches. Some researchers have found regular massage can help reduce blood pressure, insomnia, migraine headaches, and depression. There is also some evidence that massage can stimulate nerves, improve concentration, increase blood flow and the supply of oxygen to cells, and help circulation of the lymph system.

Some practitioners claim massage raises the body's production of endorphins (chemicals believed to improve overall mood) and flushes lactic acid (waste product) out of muscles. Proponents also claim massage promotes recovery from fatigue produced by excessive exercise, breaks up scar tissue, loosens mucus in the lungs, promotes sinus drainage, and helps arthritis, colds, and constipation. There is no scientific evidence to support these claims.

What does it involve?

In all forms of massage, therapists use their hands (and sometimes forearms, elbows, and instruments such as rollers) to manipulate the body's soft tissue. Massage strokes can vary from light and shallow to firm and deep. The choice will depend on the needs of the individual and the style of the massage therapist. If a patient has a particular complaint, the therapist may focus on the area of pain or discomfort.

Massage usually takes place on a soft table covered with a clean sheet. Massage therapists often play soothing music and use dim lighting to increase relaxation and comfort. The client wears minimal clothing, but is covered by a sheet or towel. Oils are often used to keep from irritating the skin. Typical massage therapy sessions last from 30 minutes to 1 hour.

What is the history behind it?

Massage has been used in many ancient cultures including those of China, India, Persia, Arabia, Greece, and Egypt. The ancient Greek physician, Hippocrates, described massage as an effective therapy for sports and war injuries. Chinese texts dating back to 2700 BC recommended massage and other types of body movements to treat paralysis, chills, and fever.

Swedish massage, one of the most common forms of massage used today in the United States, was developed by the 19th century Swedish physician Per Henrik Ling. Other current styles include deep-tissue massage, sports massage, and neuromuscular massage.

Today there is a wide range of training and certification for massage therapists. Not every state requires massage therapists to be licensed, however, organizations such as the American Massage Therapy Association do provide certification and information about training.

What is the evidence?

A growing number of health care professionals recognize massage as a useful addition to conventional medical treatment. While some evidence from research studies is positive, it is not clear whether massage therapy is responsible for measurable, long-term, physical or psychological benefits.

Results from some recent studies indicate massage may decrease stress, anxiety, depression, and pain, and increase alertness. One review article reported massage helped improve migraines, blood pressure, postoperative pain, and chronic fatigue. One small study found that back massage helped critically ill patients sleep better, while another study found that 7 cancer patients felt more relaxed and had a reduction in pain and anxiety after getting massages. These potential benefits hold great promise for people with cancer, who deal with the stresses of a serious illness and some unpleasant side effects of conventional medical treatment. However, there is no scientific evidence that massage slows or reverses the growth or spread of cancer.

A review of these studies found that massage reduced anxiety and stress, but the massage techniques and study methods for evaluating anxiety and stress were so different that it is difficult to make any comparisons across studies and draw any conclusions about massage. Large, well-controlled studies are needed to determine the long-term health benefits of massage.

Are there any possible problems or complications?

Massage conducted by a trained, licensed professional is considered safe. One concern for people with cancer is that massage might increase the risk that tissue manipulation will cause cancer cells to travel to other parts of the body, however, there is no research to indicate that this will happen. People with cancer and chronic conditions, such as arthritis and heart disease, should consult their physician before undergoing any type of therapy that involves manipulation of joints and muscles.

References

Burke C, Macnish S, Saunders J, Gallini A, Warne I, Downing J. The development of a massage service for cancer patients. *Clin Oncol (R Coll Radiol).* 1994;6:381-384.

Cassileth B. *The Alternative Medicine Handbook.* New York, NY: W. W. Norton & Co; 1998.

Cawley N. A critique of the methodology of research studies evaluating massage. *Eur J Cancer Care (Engl).* 1997;6:23-31.

Corley MC, Ferriter J, Zeh J, Gifford C. Physiological and psychological effects of back rubs. *Appl Nurs Res.* 1995;8:39-42.

Ferrell-Torry AT, Glick OJ. The use of therapeutic massage as a nursing intervention to modify anxiety and perception of cancer pain. *Cancer Nurs.* 1993;16:93-101.

Field TM. Massage therapy effects. *Am Psychol.* 1998;53:1270-1281.

Richards KC. Effect of a back massage and relaxation intervention on sleep in critically ill patients. *Am J Crit Care.* 1998;7:288-299.

Manual Healing / Physical Touch

Moxibustion

Other common name(s)	Scientific/medical name(s)
Acumoxa, Auricular Mo	None

DESCRIPTION
Moxibustion is the application of heat resulting from the burning of a small bundle of tightly bound herbs, or moxa, to targeted acupoints. It is used in conjunction with acupuncture (see Acupuncture).

OVERVIEW
There is no evidence that moxibustion is effective in preventing or treating cancer or any other disease. Oils from the herbs used in moxibustion are dangerous if consumed.

How is it promoted for use?
Moxibustion is a practice of both traditional Chinese and Tibetan medicine that treats patients holistically, stimulating acupoints in order to promote the body's ability to heal itself (see Holistic Medicine). Practitioners claim the radiant heat generated by moxibustion penetrates deeply into the body, restoring the balance and flow of vital energy or life force called qi (or chi).

Moxibustion is promoted for the advancement of general good health and for the treatment of chronic conditions such as arthritis, digestive disorders, ulcers, and for cancerous lesions. There is no scientific evidence to support these claims.

What does it involve?
Moxibustion involves the use of a moxa preparation which is created by gathering dried leaves from mugwort or wormwood plants and forming it into a small cone (see Mugwort and Wormwood). In its earliest uses, direct moxibustion was most often applied over the acupuncture point, with the cone being placed directly on the skin. However, this method produced pain and scarring. Those who still practice direct moxibustion will often place the moxa atop a thin layer of ginger, and remove the cone as soon as it feels too warm to the patient.

Indirect moxibustion, most commonly used today, involves either placing the cone on top of an acupuncture needle and burning it, or applying heat to needle points from an electrical source.

Another kind of moxibustion is burnt match moxibustion, in which the practitioner taps one or two auricular acupoints rapidly with the head of a burnt match. Thread incense moxibustion and warm needle moxibustion involve the use of needles which are heated by the practitioner with a match or lighter.

What is the history behind it?
Moxibustion evolved thousands of years ago, in early northern China. It is part of traditional Chinese medical practices and came about at the same time as acupuncture. In such a cold, mountainous region, heating the body on energetically active points was thought to be effective. Chinese medicine practitioners currently use moxibustion in some parts of the United States.

What is the evidence?
There have been no human studies on the effects of moxibustion and cancer, however, a recent study in Taiwan found that mice with tumors that had been treated with moxibustion

lived longer than mice with tumors that had not. Animal studies may show that a certain therapy holds promise as a beneficial treatment, but further studies are necessary to determine if the results apply to humans.

A recent Chinese study suggested that moxibustion may help fetuses in breech (bottom first) return to a normal (head first) presentation. Other research in China has examined the use of moxibustion in asthma and ulcerative colitis (chronic inflammation of the colon).

Are there any possible problems or complications?

Direct moxibustion can burn the skin. Oils from mugwort and wormwood can cause toxic reactions if taken internally, although their toxicity is much lower when applied externally. Mugwort is on the Commission E (Germany's regulatory agency for herbs) list of unapproved herbs. This means that it is not recommended for use because it has not been proven to be safe or effective. Relying on this type of treatment alone, and avoiding conventional medical care, may have serious health consequences.

References

Alternative Medicine: Expanding Medical Horizons. A Report to the National Institutes of Health on Alternative Medical Systems and Practices in the United States. Washington, DC: US Government Printing Office; 1994. NIH publication 94-066.

Cardini F, Weixin H. Moxibustion for correction of breech presentation: a randomized controlled trial. *JAMA*. 1998;280:1580-1584.

Cassileth B. *The Alternative Medicine Handbook*. New York, NY: W. W. Norton & Co; 1998.

Hau DM, Lin IH, Lin JG, Chang YH, Lin CH. Therapeutic effects of moxibustion on experimental tumor. *Am J Chin Med*. 1999;27:157-166.

Jarvis WT. How quackery harms. Quackwatch Web site. Available at: http://www. quackwatch.com. Accessed May 8, 2000

Medical Economics. *PDR for Herbal Medicines*. Montvale, NJ: Medical Economics Company; 1998.

Wu H, Chen H, Hua X, Shi Z, Zhang L, Chen J. Clinical therapeutic effect of drug-separated moxibustion on chronic diarrhea and its immunologic mechanisms. *J Tradit Chin Med* 1997;17:253-258.

Myofascial Release

Other common name(s)	Scientific/medical name(s)
None	None

DESCRIPTION / OVERVIEW
Myofascial Release is based on the body's fascia system, which practitioners say is a tough connective tissue system that weaves through the entire body much like a spider web. Practitioners explain that fascia surrounds all the muscles, bones, nerves, blood vessels, and organs, and any kind of tension or pressure present in this system can cause the body to malfunction. A gentle form of stretching and manual compression is said to "heal" this connective tissue and provide relief from fascial restrictions and pain. There is no scientific evidence to support this claim.

Myotherapy

Other common name(s)	Scientific/medical name(s)
Trigger Point Therapy, Pressure Point Therapy, Trigger Point Injections	None

DESCRIPTION

Myotherapy is a form of massage that targets trigger points in soft tissues of the body to relieve pain and muscle tension and promote a sense of well being (see Bodywork and Massage). Trigger points are abnormally sensitive, highly irritable spots found within muscles or around muscles that cause pain, limit range of joint motion, and constrict blood flow.

OVERVIEW

Myotherapy appears to provide muscle-related pain relief; however, the effectiveness of myotherapy has not been proven scientifically. Other types of pain, such as cancer-related pain, are best treated by conventional therapies that have been proven to be safe and effective.

How is it promoted for use?

Proponents claim myotherapy can reduce 95% of all muscle-related pain, and in some cases can replace the use of pain-relieving drugs. They say the techniques used in myotherapy relax muscles and improve muscle strength, flexibility, and coordination; relieve pain; reduce the need for pain medications; increase blood circulation; improve stamina and sleep patterns; and correct posture imbalances.

While most myotherapists do not claim they can cure illnesses, some do claim it is effective for relieving pain in people with conditions such as rheumatoid arthritis, lupus, cancer, multiple sclerosis, and AIDS. There is no scientific evidence to support the claim that myotherapy can treat disease-related pain.

What does it involve?

After an initial evaluation, a myotherapy patient lies on a massage table and the therapist then probes muscles for active trigger points that have resulted from muscle damage or stress. Direct, firm, and rhythmical pressure is applied with fingers, hands, and elbows to trigger points. Patients typically wear loose clothing during a session.

The myotherapist may choose to employ a variety of techniques, including trigger point compression (direct pressure applied to irritable points along a muscle), myo massage (muscle massage to aid healing and circulation), passive stretch (assisted flexibility movements), and corrective exercise programs that can be done at home. Many myotherapists are also licensed massage therapists. Some nurses are trained to practice myotherapy. It can also be taught to caregivers who can practice it on patients at home.

What is the history behind it?

In the 1940s, Janet Travell, MD, developed the technique called trigger point injections, in which pain-relieving drugs are injected directly into painful muscles. Dr. Travell later served as President John F. Kennedy's personal physician. Dr. Travel stayed on at the White House for President Lyndon Johnson and continued to treat other members of the Kennedy family.

In 1976, physical therapist Bonnie Prudden, while working with trigger point injection practitioner Desmond Tivy, MD, discovered she could relieve muscular pain using various patterns of external pressure rather than drugs. Because trigger-point injections can only be administered by a physician, Prudden's method opened the door for other health care practitioners, such as massage therapists and physical therapists, to treat pain and discomfort without medications. In 1979, Prudden opened a school to teach her method to other practitioners. There are currently a number of massage schools that offer training in myotherapy.

What is the evidence?

There is no scientific evidence to support the claims made for myotherapy, but many people who have undergone the treatment say that they feel better and experience less pain after a myotherapy session. Trigger point therapy is not considered a long-term method of pain relief.

Some investigators have found that myotherapy does not interfere with other medical treatments and may be done safely without the pre-approval of a surgeon or attending physician. One practitioner reported that myotherapy frequently provided temporary muscle pain relief for patients, and that the technique could easily be taught to family members.

Are there any possible problems or complications?

Myotherapy is generally considered safe. However, pressure applied to muscles improperly or in the wrong places may increase pain. Patients should choose a therapist who has undergone training from a reputable myotherapy school. People with cancer and chronic conditions, such as arthritis, should consult their physician before undergoing any type of therapy that involves manipulation of joints and muscles.

References

Witt JR. Relieving chronic pain. *Nurse Pract.* 1984;9:36-38.

Trujillo L. Trigger point relief. *Nurse Pract.* 1998;23:119.

Neural Therapy

Other common name(s)	Scientific/medical name(s)
None	None

DESCRIPTION

Neural therapy involves the injection of anesthetics (drugs to reduce pain) into various sites of the body to eliminate pain and cure illness.

OVERVIEW

Research into neural therapy has been conducted mainly in Germany where the therapy is widely used. No research is currently underway in the United States on the effectiveness of neural therapy for pain management or for any other health problems.

How is it promoted for use?

The practice of neural therapy is based on the belief that energy flows freely through the body of a healthy person. Proponents claim injury, disease, malnutrition, stress, and even scar tissue disrupt this flow, creating energy imbalances called "interference patterns." They believe interference patterns are responsible for chronic illness. Some researchers in Germany have stated that 40% of all illness and chronic pain may be caused by interference patterns in the body. However, even those who practice neural therapy acknowledge the process is not well understood.

Neural therapy is promoted mainly to relieve chronic pain. There are conflicting beliefs about its usefulness for easing cancer-related pain. Some proponents believe neural therapy can even cause reversal of cancer when applied at the right moment. However, they say if applied too early, it could cause cancer to spread. Practitioners also claim neural therapy is effective against allergies, arthritis, depression, emphysema, glaucoma, headaches, heart disease, prostate disorders, skin diseases, and ulcers. There is no scientific evidence to support any of these claims.

This method is not to be confused with the nerve blocks and local anesthesia used in conventional medicine. Nerve blocks involve injections of medication to relieve pain caused by stimulation of a peripheral nerve. Local anesthesia is medication given at a local site to relieve localized pain. For example, a local anesthetic may be given before a tooth extraction or before removing a small skin lesion. These types of anesthetics have been proven to be effective.

What does it involve?

Practitioners first locate energy flow disturbances in the body, then inject anesthetics, such as lidocaine and procaine, at key points that may be far from the pain source. These injections are intended to eliminate the interference patterns and restore the body's natural energy flow. The injections may be given into nerves, acupuncture points, glands, scars, and trigger points (see Acupuncture and Myotherapy). A course of treatment may involve one or more injections. A few practitioners use electrical current and lasers instead of injected drugs.

What is the history behind it?

The idea behind neural therapy, that the nervous system influences all bodily functions, originated in Germany in the late 1800s with a Russian physiologist named Ivan Petrov. Later, in the 1940s, Ferdinand and Walter Huneke, both physicians, carried this idea further. They believed that injecting local anesthetics could affect distant parts of the body. They based their theory on a clinical experience with a patient who complained of shoulder pain. When Ferdinand Huneke injected an anesthetic drug directly into an existing scar on the patient's leg, the patient's shoulder pain reportedly disappeared in minutes. From this experience arose the notion of interference fields and the development of neural therapy.

Today, neural therapy is only practiced at a few clinics in the United States. However, it is widely used in Europe and South America.

What is the evidence?

Most articles on neural therapy have been published in Germany (where neural therapy is widespread) and most of the literature focuses on pain relief. Many of the promoters have claimed positive results, but no clinical studies have been conducted in the United States. There is no scientific evidence that neural therapy is effective in treating cancer or any other disease.

Are there any possible problems or complications?

Since there are few studies done on the use of neural therapy, information about side effects is limited. There are many other methods for relieving acute and chronic pain that have proven to be effective. In fact, anesthetic drugs are sometimes used to treat some types of chronic pain, such as neuropathic pain. These drugs do not treat the cancer but rather the pain.

References

Cassileth B. *The Alternative Medicine Handbook*. New York, NY: W. W. Norton & Co; 1998.

Raso J. Unnaturalistic methods. Quackwatch Web site. Available at: http://www.quackwatch.com. Accessed May 8, 2000.

Ohashiatsu®

Other common name(s)	Scientific/medical name(s)
Shiatsu	None

DESCRIPTION / OVERVIEW

Using touch, exercise, meditations, and Eastern healing techniques, Ohashiatsu practitioners claim that one can achieve balance and harmony by altering the flow of vital energy or life force called qi (or chi), through the body rather than focusing on any one area. Ohashiatsu practitioners say this therapy, based on the traditional Japanese practice of shiatsu, offers physical, psychological, and spiritual healing benefits. Promoters say Ohashiatsu is a "step up" from shiatsu because it offers a more complete experience of healing and personal growth. According to its followers, successful Ohashiatsu sessions depend not only on the technical skill of the practitioner, but also on the feelings of compassion and empathy the practitioner is able to convey. A connection between the giver and receiver of Ohashiatsu therapy is said to be important to the effectiveness of this practice. There is no scientific evidence to support the claims of physical healing (see Bodywork).

Osteopathy

Other common name(s)	Scientific/medical name(s)
Osteopathic Medicine	None

DESCRIPTION

Osteopathy is a form of physical manipulation that is used to restore the structural balance of the musculoskeletal system (bone and muscles). The word osteopathy comes from two Greek words meaning bone disease.

OVERVIEW

There is little scientific evidence that osteopathy is effective in treating cancer or any other condition, except musculoskeletal problems. Research funded by the National Institutes of Health (NIH) will soon be underway.

How is it promoted for use?

Doctors of osteopathy (called DOs) use their hands to diagnose and correct muscle, tendon, and joint abnormalities, which they claim are the cause of many diseases. Osteopathy is based on the belief that all systems in the human bodywork together. Osteopaths claim that if bones and muscles are in balance and functioning properly, the body can heal itself. Practitioners most often recommend osteopathy for head, neck, and back pain, headaches, joint pain, muscle strain, repetitive strain injuries, and sports-related problems. There is some evidence that osteopathy may help relieve musculoskeletal problems.

Osteopathy is promoted as an alternative method to ease pain, improve the quality of a patient's life, minimize the side effects of treatment, enhance other types of treatments, and extend the life of some cancer patients. Some proponents claim that people with cancer, emphysema, heart disorders, high blood pressure, menstrual problems, stomach disorders, and a variety of other conditions can benefit from osteopathy. When used as a complementary method to conventional medicine, they claim osteopathy can reduce the pain from arthritis and the symptoms of asthma, chronic fatigue, and some gynecological problems. There is no scientific evidence to support these claims.

What does it involve?

In treating people with various conditions, DOs use several different forms of physical manipulation. *Articulation* involves moving the patient's joints through the normal range of motion. *Counterstrain techniques* involve placing a joint or muscle in a relaxed position and then stretching tightly. *Cranial techniques* involve the manipulation of bones in the skull to relieve pain (especially in the jaw) and treat other conditions (see Craniosacral Therapy).

Functional techniques involve gently moving the patient's joints until restrictions to movement are found. *Muscle energy techniques* involve stretching the patient's muscles and then forcing the muscles to move against resistance.

Hands-on massage may also be used in osteopathy (see Massage).

These techniques are sometimes used in combination with conventional medical treatment or after conventional treatment has failed. For example, an osteopath who treats cancer patients may use the same chemotherapy, radiation therapy, or surgical treatments as a physician, but may also look at how the disease has affected the patient's body structure and provide osteopathy to correct any abnormalities.

Some DOs limit their practice to conventional medicine only, while others may practice manipulative therapy almost exclusively. However, in recent years, the distinctions between osteopaths and doctors of conventional medical practice have begun to blur.

What is the history behind it?

Originally started in the 1800s as a reaction to conventional medicine's reliance on drug therapy, osteopathy today is quite similar to conventional medicine except for its use of osteopathic manipulative therapy. Andrew Taylor Still, MD, first expressed the philosophy and principles of osteopathy in 1874. Dr. Still rejected the contemporary reliance on drug therapy and considered surgery a last resort in treating diseases. He believed that diseases could be cured by manipulating misplaced bones, nerves, and muscles which cleared "obstructions."

In 1892 he founded the first osteopathic medical school in Kirksville, Missouri, to promote his philosophy of medicine. Today, there are 19 osteopathic medical colleges in the United States, and osteopathy has evolved to incorporate the theories and practices of conventional medicine as well. There are more than 40,000 DOs practicing in the United States today, with about half in general practice or one of the primary-care specialties—family practice, internal medicine, pediatrics, and obstetrics and gynecology. Osteopaths make up about 5% of the 700,000 doctors practicing in the United States but represent almost 10% of the primary-care specialists.

Doctors of osteopathy are allowed to do more in the United States than in any other country. Laws in every state and the military permit DOs unlimited medical practice once they are licensed by the state following training in an accredited osteopathic medical school and a one-year internship in an approved hospital. Osteopaths may also undertake residency training in any medical specialty, and become board certified by passing a certification examination.

Once barred from conventional hospitals and restricted to their own hospitals, most osteopaths now receive at least some of their training in conventional hospitals and may practice in conventional medical settings. Osteopathic medical schools have similar curriculums to conventional medical schools, with the exception of up to 300 hours of training in manipulation therapy.

What is the evidence?

There is little scientific evidence that osteopathy alone has a beneficial effect on most diseases, although some studies have indicated that the therapy may help alleviate musculoskeletal problems.

However, the NIH, through its National Center for Complementary and Alternative Medicine, is making research money available to fund scientific studies on the effectiveness of osteopathy in the management and treatment of musculoskeletal injuries and diseases, especially in children and physically disabled adults.

Are there any possible problems or complications?

As with any medical treatment, osteopathic treatments may carry risks of failure or may have serious effects. Some say that it is not recommended for anyone with bone cancer. People with cancer and chronic conditions, such as arthritis and heart disease, should consult their physician before undergoing any type of therapy that involves manipulation of joints and muscles.

References

Barrett S. Dubious aspects of osteopathy. Quackwatch Web site. Available at: http://www.quackwatch.com. Accessed May 8, 2000.

Still AT. Autobiographyówith a history of the discovery and development of the science of osteopathy. Reprinted, New York, NY: Arno Press and the New York Times; 1972.

Wood DL. Research lacking in osteopathic medical profession. *J Am Osteopath Assoc* 1997;97:23.

Zugar A. Scorned no more, osteopathy is on the rise. New York Times. Feb. 17, 1998, sec F, pg 1, col 1.

Polarity Therapy

Other common name(s)	Scientific/medical name(s)
Polarity Balancing, Polarity Energy Balancing	None

DESCRIPTION

Polarity therapy is a system of touch and movement based on the idea that a person's health and well being are determined by the natural flow of energy through the body. Polarity refers to the positive and negative charges of the body's electromagnetic energy field.

OVERVIEW

There is no scientific evidence that shows polarity therapy is effective in treating cancer or any other disease. However, it is sometimes recommended by physicians as a tool for relaxation when conducted by a trained professional.

How is it promoted for use?

Polarity therapy is based on the theory that a smooth flow of energy maintains health, while disruptions in the flow caused by trauma, stress, poor nutrition, and other factors lead to energy imbalances, fatigue, and illness (see Electromagnetic Therapy). The top and right side of the body are believed to have a positive charge, while the feet and left side of the body have a negative charge. The stomach is considered neutral.

Practitioners of polarity therapy claim they can identify the sources of energy blockages and disruptions by observing symptoms such as headaches, tight shoulders and back muscles, muscle spasms, pain, abdominal discomfort, and even tumors. They also claim it can be used to promote relaxation and range of motion, relieve tension, increase energy, and reduce pain, inflammation, and swelling. They further claim polarity therapy enhances the body's ability to fight off serious illness, including cancer. However, there is no scientific evidence to support this claim.

What does it involve?

While the patient lies on a massage table, the polarity therapist applies a variety of hands-on techniques to balance and clear the energy field paths. Some of these include twisting the torso, spinal realignment, curling toes, rocking motions, and moving crystals along the body's natural energy pathways (see Crystals). Some techniques are similar to those used by chiropractors (see Chiropractic). Other aspects of polarity therapy include deep-breathing exercises, dietary management, hydrotherapy (such as whirlpool baths), stretching, and yoga (see Hydrotherapy and Yoga). During a successful session of polarity therapy, the patient is said to reach a state of deep relaxation. A polarity therapy session lasts about 1 hour or more.

What is the history behind it?

Polarity therapy was developed late in the 1940s by Randolph Stone, a chiropractor, osteopath, and naturopath. Dr. Stone studied several forms of traditional medicine practices from India and China. He taught that each person is responsible for his or her own health, and that simple steps such as those involved in polarity therapy improve physical and spiritual well being. According to the American Polarity Therapy Association, more than 500 polarity therapists currently practice in the United States. Various schools and individuals from around the world teach polarity therapy. Some organizations have training programs to certify polarity therapists. However, these organizations are not regulated by any government agency.

What is the evidence?

Claims that polarity therapy is an effective treatment for cancer and other serious diseases have not been proven. The existence of energy field paths in the human body have also not been proven. No clinical research has been published in peer-reviewed medical journals on polarity therapy.

However, patients have reported feeling relaxed and less tense after a polarity therapy session. Some physicians encourage patients to undergo movement therapies because they make people feel better, if only for a short time. Others believe the prolonged physical contact involved in hands-on techniques is beneficial and relaxing to some people.

References

Alternative Medicine: Expanding Medical Horizons. A Report to the National Institutes of Health on Alternative Medical Systems and Practices in the United States. Washington, DC: US Government Printing Office; 1994. NIH publication 94-066.

Cassileth B. *The Alternative Medicine Handbook*. New York, NY: W. W. Norton & Co; 1998.

Manual Healing / Physical Touch

Psychic Surgery

Other common name(s)	Scientific/medical name(s)
None	None

DESCRIPTION

Psychic surgery is used to remove spirits or physical manifestations of spiritual problems from a patient by the use of bare fingers and hands without any actual surgery.

OVERVIEW

There is no scientific evidence that psychic surgery offers any value to people with cancer or any other disease. Psychic surgeons create the illusion that they can remove tumors, unhealthy tissue, and organs by making an invisible incision using only their fingers and hands.

How is it promoted for use?

Some psychic surgeons claim they can cure cancer and other serious illnesses by removing tumors or other unhealthy tissue from a patient's body without leaving an incision or wound. There is no scientific evidence to support these claims.

What does it involve?

No anesthesia or surgical instruments are used in psychic surgery. During the procedure, practitioners appear to press their fingers and hands into the patient's abdomen in order to remove tissue, tumors, or other material that is believed to be making the patient sick. The practitioners often show their hands that appear bloody to patients as proof of their ability to enter the body without surgical instruments. Critics believe the material they remove is actually dyed cotton pads or other props soaked in animal blood that they hold in a false finger or thumb.

Some psychic surgeons hold up objects such as palm leaves, glass, plastic bags, and corncobs they supposedly removed from the patient. Practitioners will then "close" the wound using their fingers and hands, then wipe the blood away. During the procedure, patients feel no pain. The patient is asked to stand and walk immediately after the procedure has ended. The skin displays no scars or wounds where the "incision" has been made.

What is the history behind it?

Psychic surgery originated in rural parts of the Philippines during the 20th century. Eleuterio Terte was reportedly the first Filipino to perform psychic surgery in the 1940s (see Shamanism). Medical anthropologists have described the development of psychic surgery as a transition from traditional shamanism. Legal authorities have convicted some psychic surgeons for practicing medicine without a license. Psychic surgery is practiced in the Philippines and Brazil, and sometimes in the United States. Some Americans travel abroad for psychic surgery where it is practiced in the original surroundings of religious and traditional healing.

What is the evidence?

There is no scientific evidence that psychic surgery has any medical value. It has never been known to remove tumors, or cure cancer or any other disease.

Are there any possible problems or complications?

Consumers should be aware that the claims made by practitioners of psychic surgery have not been proven. There is also a very slight chance of infection from HIV or hepatitis if human, instead of animal blood, is used by a psychic surgeon. There has been at least one report of a psychic surgeon in the Philippines who uses human blood for this procedure. Relying on this type of treatment alone, and avoiding traditional medical care, may have serious health consequences.

References

Barrett S, Herbert V. Questionable medical therapies. Quackwatch Web site. Available at: http://www.quackwatch.com. Accessed October 7, 1999.

Cassileth B. *The Alternative Medicine Handbook*. New York, NY: W. W. Norton & Co; 1998.

US Congress, Office of Technology Assessment. Unconventional Cancer Treatments. Washington, DC: US Government Printing Office; 1990. Publication OTA-H-405.

Reflexology

Other common name(s)	Scientific/medical name(s)
Zone Therapy	None

DESCRIPTION

Reflexology is a treatment that applies hand pressure to specific areas of the feet to heal a variety of problems and balance the flow of vital energy or life force called qi (or chi) throughout the body.

OVERVIEW

There is some evidence that reflexology may be useful for relaxation and for reducing some types of pain. However, most of the claims for reflexology are unproven. There is no scientific evidence that reflexology cures cancer or any other disease.

How is it promoted for use?

Reflexology is based on the concept of reflex points, located in the feet. Practitioners claim reflex points are directly linked to various parts of the body and organs and when manipulated, they can affect the connected organ or body part. By stimulating these reflex points, a wide variety of health problems can supposedly be treated without medication or special equipment. Reflexology is similar to other forms of body manipulation such as acupuncture and acupressure (see Acupuncture).

Proponents claim reflexology can help conditions such as respiratory infections, headaches, asthma, diabetes, back pain, premenstrual distress, and problems with the skin, and gastrointestinal tract. They also say reflexology can stimulate internal organs, boost circulation, and restore bodily functions to normal. They believe that energy travels from the foot to the spine, where it is released to the rest of the body. The practice or reflexology releases endorphins (natural pain killers) and detoxifies the body by dissolving uric acid crystals in the feet. There is no scientific evidence to support these claims.

What does it involve?

A reflexologist will first gently massage a person's feet while he or she lies on a massage table. Then the reflexologist will apply pressure to selected reflex points on the feet. A person may experience tingling sensations in areas of the body that correspond to the reflex points being manipulated; however, no pain is felt. The whole process can take from 30 minutes to 1 hour.

What is the history behind it?

Reflexology has existed for hundreds of years. It may have been used by the Egyptians, early Chinese, and North American Indian tribes. In the early 20th century, an American ear, nose, and throat specialist, William Fitzgerald, MD, decided the foot was the best place to "map" parts of the body for diagnosis and treatment. He divided the body into 10 zones and decided which section of the foot controlled each zone. Dr. Fitzgerald believed gentle pressure on a particular area of the foot would generate relief in the targeted zone. This process was originally named zone therapy.

In the 1930s, Eunice Ingham, a nurse and physiotherapist, further developed these maps to include reflex points, which were much more specific than Fitzgerald's maps. It was Ingham who changed the name of zone therapy to reflexology. Today in the United States, reflexologists learn Ingham's method of reflexology or another method developed by Laura Norman, another reflexologist.

What is the evidence?

There is no scientific evidence that reflexology cures cancer or any other disease. However, it has been shown to have some effectiveness in promoting relaxation and reducing some types of pain.

A 1993 study looked at the use of reflexology versus regular foot massage in reducing premenstrual symptoms in 35 women. The women who received reflexology treatments reported a larger decrease in their PMS symptoms than the women given the placebo treatment. This study has been criticized, however, due to a potential bias in the selection of the women. Also, since all the participants received either a reflexology treatment or a placebo massage, reduction in PMS symptoms could have been due to the relaxing nature of the massage-like treatment and not the reflexology itself.

In a Danish study in the early 1990s, 220 people suffering from migraines or tension headaches were evaluated, 81% of the participants said they were helped or cured by reflexology. Nineteen percent of those who had been taking medication were able to stop after 6 months of reflexology treatments. Scientists who conducted the study cautioned that the patients' improved well being could have been due to other factors. The scientists concluded that further study would be needed to determine the benefits, if any, of reflexology.

Most evidence regarding reflexology is anecdotal. Because reflexology resembles massage, it can be relaxing and feel good. However, further study is needed to determine if reflexology can have any benefits beyond that of massage therapy.

Are there any possible problems or complications?

There are no known harmful effects of reflexology. People with cancer and chronic conditions, such as arthritis and heart disease, should consult their physician before undergoing any type of therapy that involves manipulation of joints and muscles.

References

Botting, D. Review of literature on the effectiveness of reflexology. *Complement Ther Nurs Midwifery.* 1997;3:123-130.

Cassileth B. *The Alternative Medicine Handbook.* New York, NY: W. W. Norton & Co; 1998.

Launso L, Brendstrup E, Arnberg S. An exploratory study of reflexological treatment for headache. *Altern Ther Health Med.* 1999;5:57-65.

Oleson T, Flocco W. Randomized controlled study of premenstrual symptoms treated with ear, hand, and foot reflexology. *Obstet Gynecol.* 1993;82:906-911.

Reiki

Other common name(s)	Scientific/medical name(s)
Reiki System, Reiki Healing, Usui System of Reiki	None

DESCRIPTION

Reiki is a form of hands-on treatment used to manipulate energy fields within and around the body (believed to influence a person's physical and spiritual health) in order to liberate the body's natural healing powers. Reiki is a Japanese word meaning "universal life energy."

OVERVIEW

There are no scientific studies that show the effectiveness of reiki for treating cancer or any other disease. However, some conventional medical practitioners note it may be useful as a complementary therapy to help reduce stress and improve quality of life.

How is it promoted for use?

Proponents claim when the energy paths of the body are blocked or disturbed, the result can be illness, weakness, and pain (see also Electromagnetic Therapy). They claim reiki can realign and strengthen the flow of energy, decrease pain, ease muscle tension, speed the healing of injuries and burns, improve sleep, and generally enhance the body's natural ability to heal itself. Reiki is also said to promote relaxation, decrease stress and anxiety, and increase a person's general sense of well being.

Most practitioners explain that reiki is not used to diagnose or treat specific illnesses, but to correct any and all underlying physical and emotional problems or imbalances. They also claim it is helpful for people with cancer who suffer pain and discomfort caused by the disease or by the side effects of conventional treatments such as chemotherapy and radiation, although there is no scientific evidence to support these claims.

What does it involve?

First degree reiki may be compared to the "laying on of hands" practiced in some religious or cultural healing traditions (see Faith Healing, Qigong, Therapeutic Touch). During a reiki session, the practitioner places his or her hands on various parts of the patient's clothed body to channel (redirect) and balance energy within and around the body. The practitioner then attempts to eliminate disturbances or blockages in the patient's energy patterns, in order to promote physical healing and spiritual rejuvenation.

A reiki session usually lasts about 1 hour. Many practitioners say that they achieve the best results when patients undergo 3 reiki sessions within a relatively short time, then take a break and repeat the process. Second degree reiki practitioners claim to be able to send healing over a distance, similar to claims by qigong masters who practice traditional Chinese healing concepts (see Qigong).

What is the history behind it?

The history of reiki is uncertain, but the basis for modern-day practice may have originated in Tibet more than 2,500 years ago. Reiki was rediscovered in the 1840s by Dr. Mikao Usui, a Christian minister in Kyoto, Japan. During a lengthy period of travel and research, Dr. Usui found ancient texts that described reiki and its power to heal by manipulating the energy fields that flow through all living things. From his studies, he developed what came to be known as the Usui system of Reiki.

Today, some training programs and certification are available from reiki organizations. However, these organizations are not regulated by any government agency. A reiki master is someone who is trained in reiki and whose personal and professional life is committed to the technique.

What is the evidence?

There are many anecdotal reports and case studies about reiki's power to refresh the spirit, speed healing, and increase well being. Some patients undergoing chemotherapy have reported reduced intensity and frequency of nausea and vomiting after reiki sessions. Some conventional medicine practitioners believe reiki may be useful as a complementary method for relaxation and managing some types of pain. However, there is no scientific evidence that reiki is effective.

A small pilot study found that reiki treatment effectively relieved pain in 20 volunteers, some of whom had cancer. The investigators noted the results were difficult to interpret because there was no comparison group of similar patients who did not receive reiki. Another group of researchers concluded that a controlled clinical study to test whether subjects could tell the difference between real and "fake" reiki treatment for relieving pain would be recommended.

More clinical research is needed to determine the benefits of reiki. In June 1999, the Center for Integrative Medicine at George Washington University submitted two research proposals to the National Institutes of Health (NIH) to investigate the potential of reiki and guided imagery by patients with breast cancer and those undergoing radiation therapy (see Imagery).

Are there any possible problems or complications?

Reiki is considered safe. People with cancer and chronic conditions, such as arthritis and heart disease, should consult their physician before undergoing any type of therapy that involves manipulation of joints and muscles.

References

Federal News Service. Prepared testimony of Susan Silver, the Center for Integrative medicine, George Washington University, before the House Government Reform Committee: The role of early detection and complementary and alternative medicine in women's cancers. June 10, 1999.

Mansour AA, Beuche M, Laing G, Leis A, Nurse J. A study to test the effectiveness of placebo Reiki standardization procedures developed for a planned Reiki efficacy study. *J Altern Complement Med.* 1999;5:153-164.

Olson K, Hanson J. Using Reiki to manage pain: a preliminary report. *Cancer Prev Control.* 1997;1:108-113.

Manual Healing / Physical Touch

Rosen Method

Other common name(s)	Scientific/medical name(s)
None	None

DESCRIPTION / OVERVIEW

The Rosen Method, a kind of bodywork, combines full body massage (to relieve muscle tension) and "talk therapy" (to release unconscious thoughts and painful emotions). A physical therapist named Marion Rosen developed this treatment method in the 1970s based on the belief that repressed emotions cause muscular tension. One of the beliefs of the Rosen philosophy is that people protect themselves from a painful past by separating from their "true selves." In order to heal, proponents of this therapy claim that the "true self" must be reclaimed through touching, verbal interaction, and breathwork. There is no scientific evidence to support the claims of physical healing (see Bioenergetics, Bodywork, and Massage).

Rubenfeld Synergy® Method

Other common name(s)	Scientific/medical name(s)
None	None

DESCRIPTION / OVERVIEW

Practitioners of the Rubenfeld Synergy Method identify and massage tense body parts while encouraging their clients to talk through emotional problems they are experiencing. The Rubenfeld Synergy Method combines the Alexander Technique®, the Feldenkrais Method, Gestalt therapy, and hypnotherapy practices. Developed in the 1960s by Ilana Rubenfeld, the aim of the Rubenfeld Method is personal growth and awareness. This therapy also includes aura analysis and dreamwork. There is no scientific evidence to support the claims of physical healing (see Bodywork and Hypnosis).

Sonopuncture

Other common name(s)	Scientific/medical name(s)
None	None

DESCRIPTION / OVERVIEW

Sonopuncture is similar to acupuncture, but an ultrasound device that transmits sound waves is applied, rather than a needle, to the body's acupoints during this treatment method. Sonopuncture is also sometimes combined with tuning forks and other vibration devices. Proponents claim this approach is useful to treat many of the same disorders as acupuncture (see Acupuncture). There is no scientific evidence to support these claims.

Therapeutic Touch

Other common name(s)	Scientific/medical name(s)
Energy Field Therapy, Biofield Therapy, TT	None

DESCRIPTION

Therapeutic Touch (TT) is a technique in which the hands are used to direct human energy for healing purposes. There is usually no actual physical contact.

OVERVIEW

There is no evidence to support many of the claims made for TT, or that energy is balanced or transferred by the use of TT. However, it may be useful in reducing anxiety and increasing a sense of well being in some people.

How is it promoted for use?

The practice of TT is based on the belief that the patient's energy field can be identified and re-balanced by a healer. Harmful energy is believed to cause blockages in the patient's normal energy flow. Proponents claim TT removes blockages and other problems in the patient's energy field that cause illness and pain. TT is promoted to improve or cure conditions such as pain, fever, swelling, infections, wounds, ulcers, thyroid problems, colic, burns, nausea, PMS, diarrhea, and headaches. They also say that TT is useful in treating diseases such as measles, Alzheimer's, AIDS, asthma, autism, multiple sclerosis, stroke, comas, and cancer. There is no scientific evidence to support these claims.

What does it involve?

There are four parts required to complete an average 20 to 30 minute TT session. The first is called centering. During centering, the therapist makes an effort to clear his or her mind in order to communicate with the patient's energy field and locate areas of energy blockage that are believed to cause pain or illness.

The second part of TT involves an assessment in which the therapist's hands are held about 2 to 6 inches above the patient's body. The therapist then passes both hands, with palms down, head to toe across the patient's body. This process is used to locate irregularities or blockages in the patient's energy field that signal a health problem.

In the third step, the therapist conducts several passes of the body with his or her hands. At the end of each pass, the therapist releases the harmful energy by flicking his or her hands into the air past the toes of the patient, throwing off the bad energy. Finally, the therapist transfers his or her own excess and healthy energy to the patient. This brings the patient's energy field back into balance and removes the blockages.

What is the history behind it?

Therapeutic touch is similar to the "laying on of hands" practiced by some religious sects as a means of transferring healing energy from the minister to the believer (see Faith Healing, Qigong, and Reiki). The idea of an energy field can be traced back to the 18th century work of Franz Anton Mesmer, an Austrian doctor who believed that illness was caused by imbalances in the body's magnetic forces. He believed he could restore magnetic balance through the use of soothing words and quieting gestures, called Mesmerism.

In the 1970s, Delores Krieger, PhD, RN, who was a professor of nursing at New York University (NYU) developed TT. The dean of nursing at NYU, Martha Rogers, believed that human beings are energy fields that interact with their environment, and her ideas stimulated scientific research of TT.

Over 100 colleges and universities in 75 countries teach TT. It is promoted by many professional nursing organizations and practiced by nurses in at least 80 hospitals in the United States and Canada. There are more than 21,000 health care professionals who use TT worldwide.

What is the evidence?

There have been very few well-designed studies of TT. A recent article published in the *Journal of the American Medical Association* reported that only 1 study out of 83 confirmed positive results for TT. They stated that some clinical studies found positive effects, such as assistance with wound healing and headaches; however, most of those studies were doctoral dissertations whose study designs were questionable. When the authors tested TT, they found that the 21 practitioners being studied were not able to detect the investigator's energy field.

Research funded by the US Department of Defense to study the effect of TT on burn patients produced mixed results. Patients reported a reduction in pain and anxiety, but there was no difference in the amount of pain medication requested. A recent controlled clinical trial on the effects of dialogue and TT on breast cancer surgery patients found that 10 minutes of TT and 20 minutes of talking lowered anxiety before surgery. No effects were found after surgery.

Many researchers believe the positive results claimed for TT are due to the placebo effect. That is, the patient wants it to work and believes it will work, so the procedure may create a beneficial result. They believe the simple presence of a person who is interested in helping can promote relaxation and increase a sense of well being. There is no scientific evidence that TT can cure cancer or any other disease.

Are there any possible problems or complications?

Therapeutic touch is generally considered safe. Some of the reported side effects include nausea, dizziness, restlessness, and irritability.

References

Cassileth B. *The Alternative Medicine Handbook*. New York, NY: W. W. Norton & Co; 1998.

O'Mathna DP. TT: what could be the harm? *Sci Rev Altern Med*. Spring, 1998.

Rosa L, Rosa E, Sarner L, Barrett S. A close look at Therapeutic Touch. *JAMA*. 1998;279:1005-1010.

Samarel N, Fawcett J, Davis MM, Ryan FM. Effects of dialogue and Therapeutic Touch on preoperative and postoperative experiences of breast cancer surgery: an exploratory study. *Oncol Nurs Forum*. 1998;25:1369-1376.

Transcutaneous Electrical Nerve Stimulation

Other common name(s)	Scientific/medical name(s)
TENS	None

DESCRIPTION

Transcutaneous electrical nerve stimulation (TENS) is a method of pain relief in which a special device transmits electrical impulses through electrodes to an area of the body that is in pain (see Electromagnetic Therapy).

OVERVIEW

There is some evidence that TENS may help reduce certain types of pain, especially mild pain, for a short period of time. However, it does not appear to reduce chronic pain.

How is it promoted for use?

Supporters claim that TENS is an effective method for relieving acute and chronic pain caused by surgery, childbirth, migraines, tension headaches, injuries, arthritis, tendonitis, bursitis, chronic wounds, cancer and other sources. Some practitioners claim that TENS stimulates the production of the body's natural painkillers. Most TENS practitioners do not claim the therapy cures the underlying causes of pain. There is some evidence that it may offer short-term pain relief for some people, but the long-term benefits have not been proven.

What does it involve?

A TENS system consists of an electrical genera-tor connected by wires to a pair of electrodes. The electrodes are attached to the patient's skin near the source of pain. When the generator is switched on, a mild electrical current travels through the electrodes into the body. Patients may feel tingling or warmth during treatment. A session typically lasts from 5 to 15 minutes and treatments may be applied as often as neces-sary, depending on the severity of pain. Some practitioners refer to TENS as a sort of "electri-cal massage."

TENS is used widely by physical therapists and other medical practitioners, but can also be performed at home by patients using a portable TENS system. There are more than 100 types of TENS units approved for use by the FDA. A prescription is needed to obtain a system. In a variation of TENS called percutaneous electrical nerve stimulation, the electrical impulses are sent through acupuncture needles (see Acupuncture).

What is the history behind it?

Drs. Ronald Melzac and Patrick Wall developed the Gate Control Theory in 1965, which claims that when nerves are electrically stimulated, a gate mechanism is closed in the spinal cord preventing the awareness of pain. After the introduction of the theory, TENS was widely used to treat pain. TENS became a relatively common therapy in the early 1970s. It is still widely used by physical therapists and physiotherapists.

What is the evidence?

Research on the effectiveness of TENS therapy for cancer-related pain is limited to small clinical studies and case reports and is somewhat conflicting. Some cancer patients, particularly those with mild neuropathic pain (pain related to nerve tissue damage), may benefit from TENS for brief periods of time. TENS may also be more effective when used with analgesics (pain medicines).

One review of TENS reported that many studies have found it useful in easing pain related to acute injuries of the muscles and bones, postoperative pain, and pain caused by a variety of other origins. A second review of 15 years of TENS research found some evidence to suggest that it is a useful addition to pain relief, although a number of the studies under review failed to demonstrate pain control benefit from TENS. One recent study found that TENS was not effective for relieving postoperative or labor pain, and another determined that percutaneous electrical nerve stimulation (in which electrical current is transmitted through acupuncture needles instead of surface electrodes) was more effective than TENS for relieving low-back pain.

Overall, there is limited evidence to show TENS effectively decreases chronic pain. More clinical studies are needed to determine what benefit TENS may have for people with cancer in the management of cancer-related pain.

Are there any possible problems or complications?

TENS is generally considered safe. However, electrical current that is too intense can burn the skin. The electrodes should not be placed over the eyes, heart, brain, or front of the throat. People with heart problems should not use TENS. The effects of long-term use of TENS on fetuses is unknown, therefore pregnant women should not undergo the therapy.

References

Barrett D. Ten tips on living with fibromyalgia syndrome. Quackwatch Web site. Available at: http://www.quackwatch.com. Accessed May 8, 2000.

Ghoname EA, Craig WF, White PF, et al. Percutaneous electrical nerve stimulation for low back pain: a randomizd crossover study. *JAMA*. 1999;281:818-823.

Long DM. Fifteen years of transcutaneous electrical stimulation for pain control. *Stereotact Funct Neurosurg*. 1991;56:2-19.

McQuay HJ, Moore RA, Eccleston C, Morley S, Williams AC. Systematic review of outpatient services for chronic pain control. *Health Technol Assess*. 1997;1:1-135.

Spencer JW, Jacobs JJ. *Complementary/Alternative Medicine: An Evidence-Based Approach*. St. Louis, MO: Mosby, Inc; 1999.

Sykes J, Johnson R, Hanks GW. ABC of palliative care. Difficult pain problems. *BMJ*. 1997;315:867-869.

Manual Healing / Physical Touch

Tui-Na

Other common name(s)	Scientific/medical name(s)
None	None

DESCRIPTION / OVERVIEW

Tui-Na uses the principles of looking, listening, smelling, questioning, and palpating to diagnose areas of the body where energy flow is restricted. Tui-Na has its roots in ancient Chinese culture and actually predates the popular practice of acupuncture. The theory behind Chinese medicine is that in order to be healthy, a person's vital energy or life force called, qi (or chi) must be able to flow freely through the body in a balanced fashion. Tui-Na also attempts to free these energy pathways through 13 basic hand massage techniques that include manual pushing, pressing, pulling, and "wiping" the skin. Practitioners often target and treat the muscles that exist on either side of the spine with this technique. There is no scientific evidence to support the claims of physical healings (see Acupuncture, Bodywork, and Massage).

Watsu®

Other common name(s)	Scientific/medical name(s)
None	None

DESCRIPTION / OVERVIEW

Watsu, also known as water shiatsu, is a form of bodywork that is practiced in warm water. A Watsu practitioner stretches, cradles, and massages clients while holding them afloat. The goal of Watsu is to achieve a feeling of peace and simplicity that supposedly is felt in the womb and during early childhood and to release emotional and physical blockages of the body's energy pathways. Practitioners strive to covey a theme of gentleness, acceptance, and unconditional love through Watsu. Proponents claim it can speed both physical and emotional healing processes, although there is no scientific evidence to support the use of this for the treatment of disease (see Bodywork, Hydrotherapy, and Massage).

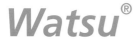

Manual Healing / Physical Touch

Chapter 7

Herb, Vitamin, and Mineral Methods

This category contains plant-derived preparations that are used for therapeutic purposes, as well as everyday vitamins and minerals. It is noted when there are instances where chemicals extracted from plants are used rather than the plant components.

Aconite

Other common name(s)	Scientific/medical name(s)
Monkshood, Wolfsbane, Fu-Tzu	*Aconitum napellus*

DESCRIPTION / OVERVIEW

Aconite is a Chinese herb used to treat pain related to arthritis, cancer, gout, inflammation, migraine headaches, neuralgia, rheumatism, and sciatica (see Chinese Herbal Medicine). Certain ingredients are extracted from the leaves, flowers, and roots of the plant. It is available as a tincture, tea, or ointment, however, it is not commercially prepared in the United States. Because it is extremely toxic and can cause irregular heartbeats, heart attack, and even death, few sources promote the use of this herb for medicinal purposes. It is dangerous even when used as an ointment. Aconite is on the Commission E (Germany's regulatory agency for herbs) list of unapproved herbs. This means that it is not recommended for use because it has not been proven to be safe or effective. This herb should be avoided, especially by women who are pregnant or breast-feeding.

Aloe

Other common name(s)	Scientific/medical name(s)
Aloe Vera, Aloe Vera Gel, T-UP	*Aloe barbadensis, Aloe capensis*

DESCRIPTION

The aloe plant, a member of the lily family, is a common household plant originally from Africa. The most common and widely known species of aloe plant is aloe vera. Aloe vera plants have dark green leaves that look like small cacti but are soft and supple. The gel from aloe vera is a thin, clear, jelly-like substance found in the inner portion of aloe leaves.

OVERVIEW

The gel inside aloe leaves may be effective in treating minor burns and skin irritations. There are mixed reports about its use as a laxative and there is no clinical evidence that aloe effectively treats any type of cancer. In fact, used as a cancer treatment, aloe is dangerous and may even be deadly.

How is it promoted for use?

Aloe is used conventionally for constipation and skin conditions. However, proponents of alternative treatments claim aloe also boosts the immune system and acts directly on abnormal cells, thus preventing or treating cancer.

The main aloe product promoted as a cancer cure is a new, unapproved drug called T-UP, which comes in an oral form or can be injected. Aloe proponents claim it is effective against all types of cancer, including liver and prostate cancer, although there is no scientific evidence to support these claims.

What does it involve?

Aloe vera is a common ingredient in many skin creams and lotions, cosmetics, and burn and wound ointments. For topical applications to minor burns or skin irritations, aloe gel is applied to the affected area 3 to 5 times a day. The aloe gel may be either purchased as a commercial gel or cream, or applied directly from a cut aloe leaf. Since some compounds in aloe gel break down quickly, fresh aloe gel (from the plant) is the best source for beneficial results.

Commission E (Germany's regulatory agency for herbs) has approved aloe for treating constipation. A common dosage is 50-200 mg of aloe latex (the residue left behind after the liquid from the gel has evaporated), taken either in liquid or capsule form, that can be used once a day for up to 10 days.

T-UP (concentrated aloe) has been promoted, in liquid form, to be taken either orally or injected directly into the tumor or bloodstream. Practitioners give T-UP injections to people with advanced cases of cancer. Aloe injections are illegal in the United States but are available at clinics in other countries.

What is the history behind it?

The earliest known references for the medicinal use of aloe come from the ancient Egyptians who used it as a treatment for cuts, burns, and skin irritations. Many other cultures have also used aloe for similar purposes. Beginning in the 1930s, aloe has been used frequently in hospitals and clinics for the treatment of minor skin ailments and for skin reactions from radiation burns.

From 1996 to 1997, a company based in Maryland began producing and selling T-UP, a concentrated form of aloe, to be used orally and by injection for the treatment of cancer, AIDS, herpes, and other autoimmune disorders. In the summer of 1999, the US Attorney's Office and the Food and Drug Administration (FDA), indicted the makers of T-UP on 20 different charges including various forms of fraud, promoting and selling an unapproved drug, and conspiracy. The makers of T-UP were charged with misleading cancer patients by making false claims including claiming FDA approval for their drug, which was never granted.

What is the evidence?

As a skin care product, aloe contains many chemicals, including carbohydrate polymers that soothe and moisturize the skin. Aloe juice also contains chemicals called anthranoids that give aloe its laxative properties. Mannans are another class of compounds found in aloe that are thought to stimulate wound healing.

There is no evidence that aloe is effective in treating people with cancer. Several people with cancer have died as a direct result of receiving aloe injections. Animal and laboratory studies have found mixed results. One study reported that aloe reduced the growth of liver cancer cells in rats but another found that it promoted the growth of human liver cancer cells in tissue culture. Another rat study reported aloe reduced precancerous liver changes in rats treated with cancer-causing chemicals. Another recent laboratory study reported that aloe promotes the growth of endothelial (blood vessel) cells, raising the concern that it might promote angiogenesis (growth of blood vessels that help "feed" a cancer).

Although aloe has been used since the 1930s in the treatment of skin reactions resulting from radiation therapy, a recent phase III clinical trial found that an aloe vera gel did not protect against radiation therapy-induced dermatitis (a skin reaction). While aloe may be effective for minor cuts and burns, more severe skin trauma may require other therapies.

Are there any possible problems or complications?

The external use of aloe for the relief of minor cuts and burns appears to be safe and effective. There are mixed reports about the safety of taking aloe internally. One report suggested that aloe taken orally might increase cancer risk to humans. Side effects of the internal use of aloe may include abdominal pain, nausea and vomiting, diarrhea, and electrolyte (chemical) imbalance, especially at high doses. It should not be used as a laxative for more than two weeks. Women who are pregnant or breast-feeding should not use aloe internally.

Aloe injections are dangerous, illegal in the United States, and have caused the deaths of several people.

References

Blumenthal M, ed. *The Complete German Commission F Monographs: Therapeutic Guide to Herbal Medicines.* Austin, Tx: American Botanical Council; 1998.

Brusick D, Mengs U. Assessment of the genotoxic risk from laxative senna products. *Environ Mol Mutagen.* 1997;29:1-9.

Corsi MM, Bertelli AA, Gaja G, Fulgenzi A, Ferrero ME. The therapeutic potential of Aloe Vera in tumor-bearing rats. *Int J Tissue React.* 1998;20:115-118.

Lee MJ, Lee OH, Yoon SH, et al. In vitro angiogenic activity of Aloe vera gel on calf pulmonary artery endothelial (CPAE) cells. *Arch Pharm Res.* 1998;21:260-265.

Lee KY, Park JH, Chung MH, et al. Aloesin up-regulates cyclin E/CDK2 kinase activity via inducing the protein levels of cyclin E, CDK2, and CDC25A in SK-HEP-1 cells. *Biochem Mol Biol Int.* 1997;41:285-292.

Lulinski B, Kapica C. Some notes on aloe vera. Quackwatch Web site. Available at: http://www.quackwatch.com. Accessed December 12, 1999.

Shamaan NA, Kadir KA, Rahmat A, Ngah WZ. Vitamin C and aloe vera supplementation protects from chemical hepatocarcinogenesis in the rat. *Nutrition.* 1998;14:846-852.

University of Texas Center for Alternative Medicine Research in Cancer. Aloe summary. University of Texas-Houston Health Science Center Web site. Available at: http://www.sph.uth.tmc.edu/utcam/summary/greentea.htm. Accessed December 12, 1999.

Williams MS, Burk M, Loprinzi CL, et al. Phase III double-blind evaluation of an aloe vera gel as a prophylactic agent for radiation-induced skin toxicity. *Int J Radiat Oncol Biol Phys.* 1996; 36:345-349.

Alsihum

Other common name(s)	Scientific/medical name(s)
Alzium™	None

DESCRIPTION / OVERVIEW

Alsihum is an herbal formula manufactured by a company in Israel that is marketed as an alternative therapy for cancer. According to the manufacturer, the compound is a liquid that consists of extracts of 11 herbs in a base of water and alcohol. The herbs include cone flower (echinacea), cayenne, burdock, myrrh, saffron, and skullcap (see Echinacea and Capsicum). The manufacturer claims that alsihum may be used by itself or along with conventional cancer treatment to help boost a patient's immune system and kill cancer cells. The company also claims alsihum may destroy cancer cells that are resistant to conventional drugs. In addition, they claim people have used alsihum successfully to treat breast infections, gout, and chronic fatigue syndrome. There is no scientific evidence to support any of these claims. The reported side effects include diarrhea, dizziness, mood swings, and dry mouth. Women who are pregnant or breast-feeding should not use this product. Relying on this type of treatment alone, and avoiding conventional medical care, may have serious health consequences.

Arnica

Other common name(s)	Scientific/medical name(s)
Arnica Root, Common Arnica, Arnica Flowers, Mountain Arnica, Mountain Tobacco, Leopardsbane, Wolfsbane	*Arnica montana*

DESCRIPTION

Arnica is a perennial plant native to Europe, the northern United States, and Canada. Its daisy-like flower and root (rhizome) are often used in herbal medicines.

OVERVIEW

This herbal remedy is used for skin wounds, infections, and inflammation. It has not been scientifically proven to be effective. If taken by mouth, it can be poisonous and has been known to cause a number of serious reactions.

Herbs / Vitamins / Minerals

How is it promoted for use?

Arnica is promoted for external use to help soothe and heal wounds, sunburn, bruises, sprains, irritation from accidental injuries and burns, arthritis, ulcers, acne, eczema, chapped lips, and irritated nostrils. Arnica contains organic substances, such as sesquiterpene lactones and flavonoid glycosides that are claimed to reduce inflammation (swelling, redness, and pain) and help heal bacterial infections. The herb is not usually recommended for internal use because it can irritate the stomach and may result in vomiting, diarrhea, and nosebleeds. However, some homeopathic practitioners claim it can be used orally to treat low grade fevers, colds, bronchitis (wheezing and a persistent cough), seasickness, inflammation of the mouth and throat, and epilepsy (see Homeopathy). There is no scientific evidence to support these claims.

Commission E (Germany's regulatory agency for herbs) has approved arnica only for external use in treating injury and effects of accidents, inflammation of the mouth and throat area, and insect bites. It is considered unsafe for internal use and can cause poisoning in people that are sensitive to the plant.

What does it involve?

Arnica is used as a whole or cut herb, powder, tea, liquid, or salve (ointment). The herb is diluted with water and made into a poultice (a soft, moist mass of herbs) that is applied directly to the skin. Arnica ointments usually contain up to 15% of arnica oil or 25% of a tincture of arnica (the herb mixed with alcohol). Blistering and inflammation may occur unless very dilute solutions are used.

What is the history behind it?

Herbal medicines made from arnica flowers and roots have been popular in homeopathy for hundreds of years. It has been said that Goethe drank arnica tea to relieve chest pains. In Germany today, the herb is used in more than 100 herbal medicines, and is promoted for treating heart conditions.

What is the evidence?

In 1998, a review of eight controlled human trials studying the effectiveness of arnica published in the *Archives of Surgery* found that arnica was no more effective than the placebo (inactive substance) it was compared with in treating injuries. The authors found the studies they reviewed had serious flaws in the methods used to evaluate the effectiveness of arnica and concluded that the human trials did not support a beneficial effect for arnica. One randomized clinical trial actually found that arnica appeared to increase pain and cause more swelling than the placebo in patients who had their wisdom teeth removed.

Are there any possible problems or complications?

Small, single doses of the herb are considered safe if applied externally. However, repeated applications can cause skin reactions, severe inflammation, itching, blisters, skin ulcers, and other allergy-related skin problems. Internal use is not recommended because arnica may cause vomiting, diarrhea, internal bleeding, rapid heartbeat, muscle weakness, nervousness, and nosebleeds in some cases. Arnica may reduce the effectiveness of high blood pressure medications and increase the risk of bleeding in people who take blood-thinning medications. Women who are pregnant or breast-feeding should not use this herb.

References

Blumenthal M, ed. *The Complete German Commission E Monographs: Therapeutic Guide to Herbal Medicines.* Austin, Tx: American Botanical Council; 1998.

Bown D. *Encyclopedia of Herbs & Their Uses.* New York, NY: DK Publishing Inc; 1995.

Ernst E, Pittler MH. Efficacy of homeopathic arnica: a systematic review of placebo-controlled clinical trials. *Arch Surg.* 1998;133:1187-1190.

Fetrow CW, Avila JR. *Professional's Handbook of Complementary and Alternative Medicines.* Springhouse, Pa: Springhouse Corp; 1999.

Gibson J, Haslam Y, Laurneson L, Newman P, Pitt R, Robins M. Double-blind trial of arnica in acute trauma patients. *Homeopathy*. 1991;41:54-55.

Kaziro GS. Metronidazole (Flagyl) and Arnica Montana in the prevention of post-surgical complications, a comparative placebo controlled clinical trial. *Br J Oral Maxillofac Surg*. 1984;22:42-49.

Medical Economics. *PDR for Herbal Medicines*. Montvale, NJ: Medical Economics Company; 1998.

Astragalus

Other common name(s)	Scientific/medical name(s)
Milk Vetch, Huang Qi, Huang Ch'i	*Astragalus membranaceus*

DESCRIPTION
Astragalus is a traditional Chinese herbal medicine taken from a plant known as Astragalus membranaceus, which is a type of bean or legume (see Chinese Herbal Medicine). The sweet-tasting root is used in herbal remedies.

OVERVIEW
Animal studies suggest that astragalus may enhance the effect of conventional immune therapy for some cancers. There is no scientific evidence that astragalus can prevent or cure cancer in humans.

How is it promoted for use?
The herb is promoted to kill cancer cells, reduce the toxic effects of chemotherapy, help the body heal burns, protect against heart disease, and fight the common cold, and overall weakness. Proponents also claim astragalus can stimulate the spleen, liver, lungs, circulatory, and urinary system, and help treat arthritis, asthma, and nervous conditions. They further claim it can lower blood sugar levels and blood pressure. Many Chinese medicine practitioners say the use of astragalus can help build the flow of vital energy or life force in the body called qi (or chi) which is essential to good health and well being. However, there is no evidence to support any of these claims.

What does it involve?
When dried, the root of the astragalus plant is used in teas, tinctures, and capsules. It is also available as a root slice and a powder. In China, healers sometimes use the dried root in soups or roast the root in honey for use as a medicinal tonic. Astragalus is often combined with other Chinese herbal remedies to enhance the effects of the herbs.

What is the history behind it?
For more than 2,000 years, Chinese herbalists have used astragalus to supposedly help the human body build up energy and resist disease. It is the most commonly used herb in Chinese medicine. Conventional medical practitioners have recently become interested in the possibility that astragalus might lessen the side effects of chemotherapy.

What is the evidence?

The scientific evidence for the ability of astragalus to enhance the immune system and fight diseases, including cancer and heart disease, comes only from laboratory and animal studies. Researchers at the University of Texas M. D. Anderson Cancer Center found that the astragalus extract enhanced the cell-destroying ability (cytotoxicity) of a conventional immunotherapy treatment (interleukin-2) by improving the immune response, and partially restored immune function of cells in test tubes. Astragalus has also been found to stimulate the production of interferon (a group of substances produced by the body as part of the normal defense mechanism against viral infections) and reduce the length of colds. Animal and laboratory studies may show a certain therapy holds promise as a beneficial treatment, but further studies are necessary to determine if the results apply to humans.

There is no scientific evidence that astragalus can prevent or cure cancer in humans or decrease the toxic effects of chemotherapy. Large-scale human trials are needed to verify the benefits, if any, of astragalus in people with cancer.

Are there any possible problems or complications?

Astragalus is generally considered safe. Side effects that have been reported include abdominal bloating, loose stools, low blood pressure, and dehydration. People with autoimmune diseases (such as rheumatoid arthritis or lupus) or people taking immune suppressing medications (such as corticosteroids or cyclosporin) should consult their physician before taking this herb.

References

Chu DT, Lepe-Zuniga J, Wong WL, LaPushin R, Mavligit GM. Fractionated extract of Astragalus membranaceus, a Chinese medicinal herb, potentiates LAK cell cytotoxicity generated by a low dose of recombinant interleukin-2. *J Clin Lab Immunol.* 1988;26:183-187.

Herb blurb: Astragalus. MCW HealthLink Web site. Available at: http://healthlink.mcw.edu/article/928273466.html. Accessed March 28, 2000.

Khoo KS, Ang PT. Extract of Astragalus membranaceus and Ligustrum lucidum does not prevent cyclophosphamide-induced myelosuppression. *Singapore Med J.* 1995;36:387-390.

Miller AL. Botanical influences on cardiovascular disease. *Altern Med Rev.* 1998;3:422-431.

Rittenhouse JR, Lui PD, Lau BH. Chinese medicinal herbs reverse macrophage suppression induced by urological tumors. *J Urol.* 1991;146:486-490.

University of Texas Center for Alternative Medicine Research in Cancer. Traditional Chinese medicine summary. University of Texas-Houston Health Science Center Web site. Available at: http://www.sph.uth.tmc.edu/utcam/therapies/tcm.htm. Accessed May 8, 2000.

Aveloz

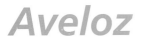

Other common name(s)	Scientific/medical name(s)
Killwart, Milkbush, Pencil Tree	*Euphorbia tirucalli, Euphorbia insulana*

DESCRIPTION

Aveloz is a large succulent shrub native to the tropical forests of Brazil, Madagascar, and South Africa. The sap, leaves, and root of various species of the shrub have been used in folk medicine for centuries.

OVERVIEW

Aveloz sap is promoted for use as an anticancer agent when placed on the skin or swallowed in liquid form. However, preliminary laboratory and animal studies have shown that aveloz sap may actually promote tumor growth, suppress the immune system, and lead to the development of certain cancers. It can also cause burning of the mouth and throat, and other serious complications.

How is it promoted for use?

The sap of the aveloz shrub has been promoted as a tumor-killing agent for people with cancer. It is also said to burn off warts, cysts, and skin cancers, especially in the face. In various parts of the world, the plant is also used to treat leprosy, earache, abscesses, toothaches, asthma, colic, cough, rheumatism, and fractures. There is no scientific evidence to support these claims.

What does it involve?

Aveloz is sold in the United States in some health food stores and by herbal practitioners in liquid form. To treat cancer, benign tumors, warts, and cysts, practitioners recommend drinking five drops of the liquid dissolved in half a glass of water or tea. Aveloz is also sold as an ointment for application directly to the skin to treat warts and tumors.

What is the history behind it?

Thousands of years ago, Amazon Indians in Brazil began applying the sap of the aveloz plant to warts and tumors on the skin. By the 1770s, African herbal practitioners were using it against cancerous tumors in folk medicine. In the 1880s, a Brazilian physician introduced the plant to conventional medicine, but it was never analyzed for its chemical composition.

In the 1970s, US supermarket tabloids began proclaiming aveloz as a cure for cancer when taken internally, saying, "One drop of sap, diluted in a glass of distilled water and taken by the tablespoon every hour, eliminates cancerous growths in one week." The craze over aveloz as a cure for cancer peaked in the 1980s, but it is still sold on the Internet as an underground, alternative treatment for cancer.

What is the evidence?

The effects of aveloz have only been studied in laboratory and animal research, but the results indicate that aveloz may actually promote tumor growth. Preliminary laboratory and animal studies have suggested that the sap, and the aveloz plant itself, may suppress the body's immune system making it less resistant to infections and some cancers. This may lead to an activation of the Epstein-Barr virus and the development of a type of cancer known as Burkitt's lymphoma, which causes tumors in the jaw and abdomen.

Are there any possible problems or complications?

Aveloz sap is caustic and harmful to skin and mucous membranes (the skin-like layer of cells that lines the mouth, throat, and other cavities in the body). It can cause burning of the mouth and throat, skin inflammation, conjunctivitis (inflammation of the eyes), diarrhea, nausea, vomiting, and stomach cramps.

References

Furstenburger G, Hecker E. On the active principles of the Euphorbiaceae, XII. Highly unsaturated irritant diterpene esters from Euphorbia tirucalli originating from Madagascar. *J Nat Prod.* 1986;49:386-397.

Imai S, Sugiura M, Mizuno F, et al. African Burkitt's lymphoma: A plant, Euphorbia tirucalli, reduces Epstein-Barr virus-specific cellular immunity. *Anticancer Res.* 1994;14:933-936.

Osato T, Mizuno F, Imai S, et al. African Burkett's lymphoma and an Epstein-Barr virus-enhancing plant Euphorbia tirucalli. *Lancet.* 1987;1:1257-1258.

Tyler VA. Aveloz. Quackwatch Web site. Available at: http://www.quackwatch.com. Accessed May 8, 2000.

Beta Carotene

Other common name(s)	Scientific/medical name(s)
Provitamin A, β-carotene	None

DESCRIPTION

Beta carotene is the major pigment in many fruits and vegetables that gives them their color. It is a carotenoid that the body converts into vitamin A. Carotenoids are a group of pigments naturally found in fruits and vegetables that also include alpha carotene, lycopene, lutein, and other compounds (see Lycopene).

OVERVIEW

Beta carotene, which occurs naturally in fruits and vegetables, is believed to be an effective cancer-preventing nutrient. As a supplement, however, there is not enough evidence to show that it prevents cancer. It may actually increase the risk of lung cancer among people already at high risk, such as smokers. Research is currently being done to examine the role of carotenoids in cancer treatment.

How is it promoted for use?

Beta carotene is an antioxidant, a compound that blocks the action of activated oxygen molecules, known as free radicals, that can damage cells. Beta carotene, found in foods, is believed to enhance the activities of natural killer cells (a type of white blood cell) and other cells in the immune system that protect the body against cancer. It is thought to work in the epithelial cells that make up the outer layers of skin and line most of the hollow structures in the body, including the mouth, throat, lungs, stomach, intestines, cervix, bladder, and glands in the breasts. Beta carotene, and sometimes other

Herbs / Vitamins / Minerals

carotenoids, are also promoted for use as dietary supplements.

What does it involve?

Fruits and vegetables are excellent sources of beta carotene and other related compounds called carotenoids that are believed to play a role in preventing cancer. Beta carotene is found in carrots, squash, sweet potatoes, dark green leafy vegetables such as spinach, and many fruits. A diet rich in green, orange, red, and yellow vegetables and fruits—at least five servings a day—is said to significantly decrease the risk of developing stomach, lung, prostate, breast, head, and neck cancer, and may slow progression of some cancers. However, these foods contain many other substances and it is not known if this decrease in risk is due to beta carotene.

Beta carotene supplements are sold in some health food stores, supermarkets, and over the Internet. The potency and dosages vary by manufacturer. Some supplements include beta carotene with other carotenoids and are sold in pill, powder, and oil form.

What is the history behind it?

In animal studies in the 1920s, researchers began to link diets deficient in vitamin A to stomach cancer and early changes that could lead to cancer in the epithelial cells lining the throat and lungs. In 1977, beta carotene was shown to delay the development of cancers and reduce cancer growth in research with animals at risk of developing tumors.

A large-scale study of humans begun in 1971 found that death from cancer was highest among people who had the lowest levels of beta carotene in their blood. Many subsequent studies confirmed the link between high beta carotene levels from dietary sources and a reduced risk of cancer. Because of the convincing evidence, the National Cancer Institute (NCI) launched a large program of randomized clinical trials in the early 1980s to study the effects of beta carotene and other retinoids on cancer. Retinoids consist of vitamin A and synthetic compounds similar to vitamin A.

What is the evidence?

Studies have found that eating foods rich in beta carotene reduces the risk of developing stomach, lung, prostate, breast, mouth, and throat cancer. However, it is not known if this is due to beta carotene alone. Evidence suggests that the combination of antioxidants in fruits and vegetables, rather than individual supplements, is most likely to be beneficial.

Population studies have shown that the risks of developing some cancers are higher in people who have diets low in vitamin A and beta carotene, although it is unclear to what extent beta carotene is responsible for the decreased risks observed. There is not enough evidence at this time to recommend beta carotene supplements for cancer prevention in the general public. Randomized clinical trials have not shown that beta carotene supplements reduce the risk of cancer. In fact, high-dose supplements may even increase the risk of developing lung cancer, especially in people who smoke cigarettes or are exposed by their occupation to carcinogens (possible cancer-causing substances), such as asbestos.

One large clinical trial in Finland sponsored by NCI found that vitamin E supplements provided no protection against lung cancer among heavy smokers, and that 18% more cases of lung cancer occurred among subjects who received beta carotene supplements. Several years later, they reported that beta carotene supplements did not protect male heart attack victims against a second heart attack. In fact, there were more deaths among the subjects who took beta carotene. The results of a second large study found no evidence that supplements of vitamin C, vitamin E, or beta carotene prevented colorectal cancer. Another large study conducted in the United States found that the risk of lung cancer and death actually increased among smokers who took beta carotene supplements.

Randomized clinical trials have not found protective effects from beta carotene supplements. Studies combining β-carotene, ∝-tocopherol, and selenium have shown some protective effects against stomach cancer. More research is needed to understand the benefits of supplemental nutrients and cancer prevention.

Are there any possible problems or complications?

Beta carotene obtained from eating fruits and vegetables is considered safe. Although not harmful, high doses of beta carotene supplements can result in a skin condition known as carotenosis in which the skin turns a yellow-orange color. In cigarette smokers and people exposed to carcinogens, beta carotene supplements can increase the risk of developing lung cancer.

References

Alpha-Tocopherol, Beta-Carotene Lung Cancer Prevention Study Group. The effect of vitamin E and beta-carotene on the incidence of lung cancer and other cancers in male smokers. *N Engl J Med.* 1994;330:1029-1035.

Cooper DA, Eldridge AL, Peters JC. Dietary carotenoids and certain cancers, heart disease, and age-related macular degeneration: a review of recent research. *Nutr Rev.* 1999;57:201-214.

Daviglus ML, Dyer AR, Persky V, et al. Dietary beta-carotene, vitamin C, and risk of prostate cancer: results from the Western Electric Study. *Epidemiology.* 1996;7:472-477.

Omenn GS. Chemoprevention of lung cancer: the rise and demise of beta carotene. *Annu Rev Public Health.* 1998;19:73-99.

Omenn GS, Goodman GE, Thornquist MD, et al. Effects of a combination of beta carotene and vitamin A on lung cancer and cardiovascular disease. *N Engl J Med.* 1996;334:1150-1155.

Paiva SA, Russell RM. Beta-carotene and other carotenoids as antioxidants. *J Am Coll Nutr.* 1999;18:426-433.

Patterson RE, White E, Kristal AR, Neuhouser ML, Potter JD. Vitamin supplements and cancer risk: the epidemiologic evidence. *Cancer Causes Control.* 1997;8:786-802.

Vainio H, Rautalahti M. An international evaluation of the cancer preventive potential of carotenoids. *Cancer Epidemiol Biomarkers Prev.* 1998;7:725-728.

Betulinic Acid

Other common name(s)	Scientific/medical name(s)
Butalin, Bet A	None

DESCRIPTION

Betulinic acid is a chemical that has a number of plant sources, but can also be made chemically from betulin. Betulin is found in the bark of white birch trees, which grow from the Arctic circle down to Florida and Texas.

OVERVIEW

Betulinic acid may hold promise as an anticancer agent. Some studies have reported antitumor activity for betulinic acid, however, these studies were done with animals and cell cultures. Additional studies are underway to determine its potential role in treating melanoma and certain brain cancers. Randomized clinical trials are needed to determine what effect, if any, betulinic acid may have in treating cancer in humans.

How is it promoted for use?

Some researchers believe that betulinic acid causes some types of tumor cells to start a process of self-destruction called apoptosis. They also believe that betulinic acid slows the progression of melanoma and other types of tumor cells and the human immunodeficiency virus (HIV), and that it has antibacterial properties. Clinical studies are now being conducted to test these claims.

Proponents claim that white birch bark (which contains betulinic acid) can be used as a remedy for eczema and other skin conditions when applied externally. Other claims for betulinic acid, obtained from birch bark, include the treatment of diarrhea, dysentery, and cholera.

What does it involve?

Betulinic acid is used internally or externally. Tea can be made by infusing a teaspoon of the birch bark in a cup of boiling water for 15 minutes. Proponents recommend from 2 to 5 cups of tea per day. Birch bark containing betulinic acid in natural form can be applied to the skin as well. Pure betulinic acid is not directly available for public use, but raw birch bark is sold in herbal medicine shops.

What is the history behind it?

White birch bark has been used by Native Americans as a folk remedy for some time. They used it in tea and other beverages to treat stomach and intestinal problems such as diarrhea and dysentery. In Russia, it has been used since 1834.

In 1994, scientists at the University of North Carolina reported that chemicals found in white birch bark slowed the growth of HIV. The following year, a researcher at the University of Illinois reported that betulinic acid killed melanoma cells in mice. Since then, a number of researchers have conducted laboratory tests on betulinic acid to determine its antitumor properties, especially with respect to melanoma cells with some promising results which may warrant future study.

What is the evidence?

Betulinic acid has not been studied in humans, but is being evaluated in laboratory studies in cultured cancer cell lines and in cancer cells taken from patients. These laboratory studies, using the pure chemical and not the birch bark, published in peer-reviewed medical journals suggest that betulinic acid holds some promise for patients with melanoma (a form of skin cancer) and certain nervous system tumors. Three German studies concluded that betulinic acid showed antitumor activity against cells from certain types of nervous system cancers in children. Two laboratory studies conducted at the University of Illinois indicated that betulinic acid may prove useful as an antitumor drug. More studies are underway. Laboratory studies may show a certain therapy or compound holds promise as a beneficial treatment, but further studies are necessary to determine if the results apply to humans.

Are there any possible problems or complications?

Researchers are still studying betulinic acid. It is not clear if it is safe for humans. Birch bark, available commercially, has not been scientifically studied and its side effects are not known.

References

Fulda S, Friesen C, Los M, et al. Betulinic Acid triggers CD95 (APO-1Fas)- and p53-independent apoptosis via activation of caspases in neuroectodermal tumors. *Cancer Res.* 1997;57:4956-4964.

Fulda S, Jeremias I, Steiner HH, Pietsch T, Debatin KM. Betulinic Acid: A new cytotoxic agent against malignant brain-tumor cells. *Int J Cancer.* 1999;82:435-441.

Fulda S, Susin SA, Kroemer G, Debatin KM. Molecular ordering of apoptosis induced by anticancer drugs in neuroblastoma cells. *Cancer Res.* 1998;58:4453-4460.

Jeong HJ, Chai HB, Park SY, Kim DS. Preparation of amino acid conjugates of betulinic acid with activity against human melanoma. *Bioorg Med Chem Lett.* 1999;9:1201-1204.

Moss R. White birch compound kills melanoma cells and HIV. The Cancer Chronicles Web site. Available at: http://www.ralphmoss.com/html/betu.shtml. Accessed May 8, 2000.

Pisha E, Chai H, Lee IS, et al. Discovery of betulinic acid as a selective inhibitor of human melanoma that functions by induction of apoptosis. *Nat Med.* 1995;1:1046-1051.

Schmidt ML, Kuzmanoff KL, Ling-Indeck L, Pezzuto JM. Betulinic acid induces apoptosis in human neuroblastoma cell lines. *Eur J Cancer.* 1997;33:2007-2010.

Herbs / Vitamins / Minerals

Black Cohosh

DESCRIPTION

Black cohosh is a woodland plant of the eastern United States and Canada that grows from 4 to 8 feet tall and has feathery white flowers. The root is used in herbal remedies.

OVERVIEW

There is some evidence that black cohosh is effective in relieving menopausal symptoms. It also appears to have some estrogen-like effects but the mechanism of action is not understood. There is no evidence that it is effective in treating cancer and should not be used for more than six consecutive months. The long-term effects are not known.

How is it promoted for use?

Black cohosh is often referred to as a "woman's remedy" because it is used primarily to relieve premenstrual discomfort, menstrual cramps, and symptoms associated with menopause such as hot flashes. Commission E (Germany's regulatory agency for herbs) has approved black cohosh for these symptoms. Black cohosh is also a source of vitamin A and pantothenic acid.

The beneficial effects of black cohosh are attributed to chemicals in the plant that resemble and mimic the effects of the female hormone called estrogen. However, the strength of the plant's estrogenic effects has been disputed, and the exact physiological mechanism by which black cohosh operates in the body is not well understood.

Because some cancers, such as breast and endometrial cancer, are stimulated by estrogen, some herbalists state that black cohosh may be dangerous for people who have cancer. But a contrary opinion holds that since the herb does not actually contain estrogen, it is safe for cancer patients. Some defenders of black cohosh state that the herb reduces the risk of breast and prostate cancer although there is no evi-

dence to support these claims.

Other conditions that black cohosh has been used to treat include pain relief before, during and after childbirth, breast pain, ovarian pain, and uterine pain. Other reported uses of black cohosh include arthritis pain relief, lowering blood pressure, sedation, treatment of bronchial infections, spasms associated with "whooping cough," and diarrhea.

What does it involve?

Black cohosh is the primary ingredient in an over-the-counter German menopausal remedy called Remifemin. Black cohosh can be found in several different forms including capsules, solutions, tablets, and tinctures. There is no standardized treatment plan for the use of the herb. The typical dose suggested is two tablets of Remifemin twice daily or 40 drops of Remifemin liquid twice daily.

What is the history behind it?

Cohosh is a Native American word that means "knobby rough roots," which describes the appearance of the plant's roots. Native Americans traditionally used black cohosh to treat uterine disorders, such as menstrual and menopausal symptoms, as well as other ailments, such as diarrhea, sore throat, and general weakness. The herb has been approved in Germany for the same purposes for more than 50 years and is commonly prescribed in other European countries.

What is the evidence?

There have been no published peer-reviewed scientific studies of black cohosh use in people or animals with cancer or even in the laboratory. Long-term studies are needed to determine the herb's safety over time.

A physician in the United States reviewed eight clinical studies of black cohosh and noted that it was effective in relieving menopausal symptoms. The author concluded that black cohosh is a safe, effective alternative to estrogen for those patients in whom estrogen replacement therapy is either refused or not advised. An article published in the magazine *Prevention* reported that five clinical trials conducted in Europe demonstrated black cohosh effectively relieved hot flashes in more than 80% of test subjects, but details of the trials were not provided.

Are there any possible problems or complications?

Not enough scientific information is available about black cohosh to determine whether it is safe. No serious reactions to moderate doses of black cohosh have been reported. However, common side effects include upset stomach, nausea, and vomiting. An excessive dose may cause slow heart rate, uterine contractions, headache, dizziness, tremors, joint pain, and light-headedness.

The Commission E recommends the herb not be taken for more than six consecutive months. It should be used with caution in individuals with high blood pressure and those taking high blood pressure medications. Women who are considering any form of hormone-replacement therapy should consult their physician before taking black cohosh. Women who are pregnant or breast-feeding should not use this herb.

References

Fetrow CW, Avila JR. *Professional's Handbook of Complementary and Alternative Medicines*. Springhouse, Pa: Springhouse Corp; 1999.

Lieberman S. A review of the effectiveness of Cimicifuga racemosa (black cohosh) for the symptoms of menopause. *J Womens Health*. 1998;7:525-529.

Medical Economics. *PDR for Herbal Medicines*. Montvale, NJ: Medical Economics Company; 1998.

Tyler VE. Five herbs that ease menopause. *Prevention*. March 1999;51:94.

Black Walnut

Other common name(s)	Scientific/medical name(s)
Black Walnut Hulls, English Walnut, Butternut, Oilnut	*Juglans nigra*

DESCRIPTION

The black walnut is a hardwood tree that grows widely in the United States, Canada, and parts of Europe. It can reach a height of more than 100 feet. The nut hulls, inner bark, leaves, and fruit are used in herbal remedies.

OVERVIEW

There is no scientific evidence that hulls from black walnuts remove parasites from the intestinal tract or that they are effective in treating cancer or any other disease.

How is it promoted for use?

A small number of herbal medicine practitioners claim that cancer is caused by a parasite. They claim that a tincture made from black walnut hulls combined with wormwood and cloves will kill the cancer-causing parasites, preventing or curing the disease without causing significant side effects. Black walnut is said to effectively kill more than 100 types of parasites. There is no scientific evidence to support these claims.

Black walnut is also promoted as a natural remedy for such wide-ranging conditions as acne, thyroid disease, colitis, eczema, hemorrhoids, ringworm, sore throats, tonsillitis, skin irritations, and wounds. Supporters claim black walnut hulls can be used as a mild laxative that eases general digestive problems. A few proponents claim that black walnuts reduce the risk of heart attacks. Because of its claimed anti-parasite properties in the stomach and intestines, proponents recommend black walnut for people who travel to areas with contaminated water supplies.

What does it involve?

The part of the black walnut tree used as a remedy is the hull of the fruit. Black walnut hull is available in tablets, capsules, and tinctures. However, some claim that only a tincture preparation with alcohol is effective.

What is the history behind it?

Ancient Greeks and Romans called black walnut fruit the "Imperial nut," and reportedly used the hull to treat intestinal ailments. Black walnut has also played a part in Russian folk medicine since the 17th century. Throughout history, every part of the tree has been used in folk medicine to treat dozens of conditions, including the bite of a mad dog. According to traditional Chinese medicine, eating black walnuts builds physical strength (see Chinese Herbal Medicine). In Texas folk medicine, black walnut extract is considered an effective treatment for scorpion bites.

Craftsmen and artists prize the tree's fine-grained wood for making furniture and carvings, and the nuts are a safe and very popular food.

What is the evidence?

There is no scientific evidence that black walnut hulls can cure any diseases, including cancer. The notion that parasites cause cancer or that they can be killed using herbal remedies is unproven. No studies have been done in humans to support any of the claims made for black walnut.

Are there any possible problems or complications?

Due to the lack of research, little is known about the potential side effects of black walnut hulls.

References

Kruger J, Savitsky K, Gilovich T. Superstition and the regression effect. *Skeptical Inquirer.* 1999;23:24.

McGuffin M, Hobbs C, Upton R, Goldberg A, eds. *Botanical Safety Handbook.* Boca Raton, FL: CRC Press; 1997.

Walsh T. Debunking the detoxification theory. *Nutrition Forum.* 1999;16:1.

Bromelain

Other common name(s)	Scientific/medical name(s)
None	None

DESCRIPTION

Bromelain is a natural enzyme found in pineapples. The pineapple is a tropical fruit native to Central and South America. Bromelain supplements are promoted as an alternative remedy for various health problems including joint inflammation and cancer.

OVERVIEW

A small clinical study conducted in Germany recently found that bromelain may have some effect on immune function. No scientific studies have evaluated whether bromelain shrinks tumors or extends the survival of people with cancer. Laboratory studies on the bromelain enzyme have shown it to be effective in treating diarrhea in some animals, but the health benefits to humans have not been proven. More research is needed before any conclusions can be made about the effectiveness of bromelain.

How is it promoted for use?

Proponents claim bromelain reduces swelling and inflammation associated with soft-tissue injuries. Some people also believe that the enzyme is an effective treatment for a number of digestive disorders because it stimulates the contraction of intestinal muscles. Some practitioners claim bromelain relieves the pain and inflammation caused by joint disorders, such as arthritis and carpal tunnel syndrome, and that it inhibits can-cer cell growth when combined with chemotherapy. Supporters also state bromelain fights bacterial and viral infections and reduces the risk of heart attacks by thinning the blood. There is no scientific evidence to support these claims.

What does it involve?

Although bromelain can be obtained naturally by eating pineapples, some people also use supplements. They are available in capsules and ointments in most health food stores. It is also often an ingredient (along with other herbs) in supplements sold for joint health. Recommended dosages vary by manufacturer.

What is the history behind it?
Christopher Columbus discovered pineapples growing on the island of Guadeloupe in 1493 and brought them back to Spain. They became very popular in Europe by the 1600s. Bromelain has been used for hundreds of years as a digestive aid, and to treat inflammation and other health problems. Recently, bromelain has been investigated for possible anticancer activity.

What is the evidence?
A recent clinical study of 16 breast cancer patients in Germany found that a bromelain drug taken orally may stimulate one aspect of immune function which might partially explain its proposed antitumor activity. Other studies suggest that bromelain increases the quantity of cytokines (immune system hormones) produced by white blood cells. No scientific data is available on bromelain's impact on survival or quality of life in people with cancer. More well-controlled research is needed to understand its role, if any, in cancer treatment.

A number of laboratory and animal studies suggest that bromelain is effective in treating diarrhea related to *E. coli* infections and helps prevent platelets from sticking together, thus preventing blood clot formation. Animal and laboratory studies may show a certain substance holds promise as a beneficial treatment, but further studies are necessary to determine if the results apply to humans.

Are there any possible problems or complications?

Bromelain is generally considered safe. Some people may be allergic to bromelain, and it may cause bleeding when taken with anticoagulant (blood thinning) medications. Some practitioners advise caution when administering bromelain to people with high blood pressure.

References
Bromelain. Monograph. *Altern Med Rev.* 1998;3:302-305.

Cassileth B. *The Alternative Medicine Handbook.* New York, NY: W. W. Norton & Co; 1998.

Chandler DS, Mynott TL. Bromelain protects piglets from diarrhea caused by oral challenge with K88 positive enterotoxigenic Escherichia coli. *Gut.* 1998;43:196-202.

Desser L, Rehberger A, Kokron E, Paukovits W. Cytokine synthesis in human peripheral blood mononuclear cells after oral administration of polyenzyme preparations. *Oncology.* 1993;50:403-407.

Eckert K, Grabowska E, Stange R, Schneider U, Eschmann K, Maurer HR. Effects of oral bromelain administration on the impaired immunocytotoxicity of mononuclear cells from mammary tumor patients. *Oncol Rep.* 1999;6:1191-1199.

Metzig C, Grabowska E, Eckert K, Rehse K, Maurer HR. Bromelain proteases reduce human platelet aggregation in vitro, adhesion to bovine endothelial cells and thrombus formation in rat vessels in vivo. *In Vivo.* 1999;13:7-12.

Calcium

Other common name(s)	Scientific/medical name(s)
Calcium Carbonate	Ca, Ca++

DESCRIPTION

Calcium is a mineral that is vital for a number of biological processes in the body, including heartbeat regulation. It is found naturally in many dairy products, leafy green vegetables, and some fish. Calcium is also the building block of bones. Because humans cannot manufacture calcium, it must be obtained from diet or supplements.

OVERVIEW

Many people, especially women, can benefit from monitoring calcium intake to prevent bone problems such as osteoporosis. Calcium supplements will not slow the growth of most cancers, although they are being studied for the treatment or prevention of precancerous changes such as adenomatous polyps of the colon. Calcium supplements may be important for some people with cancer, depending on their specific medical situation (eg, cancer type and stage, type of treatments received). Anyone considering using supplements should consult their physician to discuss the benefits for their specific situation.

How is it promoted for use?

Calcium is known to help the growth and maintenance of bones and teeth and to assist heart and other muscle contractions. There is strong evidence that low calcium intake can lead to bone fragility, high blood pressure, and certain cancers. Recent studies have shown that calcium may reduce the risk of developing colon cancer and perhaps some other cancers. When combined with vitamin D, calcium may have the potential to help prevent cancers of the breast and pancreas. Calcium has also been found to be of significant benefit in reducing certain symptoms of premenstrual syndrome. There is some preliminary evidence that calcium may play a role in helping to prevent heart disease and reducing insulin resistance in diabetic patients.

Because calcium plays a crucial role in building and maintaining bone mass and strength, its greatest benefit to people with cancer may be to reduce the risk of osteopenia

(reduced bone mass) and osteoporosis (bone fragility and a severe decrease of bone mass and strength). Both conditions are associated primarily with aging, and osteoporosis is a common problem for postmenopausal women. Osteopenia and osteoporosis can also result from poor nutrition, prolonged drug therapy, disease, and decreased mobility, all of which may apply to people with cancer.

What does it involve?

Calcium metabolism is complex and affected by many hormones and factors other than dietary intake. There are many ways to treat bone problems and calcium balance problems. The best source of calcium comes from eating a good balanced diet, which will help to avoid bone problems and decrease the risk of some cancers. Foods and beverages high in calcium include milk and other dairy products (low-fat products are more healthy), leafy green vegetables such

Herbs / Vitamins / Minerals

as broccoli and greens, nuts, seeds, beans, tofu (prepared with calcium), cheese, dried figs, kelp, oysters, and canned fish that still has bones, such as sardines and salmon.

Although direct calcium intake from healthy food is the best source, calcium supplements are also available in drug stores, grocery stores, and many health food stores. The Recommended Dietary Allowance (RDA) for calcium is 1,000 mg/day for men and women ages 19-50, and 1,200 mg/day for people over 50. Some nutritionists recommend that calcium supplements be accompanied with supplements of vitamin D and other important minerals, such as magnesium and potassium.

What is the history behind it?

The importance of calcium for maintaining overall health and promoting bone strength has been known for decades. Some scientists even believe that due to evolution, humans became accustomed to high calcium diets as far back as 35,000 years ago. Calcium's role in preventing or slowing the growth of cancer has only become a notable subject of research within the last 10 to 15 years.

What is the evidence?

A number of important studies to measure calcium's impact on cancer have been published in peer-reviewed medical journals. Preliminary research suggests that a diet rich in calcium may decrease the risk of colorectal cancer. A recent randomized clinical trial published in the *New England Journal of Medicine* involved more than 900 subjects over 4 years. The researchers found that calcium supplements moderately reduced the recurrence of colorectal adenomas (an adenoma is a polyp that may indicate future cancer growth).

One researcher reviewed several dozen studies of the effects of calcium on various diseases and concluded that long-term deficiencies in calcium and vitamin D may lead not only to bone fragility, but also to colorectal cancer and high blood pressure in some individuals. Higher calcium intake may help to prevent these conditions in certain people. For example, results from a randomized clinical trial suggested that a high calcium diet may be associated with a

reduced risk of recurrent adenomas, particularly for people with high-fat diets. An animal study conducted at Texas Tech University in Lubbock concluded that adequate calcium intake as part of a healthy diet might help to prevent the formation of colorectal cancer, whether the source of calcium is from diet or from supplements.

While further research is needed to clarify the role of calcium in preventing or reversing cancer growth, there is little doubt that adequate calcium intake is essential for preventing osteopenia and osteoporosis. For people with cancer, calcium intake may be very important for maintaining bone strength. Some chemotherapy medications can reduce appetite, create swallowing difficulties, or cause nausea and vomiting, and result in osteopenia. The chemotherapy drugs methotrexate and doxorubicin may directly damage bones. Radiation therapy can cause osteopenia within the area being treated, and the combination of both radiation and chemotherapy can cause even greater damage to bone structure. Some cancers also can harm bones.

Are there any possible problems or complications?

The greatest risk associated with calcium, as noted above, comes from not getting enough of the mineral. In rare cases, ingesting very high levels of calcium (eg, more than 2,400 mg/day) can lead to hypercalcemia, which can cause kidney stones, muscle pain, and mental confusion, and is considered a serious medical condition. People who are undergoing treatment for cancer should consult their physician before taking vitamins, minerals, or other supplements that might interact with the cancer drugs prescribed. A Harvard University study also showed indirect evidence that excessive levels of dietary or supplemental calcium should be avoided to reduce the risk of advanced prostate cancer.

References

Barger-Lux MJ, Heaney RP. The role of calcium intake in preventing bone fragility, hypertension and certain cancers. *J Nutr.* 1994;124:1406S-1411S.

Baron JA, Beach M, Mandel JS, et al. Calcium supplements for the prevention of colorectal adenomas. *N Engl J Med.* 1999;340:101-107.

Cassileth B. *The Alternative Medicine Handbook.* New York, NY: W. W. Norton & Co; 1998.

Cats A, Keibeuker JH, van der Meer R, et al. Randomized, double-blinded, placebo-controlled intervention study with supplemental calcium in families with hereditary nonpolyposis colorectal cancer. *J Natl Cancer Inst.* 1995;87:598-603.

Giovannucci E, Rimm EB, Wolk A, et al. Calcium and fructose intake in relation to risk of prostate cancer. *Cancer Res.* 1998;58:442-447.

Holt PR. Dairy foods and prevention of colon cancer: human studies. *J Am Coll Nutr.* 1999;18:379S-391S.

Holt PR, Lipkin M, Newmark H. Calcium intake and colon cancer biomarkers. *JAMA.* 1999;281:1172-1173.

Hyman J, Baron JA, Dain BJ, et al. Dietary and supplemental calcium and the recurrence of colorectal adenomas. *Cancer Epidemiol Biomarkers Prev.* 1998;7:291-295.

Lipkin M, Newmark HL. Vitamin D, calcium and prevention of breast cancer: a review. *J Am Coll Nutr.* 1999;18:392S-397S.

Neugut AI, Horvath K, Whelan RL, et al. The effect of calcium and vitamin supplements on the incidence and recurrence of colorectal adenomatous polyps. Cancer. 1996;78:723-728.

Thys-Jacobs S, Starkey P, Bernstein D, Tian J. Calcium carbonate and the premenstrual syndrome: effects on premenstrual and menstrual symptoms. Premenstrual Syndrome Study Group. *Am J Obstet Gynecol.* 1998;179:444-452.

Capsicum

Other common name(s)	Scientific/medical name(s)
Capsaicin, Chili Pepper, Hot Pepper, Red Pepper, Paprika	*Capsicum annum*

DESCRIPTION

Capsicum annum is an annual plant native to Mexico and Central America cultivated in many warmer regions of the world. Capsicum varieties include cayenne pepper, jalapeños, other hot peppers, and paprika. Capsaicin is the active ingredient in the plant and has been approved by the FDA.

OVERVIEW

Although no research has been reported using the Capsicum annum plant for people with cancer, capsaicin (the active ingredient) has been studied in oral and topical (applied to the skin) forms. Several studies have shown capsaicin may be somewhat useful for managing pain related to surgery and mouth sores due to chemotherapy and radiation, however, more research is needed to determine other uses of capsaicin.

How is it promoted for use?

Capsaicin is used primarily as a topical cream for pain caused by conditions such as arthritis and general muscle soreness. There is some evidence that capsaicin may be useful in managing post-surgical pain from mastectomy, thoracotomy, amputation, and other surgery related to conventional cancer treatment. Researchers have found that capsaicin may provide temporary relief for mouth sore pain caused by chemotherapy and radiation.

Some proponents claim that capsaicin has antioxidant properties which help to fight the carcinogen nitrosamine (a cancer causing agent). An antioxidant is a compound that blocks the action of activated oxygen molecules, known as free radicals, that can damage cells. Still others claim that it may prevent DNA damage and cancer of the lungs from cigarette smoke; however, these claims have not been proven.

Over the years, the *Capsicum annum* herb has been used by alternative medicine practitioners as a remedy for a variety of conditions, such as upset stomach, menstrual cramps, headaches, shingles (herpes zoster), diarrhea, loss of appetite, stomach ulcers, poor digestion, sore throat, itching, alcoholism, seasickness, malaria, and yellow fever. Some practitioners also claim it can prevent colds, heart disease, and stroke, increase sexual potency, and strengthen the heart, although there is no scientific evidence to support these claims.

What does it involve?

Capsaicin cream is rubbed directly onto the skin over painful areas. Depending on the concentration of the cream, applications to the skin are recommended for as little as two days or as long as two months. It is available by prescription or over the counter.

The capsicum herb is available in health food stores as a tonic, a capsule, or in tea. There are some recipes available over the Internet that advocate making a candy with cayenne pepper to relieve the pain of mouth sores from chemotherapy and radiation.

What is the history behind it?

As far back as 5000 BC, Indians in South America ate meals prepared with hot peppers. Native Mexican Indians, and some Chinese (Hunan and Szechwan) are also known to have used hot peppers in many dishes and continue to do so. These cultures have also used hot peppers in herbal medicine to treat numerous conditions over the years.

While foods made with different kinds of peppers are also popular in the United States and Europe, it is only in recent years that interest in using capsaicin from hot peppers for pain management and other symptoms or illnesses has grown. The medical community is beginning to look at the use of capsaicin to treat some side effects of conventional cancer treatment like chemotherapy and surgery.

What is the evidence?

Although there has been no research done on the use of the *Capsicum annum* herb for people with cancer, capsaicin (the active ingredient) has been studied for external use. A study in 1989 found topical capsaicin to have pain-relieving effects among 50% of a small group of women who had undergone mastectomies for breast cancer. A 1993 study found similar results, thus further research into capsaicin was encouraged.

One study done in 1991 concluded that capsaicin cream decreased the amount of pain caused by diabetic neuropathy (a nerve disorder). A more recent study of capsaicin's usefulness in the management of neuropathic pain after surgery concluded that patients preferred capsaicin cream to a placebo (an inactive substance or treatment). Neuropathic pain is often experienced by patients after removal of a malignancy and can include burning, numbness, low pain threshold, and sympathetic nerve dysfunction. In 1994, a review of previous research concluded that while topical capsaicin is not satisfactory as a therapy by itself, it may be used with other medications to ease pain.

In a pilot study conducted at the Yale University School of Medicine, oral capsaicin (mixed with taffy) produced substantial pain reduction in patients with mouth sores caused by chemotherapy or radiation therapy. For most of the patients, however, the pain relief was temporary.

Studies have also been conducted to examine capsaicin's potential to relieve itching, reduce the size of nasal polyps and protect against substances that cause cancer. However, researchers have found it difficult to conduct these studies because of the burning sensation caused by oral or topical use of capsaicin. The discomfort has caused some patients to stop using it, making it difficult for researchers to conduct placebo studies of the drug.

Are there any possible problems or complications?

The consumption of cayenne, and other peppers, is considered safe in moderate amounts, however, it can cause stomach upset or diarrhea in some cases. Women who are pregnant or breast-feeding should avoid using this remedy internally. Capsaicin cream typically causes temporary stinging, burning, or itching when applied directly to the skin or taken orally. In severe cases, blisters may result. Contact with eyes and mucous membranes should be avoided.

References
Berger A, Henderson M, Nadoolman W, et al. Oral capsaicin provides temporary relief for oral mucositis pain secondary to chemotherapy/radiation therapy. *J Pain Symptom Manage.* 1995;10:243-248.

Dini D, Bertelli G, Gozza A, Forno GG. Treatment of the post-mastectomy pain syndrome with topical capsaicin. *Pain.* 1993;54:223-226.

Ellison N, Loprinzi CL, Kugler J, et al. Phase III placebo-controlled trial of capsaicin cream in the management of surgical neuropathic pain in cancer patients. *J Clin Oncol.* 1997;15:2974-2980.

Fetrow CW, Avila JR. *Professional's Handbook of Complementary and Alternative Medicines.* Springhouse, Pa: Springhouse Corp; 1999.

Medical Economics. *PDR for Herbal Medicines.* Montvale, NJ: Medical Economics Company; 1998.

Nelson C. Heal the burn: pepper and lasers in cancer pain therapy. *J Natl Cancer Inst.* 1994;86:1381-1382.

Watson CP. Topical capsaicin as an adjuvant analgesic. *J Pain Symptom Manage.* 1994;9:425-433.

Watson CP, Evans RJ. The postmastectomy pain syndrome and topical capsaicin: a randomized trial. *Pain.* 1992;51:375-379.

Cat's Claw

Other common name(s)	Scientific/medical name(s)
Una de Gato	*Unicaria tomentosa*

DESCRIPTION
Cat's claw is a woody vine that winds its way up trees at higher elevations in the Peruvian rain forests. The plant's name comes from the claw-like thorns that grow on the plant's stem, which can reach up to 100 feet. The root (which can grow to the size of a watermelon) and the inside of the bark, are the parts of the plant used in herbal remedies.

OVERVIEW
Cat's claw has been promoted as a remedy to boost the body's immune system, but there is no scientific evidence in humans of its immune-stimulating effects. No data exist showing that cat's claw is effective in preventing or treating cancer or any other disease. There are some serious side effects associated with cat's claw although the extent of these effects is not known.

How is it promoted for use?

The most common claims for cat's claw are that it boosts the immune system and increases the body's ability to fight off infections. The herb also is promoted as a remedy for arthritis, allergies, yeast infections, herpes and other viral infections, parasitic infections, inflammatory bowel disorders, cancer, cardiovascular disease, diabetes, asthma, urinary tract infections, and menstrual disorders. South American folk medicine holds that cat's claw is a contraceptive, and some practitioners claim that it can significantly decrease AIDS-related symptoms. There is no scientific evidence to support these claims.

What does it involve?

Cat's claw is taken orally and is available in capsules, tablets, tinctures, elixirs, and tea. Sometimes it can be found as a cream. Practitioner recommendations for how much to take vary widely. Some suggest a dosage of 3,000-6,000 mg/day in pill form, or 4 strong cups of tea. Herbalists may prescribe up to 20 g/day for seriously ill patients. Because herbs are not regulated in the United States, different brands of cat's claw may contain very different amounts of active ingredients.

What is the history behind it?

For centuries, South American native tribes have used cat's claw medicinally. Awareness of the herb grew in the United States and Europe during the 1970s when an Austrian Scientist, Klaus Kiplinger, traveled to the rain forests of Peru and learned about the plant from local priests. Kiplinger eventually received patents for isolating the active medicinal ingredients within the herb. Recently, cat's claw has become an extremely popular herbal supplement among consumers in the United States and Europe.

What is the evidence?

There has been no rigorous scientific study of cat's claw in humans. All of the reported positive effects of the herb are either anecdotal or the result of laboratory and animal experiments. Animal and laboratory studies may show that a certain substance holds promise as a beneficial treatment, but further studies are necessary to determine if the results apply to humans.

Researchers have found chemicals in cat's claw called alkaloids. One Canadian study concluded that some of the alkaloids may provide a strong "immunostimulant action" in rats. Other studies found that the alkaloids increase phagocytosis, the process in which white blood cells seek out and destroy invading harmful microorganisms. Also found were antioxidants—compounds that block the action of activated oxygen molecules, known as free radicals, that can damage cells.

Some laboratory studies which focused on the alkaloids (organic compounds) present in cat's claw have found that they may reduce inflammation and heart rate, slow the growth of tumors, and lower blood pressure. Peruvian researchers in the 1970s claimed that cat's claw was an effective treatment for treating children who had leukemia, but there has been no reliable scientific evidence to back up those reports.

Research is currently underway to study the effects of cat's claw as a treatment for breast cancer. Until clinical trials are completed, however, the true value of cat's claw remains questionable.

Are there any possible problems or complications?

More research is needed to determine if cat's claw is safe. Herbalists warn people who are taking anti-ulcer, high blood pressure, anticoagulant, hormonal, or insulin medications not to take cat's claw. Other people who should not take the herb include those who receive injections of foreign proteins, have low blood pressure or an autoimmune disease (eg, multiple sclerosis or tuberculosis), or those who have had an organ or bone marrow transplant. Studies have also shown that cat's claw contains tannins which, in high concentrations, may cause gastrointestinal disturbances or even kidney damage. Women who are pregnant or breast-feeding should not use this herb.

References

Cassileth B. *The Alternative Medicine Handbook*. New York, NY: W. W. Norton & Co; 1998.

Fetrow CW, Avila JR. *Professional's Handbook of Complementary and Alternative Medicines*. Springhouse, Pa: Springhouse Corp; 1999.

Moss R. *Herbs Against Cancer*. New York, NY: Equinox Press; 1998.

Sandoval-Chacon M, Thompson JH, Zhang XJ, et al. Antiinflammatory actions of cat's claw: the role of NF-kappaB. *Aliment Pharmacol Ther*. 1998;12:1279-1289.

Spaulding-Albright N. A review of some herbal and related products commonly used in cancer patients. *J Am Diet Assoc*. 1997;97:S208-S215.

University of Texas Center for Alternative Medicine Research in Cancer. Cat's claw summary. University of Texas-Houston Health Science Center Web site. Available at: http://www.sph.uth.tmc.edu/utcam/summary/cat.htm. Accessed May 8, 2000.

Celandine

Other common name(s)	Scientific/medical name(s)
Greater Celandine, Ukrain®, Common Celandine, Tetterwort, Celandine Poppy	*Chelidonium majus*

DESCRIPTION

The celandine plant, a member of the poppy family, grows in Europe and the temperate and subarctic regions of Asia. The root and aerial parts of the plant are used in herbal remedies. Ukrain, promoted as a cancer drug, is a semisynthetic compound formed by chemically combining alkaloids (complex, biologically active, nitrogen-containing compounds) from the plant celandine with thiophosphoric acid derivatives.

OVERVIEW

There is no scientific evidence that celandine, or any synthetic compound derived from the plant, is effective in treating cancer in humans. Animal studies conducted in other countries found that Ukrain had some positive effects; however, there have been no clinical trials to determine if the results apply to humans. Celandine might cause hepatitis when used as an herbal preparation.

How is it promoted for use?

Celandine is promoted for use in the prevention of gallstones, and the treatment of gastrointestinal problems, liver disease, digestive disorders, and eye irritation. Externally, practitioners have used it to remove warts. Supporters have also used celandine as part of antiviral agents to treat herpes, HIV, and the Epstein-Barr virus. There is no scientific evidence to support these claims.

Proponents claim Ukrain improves the overall health of people with several types of cancer including lung, colon, kidney, ovarian, breast, brain, and skin cancer. They further claim it helps people with cancer live longer by boost-

Herbs / Vitamins / Minerals

ing the immune system and inhibiting tumor growth without any of the major side effects of conventional cancer treatment. Ukrain supposedly keeps cancer cells from getting air and nutrients, causing them to die, and leaves healthy cells undamaged. Proponents also claim that it protects cells from radiation damage; however, there is no scientific evidence for these claims.

What does it involve?

Celandine is on the Commission E (Germany's regulatory agency for herbs) list of approved herbs and it is sold as a whole plant, top, or just the root, and as an extract, tincture, or tea. It is also sold in health food stores and over the Internet. The average dosage is 2-5 g/day. It can be taken internally or used externally.

Ukrain is administered through injection about 3 times a week for 15 to 20 days at a dosage of 5 to 20 mg. Ukrain is available in Europe and at alternative therapy clinics in the United States, or through mail order.

What is the history behind it?

Celandine has long been believed in folk literature to have disease-fighting effects. It has been especially popular in Russia, and as early as 1931 was claimed to be effective in some cases of cancer. A tincture of lower concentrations is used in homeopathy, mainly as a liver remedy (see Homeopathy).

Ukrain, a chemical combination of compounds from the plant celandine and thiophosphoric acid, was first developed in 1978 by J. W. Nowicky, a native of the Ukraine and director of the Ukrain Anticancer Institute of Vienna, Austria. He first presented it at the 13th International Congress of Chemotherapy in Vienna in 1983. It is named after the country Ukraine.

What is the evidence?

There is no scientific evidence to support any of the claims about the benefits of celandine. Some researchers in other countries have reported success using Ukrain before radiation treatments to increase the survival rates of rats. Animal studies may show a certain substance holds promise as a beneficial treatment, but fur-ther studies are necessary to determine if the results apply to humans.

There have been some case reports suggesting that treatment with Ukrain may decrease tumor size and provide an improvement in overall health (increased appetite, reduced pain in joints, reduced fever) for people with cancer. However, response and survival rates claimed by these reports are often higher than what is actually possible with the combination of chemotherapy drugs currently available in the United States. Virtually all of the animal and human studies have been published by research affiliated with the institution where Ukrain was developed. The size and methodology of these studies are not considered by most cancer researchers to be sufficient for supporting the promoters' claims. Randomized clinical trials are needed to determine the safety and antitumor effects of Ukrain, if any, in humans.

Are there any possible problems or complications?

Researchers recently found that celandine is often prescribed as an herbal medicine for stomach problems and may be responsible for many unexplained cases of hepatitis.

There are also reports that Ukrain has produced pain, nausea, thirst, and swelling in the tumor area. Women who are pregnant or breast-feeding should not use this herb. Relying on this type of treatment alone, and avoiding conventional medical care, may have serious health consequences.

References

Benninger J, Schneider HT, Schuppan D, Kirchner T, Hahn EG. Acute hepatitis induced by greater celandine (Chelidonium majus). *Gastroenterology*. 1999;117:1234-1237.

Blumenthal M, ed. *The Complete German Commission E Monographs: Therapeutic Guide to Herbal Medicines*. Austin, Tx: American Botanical Council; 1998.

Boyko VN, Levshina YeV. The influence of the novel drug Ukrain on hemo- and immunopoiesis at the time of its maximum radioprotective effect. *Drugs Exp Clin Res*. 1998;24:335-337.

Herbs / Vitamins / Minerals

Boyko VN, Levshina YeV. A study of the influence of the novel drug Ukrain on in vivo effects of low-dose ionizing radiation. *Drugs Exp Clin Res.* 1998;24:339-341.

Medical Economics. *PDR for Herbal Medicines.* Montvale, NJ: Medical Economics Company; 1998.

Uglianitsa KN, Nefyodov LI, Brzosko W. Evaluation of the efficacy of Ukrain in the treatment of breast cancer: clinical and laboratory studies. *Drugs Exp Clin Res.* 1998;24:231-239.

Centella

Other common name(s)	Scientific/medical name(s)
Gotu Kola, Pennywort, Hydrocotyle, Talepetrako	*Centella asiatica*

DESCRIPTION

Centella is a swamp plant that grows naturally in Madagascar, India, Sri Lanka, Indonesia, and many parts of South Africa. Its dried leaves and stems are used in herbal remedies. Also known as gotu kola, centella is not related to the kola nut.

OVERVIEW

Centella is used in Ayurvedic and Chinese medicine to treat skin wounds (see Ayurveda and Chinese Herbal Medicine). There is no scientific evidence that centella is effective in treating cancer or any other disease.

How is it promoted for use?

Proponents claim that centella possesses numerous curative qualities. It has been said that the herb accelerates the healing of open wounds, burns, bedsores, and ulcers. There are claims that it can be used to relieve conditions caused by poor circulation, such as leg cramps, swelling, and phlebitis. Some practitioners maintain that centella reduces fever and relieves congestion caused by colds and upper respiratory infections. Some women use centella for birth control, and some herbalists claim that centella is an antidote for poison mushrooms and arsenic poisoning, and when applied externally, an effective treatment for snakebites, herpes sores, fractures, and sprains.

In some folk medicine traditions, centella is used to treat syphilis, rheumatism, leprosy, mental illness, and epilepsy. It is also used to stimulate urination and to relieve physical and mental exhaustion, diarrhea, eye diseases, inflammation, asthma, high blood pressure, liver disease, dysentery, urinary tract infections, eczema, and psoriasis. Some manufacturers of the herbal supplement claim centella can be used to treat cancer as well. There is no scientific evidence to support any of these claims.

What does it involve?

Centella is available in capsules, eye drops, extracts, powder, and ointments from health food stores and over the Internet. Dried centella can be made into a tea. Recommended dosage depends on the condition being treated.

What is the history behind it?

Centella has a long history in the folk medicines of India, Indonesia, Sri Lanka, and Madagascar. It has been used for generations in India to promote relaxation, improve memory, and aid meditation. In traditional Chinese medicine, the herb is believed to promote longevity. The Chinese name for centella translates to "fountain of youth." A Sri Lankan legend says that elephants live long because they eat centella. Today, centella is still widely used in these countries.

What is the evidence?

There is no clinical evidence to support the claims made for centella. A small number of laboratory studies conducted in India and Europe suggest that an ointment made from centella may speed up wound healing. One study in India reported that centella extract slowed the development of tumors in mice and increased their life span. Animal and laboratory studies may show a certain herb holds promise as a beneficial treatment, but further studies are necessary to determine if the results apply to humans. Also, extracted chemicals are not the same as the raw plant. Study results of extracts will not necessarily be consistent with studies using the raw plant.

Are there any possible problems or complications?

Centella is generally considered safe; however there are no clinical studies in humans to fully document side effects. When used directly on the skin, some possible side effects may include a burning sensation, itching, and drowsiness. Women who are pregnant or breast-feeding should not use this herb.

References

Awang DV. Gotu kola. *Can Pharm J.* 1998;131:42-46.

Babu TD, Kuttan G, Padikkala J. Cytotoxic and anti-tumour properties of certain taxa of Umbelliferae with special reference to Centella asiatica (L.) Urban. *J Ethnopharmacol.* 1995;48:53-57.

Fetrow CW, Avila JR. *Professional's Handbook of Complementary and Alternative Medicines.* Springhouse, PA: Springhouse Corp; 1999.

Medical Economics. *PDR For Herbal Medicine.* Montvale, NJ: Medical Economics Company Inc; 1998.

Cesium Chloride

Other common name(s)	Scientific/medical name(s)
High pH Therapy	CsCl

DESCRIPTION

Cesium is a rare, naturally occurring element of alkali metal similar in chemical structure to lithium, sodium, and potassium. Cesium chloride is a salt form of this element.

OVERVIEW

Radioactive cesium (cesium-137) is used in certain types of radiation therapy for cancer patients. However, there is no scientific evidence that non-radioactive cesium chloride supplements have any effect on tumors, and there have been some side effects reported.

How is it promoted for use?

Cesium can be absorbed by all cells, probably due to its similarity in chemical structure to potassium. Proponents claim the intracellular pH of tumor cells is usually very low (acidic) compared to normal cells, and that cesium chloride supplements increase the pH level of tumor cells back to a normal level, which may be detrimental to the cancer's growth. Since cesium chloride is claimed to work by raising the pH of the tumor cells, its use in therapy has been called "high pH therapy." There is no scientific evidence to support this theory.

What does it involve?

Cesium chloride supplements are available in pill form. Proponents suggest a dosage of 1-6 g/day. In a single case report describing the effect of short-term oral administration of cesium chloride in a healthy individual, 3 g of cesium chloride, dissolved in fluid, was taken after the morning and evening meals.

What is the history behind it?

Interest in cesium therapy began when scientists observed that certain regions of the world with low rates of certain cancers had a high concentration of alkali metals in the soil. As early as the 1920s, some researchers suggested cesium might be effective as an anti-tumor agent. However, further research in the 1930s suggested cesium had no effect on cancer cell growth. The use of cesium chloride for high pH therapy was first advanced in the 1980s.

What is the evidence?

There is no evidence that the intracellular pH of a cancer cell is any different than a normal cell, or that raising the pH of a malignant cell will lead to its death. Because of this, the underlining principle behind high pH therapy has not been proven. Although it was observed that certain areas with low rates of cancers had a high concentration of alkali metals in the soil, a direct benefit of dietary cesium in the protection from cancer has not been demonstrated.

Studies conducted in several experimental tumor models in the 1980s found that the administration of cesium or cesium chloride lead to reductions in tumor growth and mortality in certain tumor-bearing mice such as those with sarcoma or breast cancer. In laboratory animals, chronic ingestion of cesium caused blood and neuromuscular effects, and even death. Animal and laboratory studies may show a substance has toxic effects, but further studies are necessary to determine if the results apply to humans. More research is needed to determine the benefit of cesium, if any, for people with cancer.

Are there any possible problems or complications?

Cesium chloride is not considered toxic. However, the acute and chronic toxicity of this substance is not fully known. Consuming large amounts of cesium could result in nausea and diarrhea. Based on results of animal studies, women who are pregnant or breast-feeding should avoid taking cesium chloride supplements. Relying on this type of treatment alone, and avoiding conventional medical care, may have serious health consequences.

References

El-Domeiri AA, Messiha FS, Hsia WC. Effect of alkali metal salts on Sarcoma I in A/J mice. *J Surg Oncol.* 1981;18:423-429.

Messiha FS. Developmental toxicity of cesium in the mouse. *Gen Pharmacol.* 1994;25:395-400.

Messiha FS, Stocco DM. Effect of cesium and potassium salts on survival of rats bearing Novikoff hepatoma. *Pharmacol Biochem Behav.* 1984;21:31-34.

Neulieb R. Effect of oral intake of cesium chloride: a single case report. *Pharmacol Biochem Behav.* 1984;21:15-16.

Pinsky C, Bose R. Pharmacological and toxicological investigations of cesium. *Pharmacol Biochem Behav.* 1984;21:17-23.

Sartori HE. Nutrients and cancer: an introduction to cesium therapy. *Pharmacol Biochem Behav.* 1984;21:7-10.

Chamomile

Other common name(s)	Scientific/medical name(s)
German Chamomile, Hungarian Chamomile	*Matricaria chamomilla, Matricaria recutita, Chamomilla recutita*

DESCRIPTION

Chamomile is a daisy-like flower. The active compounds in German and Hungarian chamomile are extracted and used in herbal remedies. Other varieties of the plant, such as Roman or English Chamomile (Chamaemelum nobile), which contain similar compounds, are not used as often for herbal remedies.

OVERVIEW

Chamomile has not been found to be useful in reducing the side effects of cancer treatment. The effectiveness of chamomile for sedation, inflammation, and intestinal cramps has not been proven in human clinical trials, and its use has resulted in many allergic reactions.

How is it promoted for use?

In traditional folk medicine, chamomile has been promoted as a treatment for a long list of ailments. Today, it is most commonly promoted as a sedative to induce sleep and to soothe gastrointestinal discomfort caused by spasms and inflammation. Some proponents also claim chamomile calms the mind, eases stress, reduces pain from swollen joints and rheumatoid arthritis, speeds the healing of wounds, and can be used to reduce skin inflammation caused by sunburn, rashes, eczema, and dermatitis. The herb is also used to treat menstrual disorders, migraine headaches, eye irritation, and hemorrhoids. There is no scientific evidence to support these claims.

What does it involve?

Commission E (Germany's regulatory agency for herbs) has approved the use of German chamomile for gastrointestinal spasms, and skin and mucous membrane inflammation.

They recommend using it as a tea steeped for 5-10 minutes in hot water 3 or 4 times a day. It is also available in capsules and liquid extracts.

Bandages containing chamomile are sometimes placed over wounds.

What is the history behind it?

Chamomile has been used in herbal remedies for thousands of years. The Anglo-Saxons believed that it was one of nine sacred herbs given to humans by the god Woden. The herb has also earned a place of high regard in some systems of traditional medicine.

What is the evidence?

Research has failed to show the effectiveness of chamomile in managing the side effects of cancer treatment. In a randomized clinical trial, researchers concluded that chamomile did not decrease stomatitis (inflammation of the mouth) caused by the cancer drug 5-fluorouracil. Another randomized clinical trial found that radiation-induced skin reactions were not affected in areas treated with chamomile.

Animal studies have suggested that chamomile is effective in inducing sleep, and reducing inflammation and intestinal cramps; however, these effects have not been clearly demonstrated in humans. In a small clinical study, chamomile extract was found to be effective in inducing deep sleep in 10 of 12 people who were about to undergo cardiac catheterization. But, according to Commission E, there is no clinical evidence to support the use of German chamomile as a sedative.

Are there any possible problems or complications?

Some researchers report that allergic reactions to chamomile are relatively common and can result in abdominal cramps, airway obstruction, itching, and other symptoms. People who have severe allergies to ragweed should use it with caution. Chamomile may interact with blood thinning medications, such as warfarin. People taking these medications should consult their physician before using chamomile. It should also not be taken with alcohol or other sedatives. Women who are pregnant or breastfeeding should not use this herb.

References

Blumenthal M, ed. *The Complete German Commission E Monographs: Therapeutic Guide to Herbal Medicines.* Austin, Tx: American Botanical Council; 1998.

Fetrow CW, Avila JR. *Professional's Handbook of Complementary and Alternative Medicines.* Springhouse, Pa: Springhouse Corp; 1999.

Fidler P, Loprinzi CL, O'Fallon JR, et al. Prospective evaluation of a chamomile mouthwash for prevention of 5-FU-induced oral mucositis. *Cancer.* 1996;77:522-525.

Miller L. Herbal medicinals: selected clinical considerations focusing on known or potential drug-herb interactions. *Arch Intern Med.* 1998;158:2200-2211.

O'Hara M, Kiefer D, Farrell K, Kemper K. A review of 12 commonly used medicinal herbs. *Arch Fam Med.* 1998;7:523-536.

Chaparral

Other common name(s)	**Scientifi/medical name(s)**
Greasewood, Creosote Bush	*Larrea divericata coville,* *Larrea tridentata (DC) coville*

DESCRIPTION

Chaparral is an herb that comes from the leaves of the creosote bush, an evergreen desert shrub. The term "chaparral" refers to a plant community dominated by evergreen shrubs that have small, stiff leaves and grow in dense clusters to heights of 4-8 ft in the American West and Southwest.

OVERVIEW

Chaparral is considered a dangerous herb that can cause irreversible, life-threatening liver damage. The FDA has cautioned against the internal use of chapparal. Research has not found it to be an effective treatment for cancer or any other disease. A study of nordihydroguaiaretic acid (NDGA), one of the chemicals in chaparral, concluded that it was not useful in treating people with cancer. Researchers continue to study NDGA in laboratory experiments.

How is it promoted for use?

Proponents claim that chaparral can help relieve pain, reduce inflammation, aid congestion, increase urine elimination, and slow the aging process. It is also promoted as an anticancer agent and an antioxidant (a compound that blocks the action of activated oxygen molecules, known as free radicals, that can damage cells). There is no scientific evidence to support these claims.

Some researchers think NDGA might make other anti-cancer drugs more effective, but this theory still needs to be tested in animal studies and in clinical trials of people with cancer.

What does it involve?

Chaparral is distributed in capsule or tablet form. Chaparral is also made into a tea, which is bitter and has an unpleasant taste. Chaparral is also sometimes found in combination with other herbs in a variety of teas.

What is the history behind it?

Native Americans used chaparral as an herbal remedy. They heated the leaves and applied them to the skin to treat wounds, bronchitis, coughs, skin disorders, venereal sores, warts, blemishes, and ringworm. Heated stems were inserted into tooth cavities to relieve pain, and the leaves and stems were boiled to make tea to relieve rheumatism and other conditions, including colds, bronchitis, digestive problems, and cancer.

According to anecdotal reports, chaparral tea was used widely in the United States as an alternative anticancer agent from the late 1950s to the 1970s. Experimental studies in the 1960s showed that chaparral could cause problems with kidney and liver function. The growth of interest in alternative medicine led to increased use of chaparral in the 1980s. By the early 1990s, there had been many reports of chaparral-associated illnesses, and the FDA issued a warning, resulting in the voluntary removal of many chaparral products from stores. Despite many concerns and warnings, chaparral became more readily available again in 1998.

What is the evidence?

Chaparral does not prevent or inhibit the growth of cancer in humans. It has not been found to be an effective treatment for any other medical condition, although most research has focused on the relationship between chaparral and cancer. Some laboratory studies have indicated that one of the chemicals in chaparral, NDGA, may possess anticancer properties. However, evidence from human clinical trials has not confirmed these findings.

According to a 1990 government report, some researchers reported that NDGA inhibited cancer growth in animals, but other investigators found that low levels of NDGA actually stimulated the growth of some types of tumor cells (although higher concentrations had the opposite effect). More recent cell culture studies (using cancer cells grown in the laboratory) suggest NDGA may make other anti-cancer drugs more effective, and researchers continue to look into the potential uses of purified NDGA. Animal and laboratory studies may show that a certain substance holds promise as a beneficial treatment, but further studies are necessary to determine if the results apply to humans.

In 1970, the National Cancer Institute published results of a study on chaparral tea and NDGA. People with advanced, incurable cancer drank chaparral tea or took oral doses of pure NDGA. Of the 45 people who were evaluated, 4 experienced a decrease in the size (regression) of tumors. The regression lasted between 10 days and 20 months. However, in others, treatment with chaparral appeared to cause tumor growth. Overall, the authors concluded that chaparral tea was not an effective anticancer agent.

One case study reported that a 60-year-old woman who took chaparral for 10 months developed severe hepatitis and eventually required a liver transplant. In a subsequent review of 18 case reports of adverse reactions associated with the ingestion of chaparral, researchers concluded that the herb is linked with acute and chronic irreversible liver damage and liver failure.

Are there any possible problems or complications?

Chaparral is highly toxic and can cause severe and permanent liver disease that is sometimes fatal. In 1968, the FDA recommended that the herb not be taken internally. Other side effects of chaparral use can include fatigue, stomach pain, diarrhea, weight loss, fever, and itching. This herb should be avoided, especially by women who are pregnant or breast-feeding.

References

Ding XZ, Kuszynski CA, El-Metwally TH, Adrian TE. Lipoxygenase inhibition induced apoptosis, morphological changes, and carbonic anhydrase expression in human pancreatic cancer cells. *Biochem Biophys Res Commun.* 1999;266:392-399.

Fetrow CW, Avila JR. *Professional's Handbook of Complementary and Alternative Medicines.* Springhouse, Pa: Springhouse Corp; 1999.

Gordon DW, Rosenthal G, Hart J, Sirota R, Baker AL. Chaparral ingestion. The broadening spectrum of liver injury caused by herbal medications. *JAMA.* 1995;273:489-490.

Sheikh NM, Philen RM, Love LA. Chaparral-associated hepatotoxicity. *Arch Intern Med.* 1997;157:913-919.

Soriano AF, Helfrich B, Chan DC, Heasley LE, Bunn PA Jr, Chou TC. Synergistic effects of new chemopreventive agents and conventional cytotoxic agents against human lung cancer cell lines. *Cancer Res.* 1999;59:6178-6184.

US Congress, Office of Technology Assessment. *Unconventional Cancer Treatments.* Washington, DC: US Government Printing Office; 1990. Publication OTA-H-405.

Chinese Herbal Medicine

Other common name(s)	Scientific/medical name(s)
Traditional Chinese Medicine, Chinese Herbs	None

DESCRIPTION

Chinese herbal medicine is a major aspect of traditional Chinese medicine, which focuses on restoring a balance of energy, body, and spirit to maintain health rather than treating a particular disease or medical condition. Herbs are presumably used to restore balance by nourishing the body.

OVERVIEW

Because of the large number of Chinese herbs used and the different uses recommended by practitioners, it is difficult to comment on Chinese herbal medicine as a whole. There may be some individual herbs or extracts that play a role in the prevention and treatment of cancer and other diseases when combined with conventional treatment. However, more research is needed to determine the effectiveness of these individual substances.

Herbs / Vitamins / Minerals

How is it promoted for use?

Chinese herbal medicine is not based on Western conventional concepts of medical diagnosis and treatment. It treats patients' main complaints or the patterns of their symptoms rather than the underlying causes. Practitioners attempt to prevent and treat imbalances, such as those caused by cancer and other diseases, with complex combinations of herbs, minerals, and plant extracts.

Chinese herbal medicine uses a variety of herbs, in different combinations, to restore balance to the body (see Astragalus, Ginkgo, Ginseng, Green Tea, and Siberian Ginseng). Herbal preparations are said to prevent and treat hormone disturbances, infections, breathing disorders, and a vast number of other ailments and diseases. Some practitioners claim herbs have the power to prevent and treat a variety of cancers, including melanoma (a type of skin cancer), renal cell carcinoma (kidney cancer), lymphoma (cancer of the lymph system), leukemia (cancer of the white blood cells), osteosarcoma (bone cancer), colon and rectal cancer, lung cancer, breast cancer, ovarian cancer, and bladder cancer. There is no scientific evidence to support these claims.

Most Chinese herbalists do not claim to cure cancer. They use herbal medicine along with conventional treatment prescribed by oncologists, such as radiation therapy and chemotherapy. They claim that herbal remedies can help ease the side effects of conventional cancer therapies, control pain, improve quality of life, strengthen the immune system, and in some cases, stop tumor growth and spread.

What does it involve?

In China, there are over 3,200 herbs, 300 mineral and animal extracts, and over 400 formulas used. Herbal formulations may consist of 4 to 12 different ingredients, to be taken in the form of teas, powders, pills, tinctures, or syrups.

Chinese herbal remedies are made up of one or two herbs that are said to have the greatest effect on major aspects of the problem being treated. The other herbs in the formula treat minor aspects of the problem, direct the formula to specific parts of the body, and help the other herbs work more efficiently.

With the increase in popularity of herbal use, many Chinese herbs are sold individually and in formulas. In the United States, Chinese herbs and herbal formulas may be purchased in health food stores, some pharmacies, and from herbal medicine practitioners.

What is the history behind it?

Native cultures all over the world have traditionally used herbs to maintain health and treat illnesses. Chinese herbal medicine developed with Chinese culture from tribal roots. By 200 BC, traditional Chinese medicine was firmly established, and by the first century AD, a listing of medicinal herbs and herbal formulations had been developed.

The classic Chinese book on medicinal herbs was written during the Ming Dynasty (1152-1578) by Li Shi-Zhen. It listed nearly 2,000 herbs and extracts. By 1990, the latest edition of *The Pharmacopoeia of the People's Republic of China* listed more than 500 single herbs or extracts and nearly 300 complex formulations.

As Western conventional medicine spread to the East, some traditional Chinese medical practices began to be regarded as folklore. However, since 1949, the Chinese government has supported the use of both traditional and Western medicine. Chinese herbal medicine first came to widespread attention in the United States in the 1970s, when President Nixon visited China. Today, at least 30 states license practitioners of Oriental medicine and more than 25 colleges of Oriental medicine exist in the United States.

What is the evidence?

Some herbs and herbal formulations have been evaluated in animal, laboratory, and human studies in both the East and the West with wide-ranging results. Experts at the University of Texas Center for Alternative Medicine Research in Cancer conducted an extensive review of the research that has been done with Chinese herbs and cancer. They identified over 450 studies. Research results vary widely depending on the specific herb. A wide variety of herbs have also been studied in China.

There is some evidence from randomized clinical trials that some Chinese herbs may contribute to longer survival rates, reduction of side effects, and lower recurrence for some cancers, especially when combined with conventional treatment. Many of these studies, however, are published in Chinese, and some of them do not list the specific herbs that were tested. More controlled research is needed to determine the role of Chinese herbal medicine in cancer treatment and prevention.

Are there any possible problems or complications?

Because of the variety of herbs used in Chinese herbal medicine, there is a potential for negative interactions with prescribed drugs. Some herbal preparations contain other ingredients which are not always identified. The FDA recently issued a statement warning diabetics to avoid several specific brands of Chinese herbal products because they illegally contain the prescription diabetes drugs glyburide and phenformin. In the last five years, Chinese herbal medicines have become the leading cause of hepatotoxicity (liver damage) from herbs.

Of the more than 5,000 medicinal plant species in China, a small number are potentially toxic (poisonous) to the human body. Toxic herbs may mistakenly be harvested and shipped for herbal medicines and cause harmful reactions in those who take the medicines. In addition, the herbal formulas used are often complex and difficult for manufacturers and practitioners to formulate correctly. Women who are pregnant or breast-feeding should consult their physician before using any of the herbs.

References

Alternative Medicine: Expanding Medical Horizons. *A Report to the National Institutes of Health on Alternative Medical Systems and Practices in the United States.* Washington, DC: US Government Printing Office; 1994. NIH publication 94-066.

Boik J. *Cancer and Natural Medicine: A Textbook of Basic Science and Clinical Research.* Princeton, Minn: Oregon Medical Press; 1995.

Cassileth B. *The Alternative Medicine Handbook.* New York, NY: W. W. Norton & Co; 1998.

Miller LG. Herbal medicinals: selected clinical considerations focusing on known or potential drug-herb interactions. *Arch Intern Med.* 1998;158:2200-2211.

Shad JA, Chinn CG, Brann OS. Acute hepatitis after ingestion of herbs. *South Med J.* 1999;92:1095-1097.

University of Texas Center for Alternative Medicine Research in Cancer. Traditional Chinese medicine. University of Texas-Houston Health Science Center Web site. Available at: http://www.sph.uth.tmc.edu/utcam/therapies/tcm.htm. Accessed May 8, 2000..

Chlorella

Other common name(s)	Scientific/medical name(s)
Sun Chlorella, Green Algae	*Chlorella pyrenoidosa, Chlorella vulgaris*

DESCRIPTION

Chlorella is a single-celled freshwater algae. It reportedly contains a very high amount of chlorophyll, the chemical that gives plants their green color and is an essential component in photosynthesis, the process by which plants convert light into chemical energy.

OVERVIEW

Chlorella is widely used in Japan for a variety of health conditions; however, there have been no studies that prove its effectiveness for preventing or treating cancer or any other disease.

How is it promoted for use?

Chlorella is promoted for a wide range of herbal remedy uses. Proponents claim it kills several types of cancers, fights bacterial and viral infections, enhances the immune system, increases the growth of "friendly" organisms in the digestive tract, lowers blood pressure and cholesterol levels, and promotes healing of intestinal ulcers, diverticulosis, and Crohn's disease.

Supporters state that chlorella supplements increase the level of albumin in the bloodstream. Albumin is a protein that promoters claim is protective against diseases such as cancer, diabetes, arthritis, AIDS, pancreatitis, cirrhosis, hepatitis, anemia, and multiple sclerosis. Chlorella is said to prevent cancer through its ability to cleanse the body of toxins. There is no scientific evidence to support these claims.

Chlorella contains vitamin C and carotenoids, both of which are antioxidants (see Beta Carotene and Vitamin C). Antioxidants are compounds that block the action of activated oxygen molecules, known as free radicals, that can damage cells. According to proponents, chlorella also contains high concentrations of B-complex vitamins, which may help to relieve stress (see Vitamin B Complex). Some herbalists claim that chlorella stimulates macrophages, the immune system cells that attack and consume invading organisms; however, this has not been proven.

What does it involve?

Chlorella is available in tablets, liquid extracts, and powder. Some herbalists recommend up to 3 g/day (15 tablets). Although it may be taken on its own, many supporters suggest mixing the powder form of chlorella into foods made with flour, such as bread or cookies.

What is the history behind it?

Chlorella was discovered in the late 19th century. Due to its high protein concentration and rapid growth rate, chlorella was investigated after World War II as a possible commercial food source. In the 1950s, researchers first reported that chlorella prevented the development of liver disease in mice. A decade later, some investigators claimed that the algae decreased the side effects of chemotherapy and slowed the growth of some cancer cells. Most of the research has been conducted in Japan, where chlorella is a top-selling dietary supplement.

What is the evidence?

There is no scientific evidence showing that chlorella is effective against cancer or any other disease. Limited laboratory and animal research suggests that the algae may have some anticancer properties. One investigation concluded that a protein extract from one type of chlorella prevented the spread of cancer cells in mice. Another study in mice suggested that the extract reduced the side effects of chemotherapy treatment without affecting the potency of anticancer medications.

Extracted chemicals are not the same as the raw plant, so study results of extracts will not necessarily be consistent with studies using the raw plant. Also, animal and laboratory studies may show a certain therapy holds promise as a beneficial treatment, but further studies are necessary to determine if the results apply to humans.

Are there any possible problems or complications?

Although chlorella appears to be safe, no research has been done in humans to determine if the supplement causes any negative side effects or what can be expected from long-term use.

References

Konishi F, Mitsuyama M, Okuda M, Tanaka K, Hasegawa T, Nomoto K. Protective effect of an acidic glycoprotein obtained from culture of Chlorella vulgaris against myelo-suppression by 5-fluorouracil. *Cancer Immunol Immunother.* 1996;42:268-274.

Tanaka K, Yamada A, Noda K, Hasegawa T, et al. A novel glycoprotein obtained from Chlorella vulgaris strain CK22 show antimetastatic immunopotentiation. *Cancer Immunol Immunother.* 1998;45:313-320.

Cloves

Other common name(s)	Scientific/medical name(s)
Clove Oil, Oil of Cloves	*Syzygium aromaticum, Caryophyllum, Eugenia caryophyllata, Eugenia aromatica*

DESCRIPTION

The clove is an aromatic spice that grows as an evergreen tree in the tropical regions of Asia and South America. The oil extracted from the plant, leaves, flower buds, and fruit itself is used in herbal remedies.

OVERVIEW

There is no scientific evidence that cloves or clove oil are effective in treating or preventing cancer. Some dentists and patients report that clove oil may relieve gum and tooth pain and may be useful as a topical antiseptic in mouthwash; however, there is limited scientific evidence for this.

How is it promoted for use?

Cloves are said to have antiseptic (germ killing) and anesthetic (pain-relieving) properties. Undiluted clove oil is often applied topically to relieve pain from toothaches and insect bites. Some proponents also claim that, taken internally, cloves and clove oil combat fungal infections, relieve nausea and vomiting, improve digestion, fight intestinal parasites, stimulate uterine contractions, ease arthritis inflammation, stop migraine headaches, and ease symptoms of colds and allergies. Practitioners of traditional Chinese medicine sometimes treat hiccups and impotence with cloves (see Chinese Herbal Medicine).

One herbalist claims that a mixture of cloves, black walnut hulls, and wormwood cures cancer (see Black Walnut and Wormwood). Others claim that cloves contain antioxidants, compounds that block the action of activated oxygen molecules, known as free radicals, that can damage cells. There is no scientific evidence to support these claims.

What does it involve?

Cloves are available in capsules, powder, or as a whole herb. Pure and diluted clove oil can also be purchased.

What is the history behind it?

Cloves and clove oil were reportedly used in Chinese medicine as early as 600 AD. Since then, cloves have been a part of various folk medicine traditions around the world. Today, cloves are also used in baking and cooking, and as an ingredient in perfumes, cigarettes, and toothpaste.

What is the evidence?

Commission E (Germany's regulatory agency for herbs) approved clove oil for use as an antiseptic and topical anesthetic. However, no well-controlled clinical studies have been done to evaluate the potential antibacterial, anticarcinogenic, and pain-relieving properties of cloves or clove oil in humans.

Very limited laboratory studies conducted in other countries suggest that clove oil may fight bacteria and prevent convulsions. Another laboratory study suggested that compounds taken from cloves show promise as potential anticarcinogenic agents. However, extracted chemicals are not the same as the raw plant. Study results of extracts will not necessarily be consistent with studies using the raw plant. Also, laboratory studies may show a certain compound holds promise as a beneficial treatment, but further studies are necessary to determine if the results apply to humans.

Are there any possible problems or complications?

Cloves are generally considered safe, although a relatively small number of people may be allergic to eugenol, the main active ingredient. Excessive application of undiluted clove oil on or near the teeth may cause damage to dental pulp and other soft tissue surrounding teeth. It should be used for tooth and gum conditions only under the supervision of a dentist.

References

Fetrow CW, Avila JR. *Professional's Handbook of Complementary and Alternative Medicines.* Springhouse, Pa: Springhouse Corp; 1999.

Medical Economics Company. *PDR for Herbal Medicines.* Montvale, NJ: Medical Economics Company; 1998:1167-1168.

Perez C, Anesini C. Antibacterial activity of alimentary plants against Staphylococcus aureus growth. *Am J Chin Med.* 1994;22:169-174.

Pourgholami MH, Kamalinejad M, Javadi M, Majzoob S, Sayyah M. Evaluation of the anticonvulsant activity of the essential oil of Eugenia caryophyllata in male mice. *J Ethnopharmacol.* 1999;64:167-171.

Zheng GQ, Kenney PM, Lam LK. Sesquiterpenes from clove (Eugenia caryophyllata) as potential anticarcinogenic agents. *J Nat Prod.* 1992;55:999-1003.

Comfrey

Other common name(s)	Scientific/medical name(s)
Blackwort, Bruisewort, Knitbone, Slippery Root	*Symphtum officinale*

DESCRIPTION

Comfrey is a fast-growing herb native to Europe and temperate parts of Asia. It now grows in North America as well. The roots and leaves are used in herbal remedies.

OVERVIEW

Although comfrey has been used in folk medicine for many years to help heal wounds, sprains, and fractures, there have been no studies in humans to prove that it is useful. There is also no evidence that comfrey is effective in treating cancer. It is not safe for internal use and should not be consumed.

How is it promoted for use?

Comfrey has been promoted mainly to speed the healing of wounds, sprains, bruises, and bone fractures, and to reduce inflammation and swelling related to these injuries.

Comfrey has also been used to treat a number of other ailments, including gastrointestinal ulcers, gallstones, arthritis, colitis, pleurisy, and insect bites. A mouthwash made from comfrey is sometimes used to heal gum disease, hoarseness, and pharyngitis. Some proponents also claim comfrey has anticancer properties; however, there is no scientific evidence to support these claims.

What does it involve?

Commission E (Germany's regulatory agency for herbs) has approved comfrey for external use only to treat bruises and sprains. Ointments, compresses, and poultices are made from the crushed roots and leaves of comfrey or from liquid extracts pressed out of the plant. They are placed directly on bruises, wounds, or sprains, are covered with a dressing, and replaced daily until healing occurs. For internal use, dried comfrey is sometimes prepared as a tea, but is also available in tinctures and capsules. However, since it has the potential to cause liver damage, comfrey should not be taken internally.

What is the history behind it?

Comfrey has been used since the 16th century for wound healing, inflammation, gout, ulcers, gangrene, burns, sprains, and fractures. In folk medicine, comfrey has been used to treat conditions such as arthritis, colitis, diarrhea, gallstones, and pleurisy. A few practitioners experimented with the use of comfrey to treat cancer in the 20th century.

What is the evidence?

There is no evidence showing that comfrey is useful in treating cancer or any other disease. The herb's influence on the healing of wounds, fractures, and other injuries in humans is not known.

When taken internally, comfrey can cause severe liver damage. Several studies have shown that comfrey contains chemicals called pyrrolizidine alkaloids, which cause severe liver damage. Animal studies have also shown that these chemicals lead to the development of liver tumors.

The internal use of comfrey is not considered safe. Experts strongly warn consumers not to eat or drink any preparations that contain comfrey. This herb should be avoided, especially by women who are pregnant or breast feeding. The US Pharmacopeia reports that the use of comfrey on broken skin should also be avoided because it may be absorbed into the body's system.

References

Blumenthal M, ed. *The Complete German Commission E Monographs: Therapeutic Guide to Herbal Medicines.* Austin, Tx: American Botanical Council; 1998.

Fetrow CW, Avila JR. *Professional's Handbook of Complementary and Alternative Medicines.* Springhouse, Pa: Springhouse Corp; 1999.

Medical Economics. *PDR for Herbal Medicines.* Montvale, NJ: Medical Economics Company; 1998.

Ridker PM, McDermott WV. Comfrey herb tea and hepatic veno-occlusive disease. *Lancet.* 1989;1:657-658.

The Standard: Use of comfrey discouraged. United States Pharmacopeia Web site. Available at: http://www.usp.org/aboutusp/standard/9801/9801_05.htm. Accessed October 7, 1999.

Unconventional Cancer Therapies: Manual for Patients. British Columbia Cancer Agency Web site. Available at: http://www.bccancer.bc.ca/uctm/08.html. Accessed October 7, 1999.

Copper

Other common name(s)	Scientific/medical name(s)
None	Cu

DESCRIPTION

Copper is a trace element found naturally in foods such as seafood, organ meats, green vegetables, and nuts. It assists in the regulation of blood pressure and heart rate, and the absorption of iron in the body.

OVERVIEW

Some laboratory and animal studies have found that copper has antioxidant properties and may have some anticancer effects. Other animal studies suggest that high copper levels may promote cancer formation and growth. Human studies are needed to determine what role, if any, copper may play in the prevention or treatment of cancer.

How is it promoted for use?

Some proponents claim copper helps cells in the immune system work properly. There are claims that copper aids the body in other functions such as the healing process, expelling toxins from the body, maintaining connective tissues, forming red blood cells, and preventing heart problems. A lack of copper in the body, some practitioners say, can lead to lowered resistance to infections and a shortened life span after infection. Copper is also used in some preparations of Iscador (a species of European mistletoe) for primary tumors of the liver, gallbladder, stomach and kidneys.

There are also claims that copper actually promotes cancer growth. Proponents of this theory recommend a low copper diet and use of chelating agents that bind to copper and promote its elimination from the body (see Chelation Therapy). There is no scientific evidence to support these claims.

What does it involve?
Copper supplements are available in pill form. However, nearly all people are able to get an adequate level of copper in their bodies by maintaining a balanced diet. Fruits and vegetables can contribute up to 30% of a person's total copper intake. The estimated minimum daily requirement is 2 mg.

What is the history behind it?
While research into the antioxidant properties of copper is quite recent, healing properties have long been attributed to copper in folk medicine. Today, many multivitamins and other herbal and mineral supplements include copper.

What is the evidence?
There have been no studies in humans to determine whether copper supplements are effective in preventing or treating cancer. Animal studies have shown that copper is useful in maintaining antioxidant defenses. Antioxidant compounds block the action of activated oxygen molecules, known as free radicals, that can damage cells. While the involvement of copper in the cancer process via antioxidant effects is still unclear, copper complexes have been shown to have anticancer properties in laboratory studies. Other laboratory and animal studies suggest that high copper levels may promote formation of liver cancer and stimulate growth of brain tumors. Animal and laboratory studies may show a certain substance holds promise as a beneficial treatment, but further studies are necessary to determine if the results apply to humans.

Are there any possible problems or complications?

Copper is a necessary nutrient for absorption of iron into the body. Copper supplements are considered safe; however, most people receive adequate copper intake from a normal balanced diet and do not require supplements. People with Wilson's Disease (a genetic disorder that develops from copper poisoning) should not take copper supplements or multivitamins containing copper. Diabetics should also avoid these supplements because copper can affect blood sugar levels. Copper toxicity is rare; however, a dosage over 35 mg/day is considered toxic.

References
Cassileth B. *The Alternative Medicine Handbook*. New York, NY: W. W. Norton & Co; 1998.

Davis CD, Feng Y. Dietary copper, manganese and iron affect the formation of aberrant crypts in colon of rats administered 3,2'-dimethyl-4-aminobiphenyl. *J Nutr.* 1999;129;1060-1067.

DiSilvestro RA, Sakamoto K, Milner JA. No effects of low copper intake on rat mammary tissue superoxide dismutase 1 activity and mammary chemical carcinogenesis. *Nutr Cancer.* 1998;31:218-220.

Flint V. Contraindications and possible adverse effects of therapeutic diets and supplements. WebMD Web site. Available at: http://www.webmd.com. Accessed February 23, 2000.

Martin-Lagos F, Navarro-Alarcon M, Terres-Martos C, Lopez-G de la Serrana H, Lopez-Martinez MC. Serum copper and zinc concentrations in serum from patients with cancer and cardiovascular disease. *Sci Total Environ* 1997;204:27-35.

Renault E, Deschatrette J. Alterations of rat hepatoma cell genomes induced by copper deficiency. *Nutr Cancer* 1997;29:242-247.

Spencer JW, Jacobs JJ. *Complementary/Alternative Medicine: An Evidence-Based Approach*. St. Louis, MO: Mosby, Inc; 1999.

Strain JJ. Putative role of dietary trace elements in coronary heart disease and cancer. *Br J Biomed Sci.* 1994;51:241-251.

US Congress, Office of Technology Assessment. *Unconventional Cancer Treatments*. Washington, DC: US Government Printing Office; 1990. Publication OTA-H-405 .

Echinacea

Other common name(s)	Scientific/medical name(s)
Purple Cone Flower, Kansas Snakeroot, Black Sampson	Echinacea purpurea, Echinacea angustifolia, Echinacea pallida

DESCRIPTION

Echinacea is an herb that grows wild primarily in the Great Plains and eastern regions of North America. It is also cultivated in Europe. There are three different species of the plant used in herbal remedies. Echinacea purpurea is the most frequently used for research and treatment. Liquid extracts are made from the leaves and roots, or from the whole plant.

OVERVIEW

Although Echinacea has been widely promoted to help fight colds and flu, there is little scientific evidence that it helps boost the immune system. There is also no evidence showing that Echinacea increases resistance to cancer or alleviates the side effects of chemotherapy or radiation therapy. When used longer than eight weeks, Echinacea can cause liver damage.

How is it promoted for use?

Echinacea is promoted mainly as a treatment for colds, the flu, and other respiratory infections. In Germany, Echinacea is a common over-the-counter medication and more than 300 Echinacea products are reportedly sold. Commission E (Germany's regulatory agency for herbs) approved Echinacea for treating respiratory infections, urinary tract infections, and poorly healing wounds.

It is also claimed that Echinacea boosts the body's immune system by stimulating the activity of macrophages (immune system cells that attack and consume invading organisms), which can attack cancer cells. Some claim that the herb stimulates the anticancer activity of natural killer cells (a type of white blood cell) and therefore could be used as a supplement to chemotherapy or radiation therapy. There is no scientific evidence to support these claims.

What does it involve?

Echinacea is available in capsule and liquid form; however, there is controversy over its usefulness in liquid form. Although dosage may vary, most practitioners recommend 900 mg/day for no longer than 8 weeks to boost the immune system. An injectable form is also available outside the United States.

What is the history behind it?

Echinacea has long been used in herbal remedies by Native Americans. In the 19th century, it became a commonly prescribed tonic and was billed as a natural remedy for infections and inflammation. The herb's use in the United States has surged along with interest in natural medicine. According to one source, Echinacea was the leading herb supplement sold in the United States in 1996 and 1997. In the United States, products commonly labeled under the name Echinacea can be completely different chemical preparations, due to the different species and plant parts used, different extraction methods, and the addition of other plant extracts.

What is the evidence?

Many practitioners and patients, particularly in

Europe, but also in the United States, are convinced that Echinacea has the ability to enhance the immune system and fight off infections from colds and the flu. However, the few reliable studies that have been published have shown mixed results. Two randomized clinical studies in Germany concluded that Echinacea did not significantly reduce the number, length, or severity of colds and respiratory infections compared to placebo (an inactive substance or treatment). Another German paper, which reviewed five prior Echinacea studies, stated that two of the studies showed Echinacea had promise as an anti-infection agent, but the other three found no such properties. A Swedish study of healthy individuals with colds found that one type of Echinacea was more effective than other preparations in reducing symptoms of colds. Both, however, were an effective treatment with low risk to the individual for colds.

In terms of how people with cancer use Echinacea, there is no reliable evidence proving Echinacea increases resistance to cancer or alleviates the immune suppression resulting from chemotherapy. Clearly, more research is needed before scientists can make firm conclusions about Echinacea's effectiveness and how much or what type of preparation to use.

Are there any possible problems or complications?

It is not clear whether the use of Echinacea is safe. Practitioners caution that Echinacea may cause liver damage, or suppress the immune system if used for more than eight weeks. They urge people taking medications known to cause liver toxicity, such as anabolic steroids, amiodarone (a drug for heart rhythm problems), and the chemotherapy drugs methotrexate and ketoconazole, to avoid Echinacea use. Others who should not take Echinacea include people with autoimmune disorders such as multiple sclerosis or HIV, people with leukemia, and women who are pregnant or breast-feeding.

References

Blumenthal M, ed. *The Complete German Commission E Monographs: Therapeutic Guide to Herbal Medicines.* Austin, Tx: American Botanical Council; 1998.

Brinkeborn RM, Shah DV, Degenring FH. Echinaforce and other Echinacea fresh plant preparations in the treatment of the common cold. A randomized, placebo controlled, double-blind clinical trial. *Phytomedicine.* 1999;6:1-6.

Grimm W, Muller, HH. A randomized controlled trial of the effect of fluid extract of Echinacea purpurea on the incidence and severity of colds and respiratory infections. *Am J Med.* 1999;106:138-143.

Melchart D, Linde K, Worku F, et al. Results of five randomized studies on the immunomodulatory activity of preparations of Echinacea. *J Altern Complement Med.* 1995; 1:145-160.

Melchart D, Walther E, Linde K, Brandmaier R, Lersch C. Echinacea root extracts for the prevention of upper respiratory infections: a double-blind, placebo-controlled randomized trial. *Arch Fam Med.* 1998;7:541-545.

Miller LG. Herbal medicinals: selected clinical considerations focusing on known or potential drug-herb interactions. *Arch Intern Med.* 1998;158:2200-2211.

O'Hara M, Kiefer D, Farrell K, Kemper K. A review of 12 commonly used medicinal herbs. *Arch Fam Med.* 1998;7:523-536.

Herbs / Vitamins / Minerals

Essiac Tea

Other common name(s)	Scientific/medical name(s)
Essiac®, Flor Essence®, Tea of Life®, Herbal Essence®, Vitalitea®	None

DESCRIPTION

Essiac is a mixture of herbs that are combined to make a tea. The original formula included burdock root, slippery elm inner bark, sheep sorrel, and Turkish rhubarb. Watercress, blessed thistle, red clover, and kelp were added to later recipes.

OVERVIEW

There have been no published clinical trials showing the effectiveness of Essiac in the treatment of cancer. Some of the specific herbs contained in the mixture have shown some anti-cancer effects in laboratory experiments. However, there is no scientific evidence to support its use for the treatment of cancer in humans.

How is it promoted for use?

Promoters claim Essiac strengthens the immune system, improves well being, relieves pain, increases appetite, reduces tumor size, and extends survival. Some also claim that it cleanses the blood, promotes cell repair, restores energy levels, and detoxifies the body. The different herbs are claimed to relieve inflammation, lubricate bones and joints, stimulate the stomach, and eliminate excess mucous in organs, tissues, lymph glands, and nerve channels.

It was originally claimed Essiac worked by changing tumors into normal tissue. Proponents claimed a tumor would become larger and harder after a few doses of Essiac, then it would soften, shrink, and be discharged by the body. There is no scientific evidence to support these claims.

What does it involve?

Essiac is available in dry and liquid formulas, and there are different methods of preparation and dosage according to various manufacturers. Some recommend spring or non-fluoridated water, and most require refrigeration after brewing. A typical dose is 1 oz taken 1 to 3 times per day. Practitioners advise that Essiac tea should be taken on an empty stomach, 2 hours before or after meals for at least 1-2 years.

Essiac is sold through mail order and is available in the United States in health food stores as a nutritional supplement. In Canada, Essiac cannot be sold or marketed as a drug and is only available directly from the manufacturer or, for people with advanced cancer, through Health Canada. However, Flor Essence (a leading competitor with a similar formulation) is sold in Canadian stores as an herbal tonic (but is not promoted as a cancer cure).

What is the history behind it?

In 1922, a public health nurse named Rene Caisse from Ontario, Canada learned about Essiac from one of her patients who claimed to have recovered from breast cancer by taking an Indian herbal tea developed by an Ojibwa medicine man. She obtained the recipe and reportedly treated her aunt's stomach cancer with the tea. In 1924, Caisse opened a clinic and began to offer cancer patients the herbal mixture, which she named Essiac (her last name spelled backwards). She treated thousands of patients using her secret formula as a tea and as an injection. Canadian medical authorities investigated the clinic in 1938 and concluded that there was little evidence for the effectiveness of Essiac. Caisse gave one of her formulas to a manufacturer in Toronto in 1977, one year before her death, with the intent of having it tested and sold for a reasonable cost.

Memorial Sloan-Kettering Cancer Center tested Essiac in 1959 and in the mid 1970s but no antitumor effects were verified. In 1983, Canadian federal health officials requested that Essiac be tested by the US National Cancer Institute (NCI). NCI found that no anticancer activity occurred in animals. Also at that time, Canadian health officials reviewed 86 case studies and concluded that there was no evidence that Essiac slowed the progression of cancer. They noted that there were few serious side effects, however, and that people may have benefited psychologically from the treatment.

What is the evidence?

Although there have been many testimonials, there have been no clinical trials proving the effectiveness of Essiac. One study found reduced tumor growth after giving oral and intravenous doses of Essiac to mice injected with human cancer cells. Also, some laboratory research found anticancer effects related to the specific herbs studied separately. Animal and laboratory studies may show a certain compound holds promise as a beneficial treatment, but further studies are necessary to determine if the results apply to humans.

Are there any possible problems or complications?

Serious side effects are uncommon. Essiac may have a laxative effect or cause increased urination in some people. If taken with food, it may also cause headache, nausea, diarrhea, and vomiting.

References

Alternative Medicine: Expanding Medical Horizons. *A Report to the National Institutes of Health on Alternative Medical Systems and Practices in the United States.* Washington, DC: US Government Printing Office; 1994. NIH publication 94-066.

Ernst E, Cassileth BR. How useful are unconventional cancer treatments? *Eur J Cancer.* 1999;35:1608-1613.

Kaegi E. Unconventional therapies for cancer: 1. Essiac. The task force on alternative therapies of the Canadian Breast Cancer Research Initiative. *CMAJ.* 1998;158:897-902.

University of Texas Center for Alternative Medicine Research in Cancer. Essiac summary. University of Texas-Houston Health Science Center Web site. Available at: http://www.sph.uth.tmc.edu/utcam/summary/essiac.htm. Accessed November 15, 1999.

US Congress, Office of Technology Assessment. *Unconventional Cancer Treatments.* Washington, DC: US Government Printing Office; 1990. Publication OTA-H-405.

Evening Primrose

Other common name(s)	Scientific/medical name(s)
Evening Primrose Oil	*Oenothera biennis*

DESCRIPTION

Evening primrose is a flowering plant originally native to North America that now grows throughout much of Europe and parts of Asia. It blooms every other year and its large, fragrant yellow flowers open at dusk and remain open through the night. In Germany, the plant is called "night candle" for this reason. The oil extracted from the seeds is used in herbal remedies.

OVERVIEW

There is no scientific evidence that evening primrose oil is effective in preventing or treating cancer. While the two essential fatty acids found in evening primrose play a role in health and disease, larger clinical studies are needed to determine whether the fatty acids in evening primrose oil are useful in treating cancer or other conditions.

How is it promoted for use?

Evening primrose is promoted as an herbal remedy for a very broad range of conditions, including dermatitis, premenstrual syndrome, eczema, inflammation, hyperactivity in children, high cholesterol, asthmatic cough, upset stomach, psoriasis, rheumatoid arthritis, and diabetic nerve damage. Some proponents also believe the plant has anti-cancer properties. Claims made for evening primrose are based on the fact that oil from the seeds contains two essential fatty acids which play a key role in many biological processes (see Gamma Linolenic Acid [GLA] and Omega-3 Fatty Acids).

What does it involve?

The oil can be purchased in capsules and gelcaps, and the powdered plant can be made into a tea. Daily doses of evening primrose oil have ranged from 2 to 16 capsules of 500 mg in clinical trials, although in one study up to 36 capsules per day were used.

What is the history behind it?

In folk medicine, evening primrose has been used to treat asthma, gastrointestinal disorders, whooping cough, and symptoms associated with premenstrual syndrome. The scientific name of the plant, *Oenothera biennis*, comes from two Greek words "oinos" (wine) and "thera" (hunt), because eating the roots was once believed to increase a person's appetite for wine. Folklore also says that evening primrose counters the effects of drinking too much wine. The use of evening primrose as an herbal remedy in modern times is relatively recent. Scientific research regarding its healing properties began in the 1980s.

What is the evidence?

There is very little evidence to support claims that evening primrose oil has any effect on cancer or any other disease. Results of studies of evening primrose oil for treating eczema, rheumatoid arthritis, and premenstrual syndrome have been either mixed or not favorable. Most research has been conducted in laboratory settings or involved small numbers of patients. One recent laboratory study concluded that evening primrose oil might help slow the growth of breast cancer in animal tumor models. Other laboratory studies have found that evening primrose oil slowed the growth of skin cancer cells, and a diet enriched with evening primrose oil was thought to enhance the body's ability to fight tumors. Animal and laboratory studies may show a certain substance holds promise as a beneficial treatment, but further studies are necessary to determine if the results apply to humans. Large-scale clinical trials involving humans are needed to determine the value of evening primrose or its constituent fatty acids in treating any specific condition.

Are there any possible problems or complications?

No significant health hazards have been identified with taking evening primrose. Headaches are reported as a possible side effect. One article reported that the acid in primrose oil (GLA) might lower seizure thresholds, so it should not be used with anticonvulsant medication. Women who are pregnant or breast-feeding should not use this herb.

References

Bown D. *Encyclopedia of Herbs & Their Uses.* New York, NY: DK Publishing Inc; 1995.

Fetrow CW, Avila JR. *Professional's Handbook of Complementary and Alternative Medicines.* Springhouse, Pa: Springhouse Corp; 1999.

Kleijnen J. Evening primrose oil. *BMJ.* 1994;309:824-825.

Medical Economics. *PDR for Herbal Medicines.* Montvale, NJ: Medical Economics Company; 1998.

Miller LG. Herbal medicinals: selected clinical considerations focusing on known or potential drug-herb interactions. *Arch Intern Med.* 1998;158:2200-2211.

Munoz SE, Lopez CB, Valentich MA, Eynard AR. Differential modulation by dietary n-6 or n-9 unsaturated fatty acids on the development of two murine mammary gland tumors having different metastatic capabilities. *Cancer Lett.* 1998.126:149-155.

Munoz SE, Piegari M, Guzman CA, Eynard AR. Differential effects of dietary Oenothera, Ziziphus mistol, and corn oils, and essential fatty acid deficiency on the progression of a murine mammary gland adenocarcinoma. *Nutrition.* 1999;15:208-212.

Flaxseed

Other common name(s)	Scientific/medical name(s)
Flaxseed Oil, Linseed, Lint Bells, Linum	*Linum usitatissimum*

DESCRIPTION
Flax is an annual plant cultivated for its fiber, which is used in making linen. Flaxseed and its oil are used in herbal remedies.

OVERVIEW
Flaxseed and its oil have been promoted since the 1950s as a dietary nutrient with anticancer properties. However, the only evidence for its possible ability to prevent cancer from occurring or growing comes from a limited number of animal studies. There is no scientific evidence that it is effective in preventing or treating cancer in humans.

How is it promoted for use?

Herbalists promote the use of flaxseed for constipation, abdominal problems, respiratory problems, sore throat, eczema, menstrual problems, and arthritis. The oil extracted from flaxseeds is said to lower cholesterol levels, boost the immune system, and prevent cancer. Flaxseed oil is high in alpha-linolenic acid, an omega-3 fatty acid, which is thought to have beneficial effects against cancer when consumed (see Omega-3 Fatty Acids).

Recently, attention has focused on the flaxseed itself, which is a rich source of lignans, compounds that can act as antiestrogens or as weak estrogens, which may play a role in preventing estrogen-dependent cancers, such as breast cancer, and other cancers. Lignans may also function as antioxidants and may slow cell growth by mechanisms not yet understood. When flaxseeds are consumed, the lignans are chemically converted into active forms by bacteria in the intestine.

What does it involve?

Flaxseed is available in flour, meal, and seed form. It may be found in some multi-grain breads, cereals, breakfast bars, and muffins. The toasted seeds are sometimes mixed into bread dough or sprinkled over salads, yogurt, or cereal. Flaxseed meal can be used in the same way. Flaxseed oil is available in many health food stores in liquid form and is sometimes mixed into cottage cheese. The oil is also available in softgel capsules.

What is the history behind it?

Flaxseed was cultivated by the Babylonians in 3000 BC. A German biochemist, Johanna Budwig, first brought attention to flaxseed oil as a treatment in the 1950s through a diet she devised for cancer patients. The diet was a strict regimen that avoided sugar, animal fats, salad oil, meats, butter, and margarine. The patients were given flaxseed oil mixed with cottage cheese and milk and meals high in fruits, vegetables, and fiber. She claimed that within three months, some patients on this diet had smaller tumors, some had no tumors left, and all felt better.

What is the evidence?

The evidence for an anticancer effect of flaxseed and flaxseed oil comes only from animal research, done primarily in mice and rats. No scientific, controlled human studies have been conducted. Researchers have found rats or mice fed flaxseed had significantly smaller and fewer tumor growths after they were injected with skin cancer or colon cancer cells. Other studies have shown flaxseed in the diet may reduce the risk of developing colon cancer and breast cancer among rats exposed to carcinogens. Animal and laboratory studies may show a certain substance holds promise as a beneficial treatment, but further studies are necessary to determine if the results apply to humans.

Are there any possible problems or complications?

Flaxseeds and flaxseed oil can spoil if they are not kept refrigerated. Some possible side effects include diarrhea, gas, and nausea. Flaxseed oil should not be used with other laxatives or stool softeners. People who have inflammatory disease of the intestine, esophagus, or stomach should avoid flaxseed. The immature pods of flaxseed are poisonous.

References

Cancernet. Just the flax, ma'am: researchers testing linseed. National Cancer Institute Web site. Available at: http://www.cancernet.nci.nih.gov. Accessed October 4, 1999.

Haggans CJ, Hutchins AM, Olson BA, Thomas W, Martini MC, Slavin JL. Effect of flaxseed consumption on urinary estrogen metabolites in postmenopausal women. *Nutr Cancer.* 1999;33:188-195.

Yan L, Yee JA, Li D, McGuire MH, Thompson LU. Dietary flaxseed supplementation and experimental metastasis of melanoma cells in mice. *Cancer Lett.* 1998;124:181-186.

Flower Remedies

Other common name(s)	Scientific/medical name(s)
Bach Remedies	None

DESCRIPTION

Flower remedies are essences from flowers that have been diluted in water and brandy. Essences are oils in a flower that contain its scent. There are 38 different formulas used that contain various combinations of flowers.

OVERVIEW

There is no scientific evidence that flower remedies are effective in treating cancer or any other disease. Numerous testimonials state that flower remedies are particularly effective for stabilizing emotions. However, no scientific studies have been conducted to determine if they provide any health benefits.

How is it promoted for use?

Proponents claim that flower remedies ease stress and reduce negative emotions, which in turn stimulates the body's healing processes to help fight illness. They believe that physical illness is caused by underlying emotional problems or disorders. They do not claim that flower remedies cure diseases, only that they assist the body's natural defenses. Supporters suggest that flower remedies can help improve sleep, reduce stress, calm fears, ease childbirth, reduce alcoholic tremors, and lessen skeletal and muscular pain. There is no scientific evidence to support these claims.

Particular flowers are believed to be associated with seven categories of emotional problems that include fear, uncertainty, general disinterest, loneliness, over-sensitivity, despondency, and relationship problems.

What does it involve?

Drops of flower essence preparations are placed directly under the tongue or in a glass of water or juice. The flowers are collected early in the morning when they are in full bloom and soaked in spring water in bright sunlight for three hours. The blossoms are removed from the flowering plant and the blossom-soaked water is placed in a sterile bottle and mixed with an equal amount of brandy. The liquid is then highly diluted, so very small amounts remain in the final remedy formula (see Homeopathy). Practitioners determine which combination of flower essences to prescribe based on the patient's emotional condition, not on specific diseases that are present.

What is the history behind it?

In the 1930s, Edward Bach, an English homeopathic physician, developed the theory that the successful treatment of negative emotions would heal illness. His ideas in this area were shared by others who believed in the existence of a connection between the mind and body, and that emotional health influenced physical health. Bach believed flowers were one key to strengthening the mind-body link, and that flower essences could soothe emotions. Today, selection of the appropriate remedy is done by completing a 116-item questionnaire.

What is the evidence?

Despite numerous anecdotal reports claiming

flower remedies improve health, there is no scientific evidence showing the treatment results in any measurable positive results. They may produce a placebo effect, in which believing that something can or will happen generates a positive result.

Are there any possible problems or complications?

There are no known harmful effects reported with the ingestion of flower remedies.

References
Complementary and Alternative Methods. Flower remedies. American Cancer Society Web site. Available at: http://www.cancer.org. Accessed February 24, 2000.

Questionable self-help products. Quackwatch Web site. Available at: http://www.quackwatch.com. Accessed December 11, 1999.

Folic Acid

Other common name(s)	Scientific/medical name(s)
Folate, Folacin, Vitamin B Complex	Pteroylmonoglutamic Acid

DESCRIPTION
Folic acid is a B-complex vitamin found in many vegetables, beans, fruits, whole grains, and some fortified breakfast cereals (see Vitamin B Complex). It helps in the metabolism of DNA, and is especially important for the development of blood cells.

OVERVIEW
Folic acid may reduce the risk of some cancers, although the amount needed to lower the risk is unknown. Low levels of folic acid have been associated with higher rates of colorectal cancer and some birth defects. High doses of folic acid can interfere with the effectiveness of the chemotherapy drug methotrexate.

How is it promoted for use?
Folic acid is promoted primarily as a nutritional requirement for a healthy diet to reduce the risk of some types of cancer, birth defects (eg, spina bifida and anencephaly), and peripheral blood vessel disease.

What does it involve?
Folic acid is found in dark leafy green vegetables, citrus fruit, poultry, liver, and fortified grain-based cereals. Folic acid supplements are available in tablet and powder form in drug stores and health food stores. The RDA is 400 micrograms (μg) per day.

What is the history behind it?
The first studies that looked at the connection between folic acid and cancer took place in the 1960s. Dr. W. Van Niekerk noted several similarities between cells from the cervix in folate-deficient women and cervical cells showing early signs of cancer development. A decade later,

investigators suspected an association between the two types of cells. A study at the University of Alabama in the 1980s suggested a connection between folic acid and abnormal cell development in the cervix. By the early 1990s, studies found that cervical cancer was more likely to develop in people with lower levels of folic acid.

The Food and Nutrition Board lowered the RDA of folate in 1989 to 180 µg/day, but the FDA did not adopt this standard. So, bottles labeled "100% folic acid" usually contain 400 µg of folic acid. Most recently, in 1998, the FDA began to require that grain-based foods, cereals, and dietary supplements be enriched with folate.

What is the evidence?

Research has shown a connection between lower intake of folic acid and a greater risk of colorectal cancer. One study found that patients with ulcerative colitis (chronic inflammation of the colon) who were taking a drug that was known to inhibit the absorption of folic acid had a 50% increased risk of abnormal cell development that could lead to cancer. Other studies involving a general population also supported the idea that low levels of folic acid result in increased rates of colorectal cancer. A Harvard study published in the *Annals of Internal Medicine* that tracked nurses in the United States from 1976 to 1994 reported that the women with a high intake of folic acid were 75% less likely to get colon cancer than those with a lower intake. Other investigations have reported a connection between low levels of folic acid and cancer of the breast, lung, esophagus, and stomach.

The exact way low levels of folic acid can promote the development of cancer is unknown. However, folic acid is essential for the production of chemicals that form DNA during cell reproduction and cell repair. Scientists believe low levels of folic acid can lead to a change in the chemicals that affect DNA, which can lead to cancer. Other theories suggest low folic acid levels impair the ability to ward off cancer-producing cells.

Folate has also been studied in relation to birth defects. A randomized clinical trial found that folic acid supplements reduced the risk of spina bifida and other neural tube defects in infants. Based on this study, the US Public Health Service recommended in 1992 that all women who might become pregnant should take 400 µg of folic acid every day.

The amount of folic acid needed to reduce cancer risk has still not been determined. Some scientists and dieticians favor fortifying grain-based foods with folic acid, noting that only 9% of all Americans consume the recommended servings of fruit and vegetables. A 1993 study stated men and women of all ages should consume approximately 400 µg/day, which would be comparable to six servings of fruit or vegetables and fortified cereal. Many scientists believe that few people eat enough green vegetables and fruit to give them adequate protection. Instead, they support a balanced diet, including large amounts of fruit and vegetables, with a multivitamin supplement containing folic acid, to ensure that 400 µg of folic acid is consumed daily. Other nutritionists have recently suggested a dose of 800 µg daily.

Are there any possible problems or complications?

Folic acid is considered a safe and necessary dietary nutrient. However, if taken in extremely large doses, it can be toxic. High doses of folate also interfere with the effectiveness of the chemotherapy drug methotrexate.

References

Alternative Medicine: Expanding Medical Horizons. *A Report to the National Institutes of Health on Alternative Medical Systems and Practices in the United States.* Washington, DC: US Government Printing Office; 1994. NIH publication 94-066.

Campbell NR. How safe are folic acid supplements? *Arch Intern Med.* 1996;156:1638-1644.

Giovannucci E, Stampfer MJ, Colditz GA, et al. Multivitamin use, folate, and colon cancer in women in the Nurses' Health Study. *Ann Intern Med.* 1998;129:517-524.

Grunwald HW, Rosner F. Folic acid fortification of food. *JAMA.* 1996;275:682-683.

Mason JB, Levesque T. Folate: effects on carcinogenesis and the potential for cancer chemoprevention. *Oncology (Huntingt)*. 1996;10:1727-1744.

MRC Vitamin Study Research Group. Prevention of neural tube defects: results of the Medical Research Council Vitamin Study. *Lancet*. 1991;338:131-137.

Oakley GP Jr. Eat right and take a multivitamin. *N Engl J Med*. 1998;338:1060-1061.

Willett WC. Folic acid and neural tube defect: can't we come to closure? *Am J Public Health*. 1992;82:666-668.

Zhang S, Hunter DJ, Hankinson SE, et al. A prospective study of folate intake and the risk of breast cancer. *JAMA*. 1999; 281:1632-1637.

Fu Zhen Therapy

Other common name(s)	Scientific/medical name(s)
None	None

DESCRIPTION / OVERVIEW

Fu Zhen therapy is a Chinese herbal remedy promoted to enhance the immune system, improve digestion, and stimulate energy levels (see Chinese Herbal Medicine). The herbs reportedly used most often in Fu Zhen include astragalus, ligustrum, ginseng, codonopsis, atractylodes, and ganoderma. Proponents claim that Fu Zhen is effective for treating cancer when used as a complementary therapy along with chemotherapy and radiation treatments. There is no scientific evidence to support these claims.

Germanium

Other common name(s)	Scientific/medical name(s)
Germanium Sesquioxide	Ge

DESCRIPTION

Germanium is a trace mineral. Inorganic germanium is mined and widely used as a semiconductor in the electronics industry. Organic germanium is found in some plants. Both forms of germanium may be included in dietary supplements, though the organic form is more commonly used.

OVERVIEW

There is no scientific evidence that germanium supplements are effective in preventing or treating cancer, and there is some information to suggest that they may be harmful. A study *conducted by the FDA reported that products containing germanium present a potential hazard to humans.*

How is it promoted for use?

Proponents claim germanium effectively combats leukemia and cancers of the lung, bladder, larynx, breast, and uterus. They also claim it can be used to treat neurosis, asthma, diabetes, hypertension, cardiac insufficiency, sinus inflammation, neuralgia, and cirrhosis of the liver. Supporters contend that germanium stimulates the body's production of interferon, a naturally occurring anticancer agent, and boosts the immune system by enhancing the activity of natural killer cells (a type of white blood cell), which attack invading microorganisms. There is no scientific evidence to support these claims.

What does it involve?

Germanium supplements are available in capsules ranging from 250 mg to 325 mg. There is no standardized dose. These supplements are available in health food stores and over the Internet.

What is the history behind it?

The late Dr. Kazuhiko Asai of Japan began investigating the biological properties of Germanium after reading reports from Russia, which said that the mineral had tremendous therapeutic value. In 1969, Dr. Asai founded the Asai Germanium Research Institute. He reportedly developed a process for producing germanium that was chemically identical to the germanium extracted from plants. Dr. Asai also found that germanium was present in many common herbal remedies, including ginseng, garlic, comfrey, and aloe (see Aloe, Comfrey, Garlic, and Ginseng).

Dr. Otto Warburg, a Nobel Prize winning biochemist, stated that germanium helped to increase the delivery of oxygen to cells. He believed that boosting the oxygen supply to healthy cells slowed the growth of tumors (see Oxygen Therapy).

What is the evidence?

There is no scientific evidence to show that germanium supplements promote health or increase the body's production of interferon. Germanium is not an essential element in animals or humans and does not play a role in biological processes.

Based on an animal study, one researcher in Belgium concluded that inorganic germanium is not toxic to humans and may even inhibit the growth of or destroy tumor cells. However, according to a study conducted by the FDA, at least 31 cases of kidney failure and death have been linked to products containing inorganic germanium. The FDA study did not conclusively show that organic germanium is toxic; however, because organic germanium could be contaminated with the dangerous inorganic germanium, products containing germanium present a potential hazard to humans.

Are there any possible problems or complications?

Although it is not clear if germanium supplements pose any danger for humans, some scientists warn that inorganic germanium (present in some supplements) may cause kidney failure and even death. Other adverse effects have included anemia, muscle weakness, and peripheral neuropathy (a disturbance in the nervous system). Women who are pregnant or breast-feeding should not use this mineral.

References

Gerber GB, Leonard A. Mutagenicity, carcinogenicity and teratogenicity of germanium compounds. *Mutat Res.* 1997;387:141-146.

Tao S-H, Bolger P. Hazard assessment of germanium supplements. *Regulat Toxicol Pharmacol.* 1997;25:211-219.

Herbs / Vitamins / Minerals

Ginger

Other common name(s)	Scientific/medical name(s)
Ginger Root	*Zingiber officinale*

DESCRIPTION

Ginger is a plant native to southeast Asia that is also grown in the United States, China, India, and various tropical regions. The root is usually the part of the plant used in herbal remedies.

OVERVIEW

Ginger has a long history as a pungent spice for cooking and as an herbal remedy for upset stomach, travel sickness, and loss of appetite. Some controlled studies in humans show ginger reduces nausea and vomiting. However, it may interfere with blood clotting and should only be used with a physician's approval by cancer patients attempting to control nausea related to chemotherapy.

How is it promoted for use?

Ginger has been used to control or prevent nausea, vomiting, and motion sickness; as an anti-inflammatory (a drug that reduces pain and swelling as in arthritis), a cold remedy, an aid to digestion; and a remedy for intestinal gas. Some research findings show that ginger can be taken to relieve nausea in cancer patients who are receiving chemotherapy. Some proponents have claimed ginger is able to prevent tumors from developing; however, this has not been scientifically proven.

What does it involve?

Ginger has been approved by Commission E (Germany's regulatory agency for herbs) for indigestion and the prevention of motion sickness. Ginger is available as a tea, in powder form, in tablets, in capsules, and in candied form in Asian food stores. Many mothers give their children ginger ale to settle an upset stomach, but the soft drink often does not contain much ginger and some ales have artificial flavoring in them rather than ginger.

Ginger root (fresh or dried) is used in cooking and preparing herbal remedies and soft drinks. A broad range of daily doses of ginger are reported, from 250 mg to 1 g. For nausea, the usual dose is 250 mg-1 g of powdered ginger taken with a liquid several times per day.

What is the history behind it?

The root of the ginger plant has been used in cooking and as a herbal remedy since ancient times. The ancient Greeks ate ginger wrapped in bread to prevent nausea from a huge feast. For many centuries, Chinese sailors have taken ginger to avoid sea sickness. A proverb from ancient India maintains that everything good can be found in ginger. It has been used as a spice in cooking for centuries. Its traditional role in herbal medicine has been as a remedy for nausea, motion sickness, heartburn, vomiting, stomach cramps, and loss of appetite.

What is the evidence?

There have been no human studies of ginger's ability to stop tumor growth. Recent preliminary results in animals showing some effect in slowing or preventing tumor growth are not well understood but warrant further investigation. However, it is too early in the research process to say if ginger will have the same effect in humans.

Ginger reduces nausea, according to some, but not all, controlled studies in humans. Studies also show that ginger reduces motion sickness and severe vomiting in pregnancy. Studies of ginger's ability to reduce nausea and vomiting associated with surgery have had mixed results. At least one study found ginger had no effect after surgery, while other studies have found a significant decrease in nausea and vomiting after surgery when ginger was given before the operation. These inconsistencies may be due to the difficulty in measuring symptoms of nausea.

Cisplatin is one of the chemotherapy drugs associated with nausea, vomiting, and delayed emptying of the stomach. Researchers from India found that extracts from ginger helped to speed up this process in dogs and rats that were given cisplatin chemotherapy. However, extracted chemicals or substances are different from the raw plant. Thus, study results of extracts will not necessarily be consistent with studies using the raw plant. While ginger may be an effective herb in treating nausea and vomiting associated with some cancer therapies, it may also interfere with blood clotting which could be life threatening to some patients receiving chemotherapy.

Experts from the US Pharmacopeial Convention (USP) have determined that there is not enough medical and scientific evidence to support recommending ginger for the prevention of nausea and vomiting. Although there has been a lack of reported harmful side effects, the USP encourages more research on ginger.

Are there any possible problems or complications?

People with cancer should consult their physician before taking ginger because it has the potential to interfere with blood clotting and prolong bleeding time. Published studies are in disagreement about the likelihood of this side effect. The risk of serious bleeding may be increased if the person is also taking medication that can lower platelet (blood cells that help the blood to clot) counts or an anticoagulant (a drug that interferes with blood clotting such as warfarin). In rare cases, some people have experienced an allergic reaction to ginger and occasional mild upset stomach. People should also consult their physician for the use of ginger for morning sickness or for gallstone problems.

References

Blumenthal M, ed. *The Complete German Commission E Monographs: Therapeutic Guide to Herbal Medicines.* Austin, Tx: American Botanical Council; 1998.

Fetrow CW, Avila JR. Professional's *Handbook of Complementary and Alternative Medicines.* Springhouse, Pa: Springhouse Corp; 1999.

Janssen PL, Meyboom S, van Staveren WA, de Vegt F, Katan MB. Consumption of ginger (Zingiber officinale roscoe) does not affect ex vivo platelet thromboxane production in humans. *Eur J Clin Nutr.* 1996;50:772-774.

Lumb AB. Effect of dried ginger on human platelet function. *Thromb Haemost.* 1994;71:110-111.

Medical Economics. *PDR for Herbal Medicines.* Montvale, NJ: Medical Economics Company; 1998.

Miller LG. Herbal medicinals: selected clinical considerations focusing on known or potential drug-herb interactions. *Arch Intern Med.* 1998;158:2200-2211.

O'Hara MA, Kiefer D, Farrell K, Kemper K. A review of 12 commonly used medicinal herbs. *Arch Fam Med.* 1998;7:523-536.

Pharmacopeial Forum. USP urges further study of ginger; creates NF monograph. US Pharmacopeia Web site. Available at: http://www.usp.org. Accessed May 8, 2000.

Sharma SS, Gupta YK. Reversal of cisplatin-induced delay in gastric emptying in rats by ginger (Zingiber officinale). *J Ethnopharmacol.* 1998;62:49-55.

Spaulding-Albright N. A review of some herbal and related products commonly used in cancer patients. *J Am Diet Assoc.* 1997;97:S208-S215.

Ginkgo

Other common name(s)	Scientific/medical name(s)
Ginkgo Biloba	*Ginkgo biloba*

DESCRIPTION

Ginkgo is an extract of leaves from a ginkgo tree, the world's oldest surviving species of tree, which comes from China, Japan, and Korea.

OVERVIEW

Ginkgo has shown some benefit in the treatment of mild to moderate dementia (decline in mental ability). Other studies have shown that it can help improve blood circulation and flow to the brain. Few side effects have been reported with its use, however it has the potential to interfere with blood clotting. There is no scientific evidence that it is effective in preventing or treating cancer.

How is it promoted for use?

Ginkgo is promoted as an aid to memory and concentration. Ginkgo is believed to stimulate blood circulation and the flow of oxygen to the brain. Widely used in Europe, the extract has recently become popular in the United States. Recent claims include an improvement of memory and vision in the elderly and a slowing of the progression of Alzheimer's disease or dementia.

Ginkgo is sometimes promoted for tinnitus (ringing in the ears), dizziness, motion sickness, and intermittent claudication (a cramp-like pain in the lower leg). In addition, it has been used as a treatment for a blood vessel disorder known as Raynaud's disease, in which the toes or fingers turn pale when exposed to cold because of an insufficient blood supply. European physicians have also used ginkgo in stroke patients to limit tissue damage to the heart.

Although not usually promoted as a cancer treatment, herbalists note that ginkgo contains a compound called ginkgolide B that may counteract a body chemical (called the platelet-activating factor) thought to promote tumor growth. There is no scientific evidence to support this claim.

What does it involve?

Ginkgo leaf extract is on the Commission E (Germany's regulatory agency for herbs) list of approved herbs, and can be taken in pill or liquid form by mouth. The average dose of ginkgo extract is 120-240 mg/day for up to 3 months. Proponents do not recommend the crude, dried leaf preparations because they claim they do not contain an adequate amount of the active ingredients.

What is the history behind it?

Chinese herbalists have used the fruit of the ginkgo tree for about 4,000 years as a remedy for asthma, coughs, and allergic reactions. In the past few decades, an extract of ginkgo leaves has been used in Western medicine, first in Europe and more recently in the United States, for its enhancement of memory, cognitive function, and blood circulation.

What is the evidence?

Some studies have found positive results from ginkgo extract. A 1996 laboratory study of aging mice found that ginkgo extracts improved short-term memory, fluidity within cell membranes of neurons, and passive avoidance learning. A 1997 controlled human study published in the *Journal* of the *American Medical Association* found evidence that ginkgo extract could improve cognitive and social function in some patients with mild to moderate forms of dementia resulting from Alzheimer's disease or multiple heart attacks. Other clinical trials have shown improved blood circulation and flow to the brain and other parts of the body with use of the extract. There have been no scientific studies on ginkgo related to cancer or tumor growth.

Are there any possible problems or complications?

Ginkgo is generally considered safe. Some possible side effects include headache and mild stomach upset. Because of its potential to inhibit the platelet-activating factor, ginkgo is not recommended for people using aspirin, non-steroidal anti-inflammatory drugs (eg, ibuprofen), or anticoagulants (drugs that inhibit abnormal blood clotting). People with seizure disorders are advised to avoid using ginkgo because it may reduce the effects of seizure medication. Women who are pregnant or breast-feeding should not use this herb.

References

Blumenthal M, ed. *The Complete German Commission E Monographs: Therapeutic Guide to Herbal Medicines.* Austin, Tx: American Botanical Council; 1998.

Le Bars PL, Katz MM, Berman N, et al. A placebo-controlled, double-blind, randomized trial of an extract of Ginkgo biloba for dementia. North American Egb Study Group. *JAMA.* 1997;278:1327-1332.

Miller LG. Herbal medicinals: selected clinical considerations focusing on known or potential drug-herb interactions. *Arch Intern Med.* 1998;158:2200-2211.

O'Hara M, Kiefer D, Farrell K, Kemper K. A review of 12 commonly used medicinal herbs. *Arch Fam Med.* 1998;7:523-536.

Stoll S, Scheuer K, Pohl O, Muller WE. Ginkgo biloba extract (EGb 761) independently improves changes in passive avoidance learning and brain membrane fluidity in the aging mouse. *Pharmacopsychiatry.* 1996;29:144-149.

Ginseng

Other common name(s)	Scientific/medical name(s)
None	*Panax ginseng* C. A. Meyer, *Panax quinquefolius*

DESCRIPTION

Ginseng is a perennial plant that grows in China, Korea, Japan, Russia (Panax ginseng), and the United States (Panax quinquefolius). The part of the plant used in herbal remedies is the dried root.

OVERVIEW

There is no scientific evidence that ginseng is effective in preventing or treating cancer. Although some population studies suggest it may have a protective effect, clinical trials are needed to determine if it is useful. Ginseng has been known to produce undesirable side effects and may even be dangerous when taken with certain medications.

How is it promoted for use?

Ginseng is promoted as an ancient herb that, due to its complex physical nature, can help the body prevent and fight diseases, including cancer. Promoters claim ginseng helps provide energy to people who are fatigued and is sometimes used during recovery from illness. There are also claims ginseng relieves anxiety, protects the heart, strengthens stomach functions, prevents arteriosclerosis, stabilizes blood pressure and insulin levels, and even delays the effects of aging. There is no scientific evidence to support these claims.

What does it involve?

Ginseng is available as a powder, capsule, tea, or is sometimes mixed with foods. There is no standard dosage; however Commission E (Germany's regulatory agency for herbs) suggests 1-2 g/day of ginseng root for up to 3 months.

There is a lot of variation among ginseng products. Since it is expensive, some packagers dilute it or substitute less expensive ingredients to make it affordable to the consumer. Some ginseng products from areas of the world such as Siberia, Alaska, and Brazil are mislabeled. True ginseng has the word *Panax* as part of its Latin (scientific) name. A 1978 study of 54 ginseng products found that one quarter of the products contained no ginseng at all.

What is the history behind it?

The Chinese have been using ginseng since at least 48 BC as an herbal remedy. Early books from China listing curative foods claim ginseng could enlighten the mind and increase wisdom. Also, the Chinese used ginseng to treat ailments of the digestive and respiratory systems, nervous disorders, diabetes, to keep the elderly warm in winter, and to increase energy and improve memory. Life-prolongation effects of ginseng were first described during China's Liang Dynasty (220-589 AD). North American ginseng was discovered growing in the mountains of Quebec by a Jesuit priest in the early 1700s. It was soon exported to China where its medicinal value was appreciated. Other variations of ginseng are grown in Korea and Japan.

Ginseng was not used in Western medicine until the 1950s when scientists in the Soviet Union began studying its health benefits and concluded that it was an "adaptogen," that is, something that helps the body adapt to outside stresses and ward off disease. The Viet Cong used it extensively to treat gunshot wounds during the Vietnam War.

In 1978, Taik-Koo Yun, MD, from the Korea Cancer Center Hospital in Seoul, began to conduct population-based studies to investigate whether ginseng had anticancer properties. By 1986, he had published an article arguing that ginseng prevented most cancers, but he was not certain how this occurred. Consequently, he encouraged more worldwide analysis of this herb.

What is the evidence?

Ginseng has been known for 3,000 years, but despite research, scientists still are not certain whether the herb has cancer-prevention properties. The medicinal effects of ginseng are thought to be connected to a molecular part of the root called "ginsenosides," which resemble steroids. Most of the studies with ginseng have been done in China and Korea, and only recently in the United States.

A few case-control studies conducted in Korea found that people who took fresh ginseng extract, white ginseng extract, or white ginseng powder were found to have decreased risk of cancer. However, the authors point out that further research is needed to determine the true benefit of ginseng in cancer prevention.

Some investigations have suggested that ginseng can inhibit cancer formation by enhancing DNA repair at the cellular level or by bolstering the immune system. But many studies of this herb have suffered from design problems, and results have been contradictory. Some scientists have found that it raises blood pressure while others have reported that it lowers blood pressure. In some studies, ginsenosides seem to act as stimulants but in others, they seem to work like sedatives. The only conclusions that can be reached with any certainty at this time are that ginseng is a complex herb and its medicinal effects are not clearly defined.

A recent systematic review of randomized clinical trials evaluated the current evidence related to the effectiveness of ginseng root extract. Based on the data from 16 trials, the researchers concluded that ginseng root extract did not have an effect on physical performance, diabetes mellitus, herpes simplex type-II infections, psychomotor performance, cognitive function, or the immune system.

The University of Texas Center for Alternative Medicine Research in Cancer designed laboratory experiments to test Korean ginseng on preventing the development of cancer. The results of their first study suggested that ginseng had no protective effect on developing tumors. It is clear that more research is needed to determine the benefit of ginseng, if any, for people with cancer.

Are there any possible problems or complications?

There are several known side effects associated with the use of ginseng. Ginseng has been known to cause hypertension, headaches, insomnia, restlessness, and in women, swollen breasts and vaginal bleeding. Because of it's estrogen-like effects, women who are pregnant or breast-feeding should not use ginseng. In fact, some physicians believe it can cause breast cancer to re-occur in women who have had the disease previously.

If used with warfarin, or any other anticoagulant (a drug that interferes with blood clotting), ginseng can alter bleeding times. If used with phenelzine sulfate, an antidepressant, ginseng can cause headaches, tremors, and manic episodes. People with cancer should consult their physician before taking this herb.

References

Blumenthal M, ed. *The Complete German Commission E Monographs: Therapeutic Guide to Herbal Medicines.* Austin, Tx: American Botanical Council; 1998.

Duda RB, Taback B, Kessel B, et al. pS2 expression induced by American ginseng in MCF-7 breast cancer cells. *Ann Surg Oncol.* 1996;3:515-520.

Miller LG. Herbal medicinals: selected clinical considerations focusing on known or potential drug-herb interactions. *Arch Intern Med.* 1998;158:2200-2211.

O'Hara M, Kiefer D, Farrell K, Kemper K. A review of 12 commonly used medicinal herbs. *Arch Fam Med.* 1998;7:523-536.

Spaulding-Albright N. A review of some herbal and related products commonly used in cancer patients. *J Am Diet Assoc.* 1997;97:S208-S215.

University of Texas Center for Alternative Medicine Research in Cancer. Traditional Chinese medicine summary. University of Texas-Houston Health Science Center Web site. Available at: http://www.sph.uth.tmc.edu/utcam/therapies/tcm.htm/. Accessed May 8, 2000.

Vogler BK, Pittler MH, Ernst E. The efficacy of ginseng. A systematic review of randomised clinical trials. *Eur J Clin Pharmacol.* 1999;55:567-575.

Yun TK, Choi SY. Preventive effect of ginseng intake against various human cancers: a case-control study on 1987 pairs. *Cancer Epidemiol Biomarkers Prev.* 1995;4:401-408.

Yun TK, Choi SY. Non-organ specific cancer prevention of ginseng: a prospective study in Korea. *Int J Epidemiol.* 1998;27:359-364.

Goldenseal

Other common name(s)	Scientific/medical name(s)
Eye Balm, Eye Root, Goldsiegel, Ground Raspberry, Indian Dye, Indian Turmeric, Jaundice Root, Yellow Paint, Yellow Puccoon, Yellow Root	*Hydrastis canadensis*

DESCRIPTION

Goldenseal is an herb native to the United States and cultivated elsewhere. Goldenseal takes its name from the golden-yellow scars that appear at the top of the root when the stem is broken off and which resembles an old-fashioned wax letter seal. The roots of the plant are used in herbal remedies.

OVERVIEW

There is no evidence that goldenseal is effective in treating cancer or other disease. Some components of the herb (berberine and hydrastine) have been studied for potential pharmacological uses. Goldenseal can have toxic side effects, and high doses can be lethal.

How is it promoted for use?

Practitioners promote the use of goldenseal for a wide variety of conditions, including digestive problems (eg, peptic ulcers, colitis), urinary tract inflammation, constipation, anorexia, hemorrhage after childbirth, painful menstruation, eczema, itching, ringing in the ears, tuberculosis, and cancer. Some claim goldenseal stimulates the immune system. Externally, goldenseal has been used to treat skin conditions, wounds, and herpes sores.

Berberine, a chemical contained in goldenseal, is said to have the ability to fight off infection caused by some bacteria, fungi, and yeast, and can act as a mild sedative. Some claim that berberine stimulates the heart and is more effective than aspirin for reducing fevers. Another chemical in goldenseal, hydrastinine, is said to reduce blood pressure. There is no scientific evidence to support these claims.

What does it involve?

Goldenseal can be taken internally in the form of capsules, extracts, tinctures, and teas. The ground root powder can also be purchased. The amount of goldenseal used varies depending on the way it is ingested (eg, tincture versus dried root).

Proponents use tooth powder and gargle made from goldenseal to treat tooth and gum infections and also apply the powder to herpes lesions and skin wounds. They also use solutions made from goldenseal in eyedrops for conjunctivitis (inflammation of the eye), and also as eardrops and douches.

What is the history behind it?

For centuries, some Native American tribes have used goldenseal for medicinal purposes, as a face paint, and as a dye for clothing (see Native American Healing). The herb became an important ingredient in American folk medicine. It was used as tea to treat sores in the mouth and throat and as a wash for eye infections. By 1900, it was nearly harvested to extinction. It is currently grown in the United States in limited quantities.

What is the evidence?

There is no clinical evidence to support the use of the herb for cancer or any other medical condition. In one recent animal study, goldenseal appeared to stimulate the immune system. Berberine, a chemical component of goldenseal, has been studied for its blood-thinning and cardiac stimulant properties in animals. Some other effects such as reductions in fever and bacteria have also been noted in laboratory experiments on berberine. Hydrastinine, another component of goldenseal, has been found to produce severe changes in blood pressure. Animal and laboratory studies may show a certain compound holds promise as a beneficial treatment, but further studies are necessary to determine if the results apply to humans.

The National Center for Complementary and Alternative Medicine (part of the National Institutes of Health) reported that a recommendation was made for the National Toxicology Program to test goldenseal for its potential to cause developmental problems and/or cancer of the reproductive system.

Are there any possible problems or complications?

Goldenseal may produce toxic effects, including digestive complaints, nervousness, depression, constipation, rapid heartbeat, diarrhea, gastrointestinal cramps and pain, mouth ulcers, nausea, seizures, and vomiting, and central nervous system depression. High doses may cause respiratory problems, paralysis, and even death. Long-term use may lead to vitamin B deficiency, hallucinations, and deliria. Women who are pregnant or breast-feeding should not use this herb in any form. Due to the potential harmful effects of goldenseal, a physician should be consulted before taking the herb for any condition, including cancer.

References

Fetrow CW, Avila JR. *Professional's Handbook of Complementary and Alternative Medicines.* Springhouse, Pa: Springhouse Corp; 1999.

Medical Economics. *PDR for Herbal Medicines.* Montvale, NJ: Medical Economics Company; 1998.

National Institutes and Health News and Research Grants. Review recommended on three herbs. National Center for Complementary and Alternative Medicine Web site. Available at: http://nccam.nih.gov/nccam/cam/1998/spring/3.htm. Accessed November 23, 1999.

Rehman J, Dillow JM, Carter SM, Chou J, Le B, Maisel AS. Increased production of antigen-specific immunoglobulins G and M following in vivo treatment with the medicinal plants Echinacea angustifolia and Hydrastis canadensis. *Immunol Lett.* 1999;68:391-395.

Green Tea

Other common name(s)	Scientific/medical name(s)
Black Tea, Chinese Tea	*Camellia sinesis*

DESCRIPTION

Green tea is a drink made from the steamed and dried leaves of the Camellia sinesis plant, a shrub native to Asia. Black tea is also made from this plant, but unlike green tea, it is made from leaves that have been dried and fermented.

OVERVIEW

Some researchers believe green tea may have a protective effect against some cancers because it contains antioxidants. However, results from human studies have been mixed. More research is needed to determine its role in cancer prevention.

How is it promoted for use?

Green tea is widely consumed in Japan, China, and other Asian nations and is becoming more popular in Western nations. Some reports indicate green tea may have the ability to help prevent certain cancers from developing, including prostate, stomach, and esophageal cancers. Green tea contains chemicals known as polyphenols, which have antioxidant properties. An antioxidant is a compound that blocks the action of activated oxygen molecules, known as free radicals, that can damage cells. One major element in green tea is epigallocatechin-3-gallate (EGCG), a compound that is believed to block production of an enzyme required for cancer cell growth. EGCG may work by suppressing the formation of blood vessels, a process called angiogenesis, thereby cutting off the supply of blood to cancer cells.

Herbalists use green tea and extracts of its leaves for stomach problems, vomiting, and diarrhea, and to reduce tooth decay, blood pressure, cholesterol levels, and blockages of the blood vessels in the heart that can lead to heart attacks. Green tea is also promoted as an herb that can prevent certain bacterial infections. In the past five years, some researchers have sug-gested that black tea may also be effective in cancer prevention. These claims are currently under investigation.

What does it involve?

Three cups a day or more is the amount typically taken in Asian countries. Green tea is usually brewed using 1 to 2 teaspoons of the dried tea in a cup of boiling water, or is steeped for 3 to 15 minutes. Green tea extracts are also available in capsule form. Three capsules of green tea extract a day are recommended by proponents, but this dosage and its effects remain uncertain.

What is the history behind it?

The Chinese have been drinking green tea to promote good health for at least 3,000 years. In recent years, scientists have begun to study its health effects in animal, laboratory, and observational human studies.

What is the evidence?

Although animal and laboratory studies have shown a positive benefit of green tea consumption in protecting against cancer, studies in humans have been mixed. Researchers from the Shanghai Cancer Institute and the NCI conducted a large population study in 1994 comparing green tea drinkers to non-green tea drinkers. They found that green tea drinking was associated with 60% fewer cancers of the esophagus for people who did not smoke. However, a review of 31 human studies and four review articles found mixed results. These studies reported on colon, urinary bladder, stomach, lungs, and esophageal cancer. Controlled, randomized clinical trials are needed to determine the effectiveness of green tea in protecting against cancer. Studies are currently underway at NCI and the National Institutes of Health Office of Alternative Medicine.

Are there any possible problems or complications?

Green tea is generally considered safe. Asians have consumed this tea for thousands of years with few dangerous side effects. However, some people may develop allergic reactions and should stop drinking it. Drinking large amounts of tea may cause nutritional and other problems because of the caffeine content and the strong binding activities of the polyphenols. Because caffeine acts as a stimulant, people with irregular heartbeats or who have anxiety attacks should not drink more than 2 cups a day. Women who are pregnant or breast-feeding should not drink green tea in large amounts.

References

Bushman JL. Green tea and cancer in humans: a review of the literature. *Nutr Cancer.* 1998;31:151-159.

Gao YT, McLaughlin JK, Blot WJ, Ji BT, Dai Q, Fraumeni JF Jr. Reduced risk of esophageal cancer associated with green tea consumption. *J Natl Cancer Inst.* 1994;86:855-858.

Ji BT, Chow WH, Hsing AW, et al. Green tea consumption and the risk of pancreatic and colorectal cancers. *Int J Cancer.* 1997;70:255-258.

Lyn-Cook BD, Rogers T, Yan Y, Blann EB, Kadlubar FF, Hammons GJ. Chemopreventive effects of tea extracts and various components on human pancreatic and prostate tumor cells in vitro. *Nutr Cancer.* 1999;35:80-86.

Mayo Clinic. Prostate cancer and green tea. Mayo Clinic Health Oasis Web site. Available at: http://www.mayohealth.org/mayo/9901/htm/tea.htm. Accessed May 8, 2000.

Medical Economics. *PDR for Herbal Medicines.* Montvale, NJ: Medical Economics Company; 1998.

Steele VE, Kelloff GJ, Balentine D. Comparative chemopreventive mechanisms of green tea, black tea and selected polyphenol extracts measured by in vitro bioassays. *Carcinogenesis.* 2000;21:63-67.

University of Texas Center for Alternative Medicine Research in Cancer. Green tea summary. University of Texas-Houston Health Science Center Web site. Available at: http://www.sph.uth.tmc.edu/utcam/summary/greentea.htm. Accessed May 8, 2000.

Yang CS. Tea and health. *Nutrition.* 1999;15:946-949.

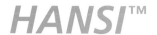

HANSI™

Other common name(s)	Scientific/medical name(s)
None	None

DESCRIPTION / OVERVIEW

HANSI is an herbal preparation consisting of very small dilutions from plants of the desert and rain forests such as cactus (Cacti grandiflora), aloe, arnica, lachesis, and licopodium in a 2% to 8% alcohol base (see Homeopathy). Proponents claim that HANSI enhances the immune system, prevents and stops the progression of some cancers, increases tolerance of side effects from chemotherapy and radiation therapy, and effectively treats chronic fatigue syndrome, AIDS, and asthma. HANSI is taken orally or delivered by injection for up to two years. The basic formula includes about 10 components whose proportions are adjusted according to the condition being treated and whether the drug will be delivered orally or by injection. The FDA has not approved HANSI injections.

HANSI was developed by an Argentine biologist Juan Jose Hirschmann, PhD, who introduced his formula in Buenos Aires in 1990. He and his colleagues claim to have used HANSI to successfully treat more than 100,000 people with cancer. There is no scientific evidence that HANSI is effective in treating cancer or any other disease. Not enough is known about HANSI to determine if it is safe or if it poses any dangers to humans. Relying on this type of treatment alone, and avoiding conventional medical care, may have serious health consequences.

Hoxsey Herbal Treatment

Other common name(s)	Scientific/medical name(s)
Hoxsey Method, Hoxsey Treatment, Hoxsey Herbs, Hoxsey Formula	None

DESCRIPTION

The Hoxsey herbal treatment is an herbal mixture taken internally or applied externally. The pastes or salves that are applied externally contain antimony trisulfide, zinc chloride, and blood root, and a yellow powder consisting of arsenic sulfide, sulfur, and talc. Both the paste and powder are escharotics, which means they can burn the skin (see Cancer Salves).

OVERVIEW

There is no scientific evidence that the Hoxsey herbal treatment is effective in treating cancer and there have been no clinical trials of the treatment. In some animal studies, a few of the *herbs contained in the Hoxsey formula were studied separately and showed some anticancer activity. It is not known if there are harmful effects of the combination of the herbs taken together. The paste made for external application can severely burn, disfigure and scar the skin.*

How is it promoted for use?

The Hoxsey herbal treatment is specifically promoted to treat people with cancer. Its proponents claim the internal formula eliminates toxins from the body, strengthens the immune system, and enhances its ability to slowly absorb and excrete tumors. The external treatment is used to treat skin cancer. It allegedly keeps cancer from spreading and helps destroy cancer cells. The goal of treatment is to restore the body's chemistry to a normal state. There is no scientific evidence to support these claims.

What does it involve?

The herbal mixture used internally is a liquid that contains a combination of numerous herbs including pokeweed, burdock root, licorice, barberry, buckthorn bark, stillingia root, red clover, prickly ash bark, potassium iodide, and cascara and sometimes other ingredients (see Pokeweed, Licorice, and Red Clover). The external preparation, usually a paste or salve, is rubbed directly onto cancerous tumors. Internal and external dosages vary depending on the patient and whether the tumor is inside the body or on the skin. The Hoxsey herbal treatment is currently illegal in the United States, although it can be obtained through clinics in Mexico.

The Hoxsey treatment now also includes antiseptic douches and washes, laxative tablets, nutritional supplements, and dietary restrictions that prohibit pork, vinegar, tomatoes, pickles, carbonated drinks, alcohol, bleached flour, sugar, and salt.

What is the history behind it?

The Hoxsey herbal treatment is one of oldest alternative cancer treatments in the United States. Its controversial history dates back to the 1920s, when Harry Hoxsey, who had no medical training, marketed a mixture of herbs that he believed would effectively treat cancer. Hoxsey claimed that his great grandfather, John Hoxsey, developed the first version of the herbal formula in 1840 when he noticed one of his horses had developed cancer on its leg. The animal began eating some of the wild plants growing in the meadow, and within a short time the tumor disappeared. John Hoxsey gathered the herbs and mixed them with old home remedies used for cancer.

Although it was Harry's father, a veterinarian, who first used the herbal formula to treat people with cancer, Harry was the one who attracted fame and fortune through self-promotion, publicity, and sensational claims. He even conducted public healing sessions using his herbal concoction. Hoxsey opened his first clinic in Taylorville, IL in the 1920s, and at one point operated clinics in 17 states. He claimed that at their peak, his clinics treated tens of thousands of cancer patients every year. Hoxsey was convicted and fined numerous times for practicing medicine without a license and kept moving his clinics from state to state to avoid legal problems.

In 1936, Hoxsey opened a clinic in Dallas that became one of the largest privately owned cancer centers in the world. In 1949, Hoxsey sued the editor of the prestigious *Journal of the American Medical Association* for libel and slander after the journal called him a fraud. Hoxsey won the case, but the judge awarded him only $1.

By 1960, after battling Hoxsey for a decade, the FDA finally banned the sale of the Hoxsey herbal treatment in the United States and forced Hoxsey to close all of his clinics in the United States. In 1963, one of Hoxsey's nurses set up a clinic in Tijuana, Mexico. It still operates today, and an estimated 1,200 new patients visit the Tijuana clinic every year. Hoxsey developed prostate cancer in 1967. When he did not respond to his own treatment, Hoxsey underwent conventional surgery. He died seven years later.

What is the evidence?

There is no evidence that the Hoxsey herbal treatment has any value in the treatment of cancer in humans. In 1946, the National Cancer Institute reviewed 77 case reports of Hoxsey's patients and concluded that none of them met the criteria for scientific evaluation.

Only 2 human studies of the Hoxsey herbal treatment have been published. One was published in a pamphlet provided by the Tijuana clinic and simply contains a description of 9 patients who received the treatment. It concluded that the treatment is effective. The other study published in the *Journal of Naturopathic Medicine* involved 39 people with various types of cancer who took the Hoxsey herbal treatment. Ten patients died after an average of 15 months and 23 never completed the study. Only 6 patients were disease-free after 48 months. In some animal studies, a few of the herbs contained in the treatment showed some anti-cancer activity. Animal studies may show a certain substance holds promise as a beneficial treatment, but further studies are necessary to determine if the results apply to humans.

Are there any possible problems or complications?

The paste made for external application can severely burn, disfigure, and scar the skin. Some of the ingredients in the internal formula, such as buckthorn, can cause nausea, vomiting, and diarrhea when taken in large quantities. Cascara can also cause diarrhea. Pokeweed is a poisonous plant that can also cause undesirable side effects such as nausea, vomiting, diarrhea, and abdominal cramps. Red clover may increase the risk of bleeding for people who take anticoagulant (blood thinning) medications. It also has estrogenic activity, which means it should be avoided by women with estrogen-positive breast tumors. Women who are pregnant or breast-feeding should not use this treatment in any form. Relying on this type of treatment alone, and avoiding conventional medical care, may have serious health consequences.

References

Alternative Medicine: Expanding Medical Horizons. *A Report to the National Institutes of Health on Alternative Medical Systems and Practices in the United States.* Washington, DC: US Government Printing Office; 1994. NIH publication 94-066.

American Cancer Society. Questionable methods of cancer management: 'nutritional' therapies. *CA Cancer J Clin.* 43;5:309-319.

American Cancer Society. Unproven methods of cancer management: hoxsey method/bio-medical center. *CA Cancer J Clin.* 1990;40:51-55.

Austin S, Ellen D, DeKadt S. Long-term follow-up of cancer patients using Contreras, Hoxsey and Gerson therapies. *J Naturopathic Med.* 1994;5:74-76.

Spaulding-Albright N. A review of some herbal and related products commonly used in cancer patients. *J Am Diet Assoc.* 1997;97:S208-S215.

University of Texas Center for Alternative Medicine Research in Cancer. Hoxsey summary. University of Texas-Houston Health Science Center Web site. Available at: http://www.sph.uth.tmc.edu/utcam/summary/hoxsey.htm. Accessed October 12, 1999.

US Congress, Office of Technology Assessment. *Unconventional Cancer Treatments.* Washington, DC: US Government Printing Office; 1990. Publication OTA-H-405.

Indian Snakeroot

Other common name(s)	Scientific/medical name(s)
Snakeroot, Rauwolfia, Serpentwood, Reserpine	*Rauwolfia serpentina*

DESCRIPTION

Indian snakeroot is a plant that grows in India, Thailand, and other parts of Asia, South America, and Africa. There are more than 100 species of Indian snakeroot. Rauwolfia serpentina is the one most commonly used in herbal remedies. Reserpine, a chemical found in the roots, is responsible for most of the plant's therapeutic effects.

OVERVIEW

The drug reserpine is used in conventional medicine to treat high blood pressure and anxiety. There is no scientific evidence, however, that Indian snakeroot is effective in treating cancer, liver disease, or mental illness. It also has many dangerous side effects.

How is it promoted for use?

According to proponents, Indian snakeroot lowers high blood pressure, eases anxiety and tension, reduces fever, stops diarrhea and dysentery, and can be used to treat some psychiatric illnesses. Some believe that Indian snakeroot inhibits the reproduction of cancer cells, however there is no scientific evidence to support this claim.

What does it involve?

Indian snakeroot is on the Commission E (Germany's regulatory agency for herbs) list of approved herbs for treating mild hypertension. The supplements are available as tablets or in liquid form. Powdered Indian snakeroot can also be brewed as a tea. An average daily dose is 600 mg. Reserpine, which is a prescription medicine approved by the FDA, is given as pills or injections.

What is the history behind it?

References to Indian snakeroot were found in Hindu texts dating back to 600 BC. A tea made from the plant has been used for centuries in India for treating insanity, hysteria, and restlessness. Mahatma Gandhi reportedly drank Indian snakeroot tea regularly.

In Western medicine, reserpine was commonly prescribed by physicians for many years to treat high blood pressure and to reduce anxiety. However, other drugs, which are equally effective and cause fewer side effects, have since taken its place.

In India, extracts from the plant are used as antidotes to bites from venomous reptiles, including snakes, and sometimes as a remedy for constipation, liver diseases, and rheumatism. African serpentwood (*Rauwolfia vomitoria*), a plant that is in the same family as Indian snakeroot, has long been used in traditional African medicine to calm mentally disturbed patients.

What is the evidence?

The drug reserpine, which is extracted from Indian snakeroot, is widely known to be an effective drug for lowering blood pressure and as a tranquilizer. But there is little or no evidence to suggest that reserpine or other chemicals found in Indian snakeroot are effective treatments for mental illness, liver disease, or cancer.

Indian snakeroot is associated with many adverse side effects, including depression, decreased heart rate, low blood pressure, decreased sex drive and performance, increased appetite, weight gain, swelling, stomach complaints, diarrhea, nasal congestion, nightmares and hallucinations, gastrointestinal ulcers, decreased motor coordination, and dry mouth. Indian snakeroot can also impair physical abilities and coordination.

People with a history of depression, peptic ulcers or ulcerative colitis, and women with a history of breast cancer, should not take Indian snakeroot. Indian snakeroot should also be avoided by people taking sleeping pills, appetite suppressants, heart medications, and antipsychotic drugs due to the potential for increased blood pressure, increased heart rate, or uncontrollable muscle movements. The use of alcohol should also be avoided due to the reduction of physical reflexes. Women who are pregnant or breastfeeding should not use this herb.

References

Blumenthal M, ed. *The Complete German Commission E Monographs: Therapeutic Guide to Herbal Medicines.* Austin, Tx: American Botanical Council; 1998.

Bown D. *Encyclopedia of Herbs & Their Uses.* New York, NY: DK Publishing Inc; 1995.

Fetrow CW, Avila JR. *Professional's Handbook of Complementary and Alternative Medicines.* Springhouse, Pa: Springhouse Corp; 1999.

Medical Economics. *PDR for Herbal Medicines.* Montvale, NJ: Medical Economics Company; 1998.

Kampo

Other common name(s)	Scientific/medical name(s)
Kampoyaku, Juzen-taiho-to, Hochu-ekki-to, Sho-Saiko	None

DESCRIPTION

Kampo is the name for traditional Japanese herbal medicine that involves the use of more than 210 different herbal preparations. Three common kampo preparations are Juzen-taiho-to, Hochu-ekki-to, and Sho-saiko.

OVERVIEW

Despite the popularity of kampo among Japanese physicians and patients, there is no scientific evidence that Japanese herbal preparations are effective in preventing or treating cancer or any other disease.

How is it promoted for use?

Proponents claim that the kampo preparations Juzen-taiho-to and Hochu-ekki-to boost the anticancer activities of cells called natural killer cells (a type of white blood cell). Sho-saiko is claimed to enhance the function of macrophages, which attack cancer cells. They also say that some kampo remedies are more effective than conventional methods for treating chronic prostatitis (inflammation of the prostate gland). Practitioners of kampo claim that specific herbal formulas can be used to treat other conditions, such as constipation, gastritis, irritable bowel syndrome, allergies, asthma, arthritis, and hypertension. There is no scientific evidence to support these claims.

What does it involve?

Kampo practitioners may prescribe one or more herbal mixtures that are prepared by hand. The formula depends on the patient's particular complaint or condition. Unlike Western medicine, kampo does not give names to diseases. Patients are diagnosed based on a concept called "sho" which involves visual and auditory observations, detailed questioning, and physical examination. Signs and symptoms are then interpreted according to the ancient Chinese theories of yin and yang, which depends a great deal on the intuition of the practitioner.

What is the history behind it?

Kampo, which evolved from traditional Chinese herbal medicine, dates back more than 800 years (see Chinese Herbal Medicine). When Western medicine was introduced in Japan between 1868 and 1912, the popularity of kampo declined, but it began to revive in 1928. By 1988, the Japanese herbal medicine industry began to regulate the production of kampo preparations to ensure quality and consistency. In 1993, the Ministry of Education in Japan approved the establishment of the Department of Japanese Oriental (Kampo) Medicine, at Toyama Medical and Pharmaceutical University which grants university degrees in kampo. Today about 70% of the physicians in Japan prescribe kampo medications. There are over 210 prescription and over-the-counter kampo drugs that the Japanese government has officially approved, some of which are covered by Japanese health insurance.

What is the evidence?

Very little research has been conducted on kampo as a cancer therapy, and there is no scientific evidence to show that Japanese herbal preparations cure cancer or slow its growth. In one laboratory animal study conducted in Japan, researchers concluded that the kampo preparations Juzen-taiho-to and Shimotsu-to significantly reduced the spread of colon cancer cells to the liver, and of melanoma (skin cancer) cells to the lungs. Several other Japanese studies found that kampo remedies did nothing to stop or slow the spread of cancer.

In one case study, a 59-year-old man with cancer of the urinary tract took oral cancer treatment drugs along with kampo medications. After 61 months, he was disease free. However, it is not known whether the effect was from the conventional cancer treatment, the kampo, or the combination of both. Randomized clinical trials are needed to test the claims that kampo is effective against cancer and other diseases, or that it improves general health and well being.

Are there any possible problems or complications?

It is not known whether kampo is safe. No research has been done to determine the possible side effects. Women who are pregnant or breast-feeding should not use these herbs.

References

Alternative Medicine: Expanding Medical Horizons. *A Report to the National Institutes of Health on Alternative Medical Systems and Practices in the United States.* Washington, DC: US Government Printing Office; 1994. NIH publication 94-066.

Onishi Y, Yamaura T, Tauchi K, et al. Expression of the anti-metastatic effect induced by Juzen-taiho-to is based on the content of Shimotsu-to constituents. *Biol Pharm Bull.* 1988;21:761-765.

Ross C. New life for old medicine. *Lancet.* 1993;342:485-486.

Herbs / Vitamins / Minerals

Kampo 231

Kava

Other common name(s)	Scientific/medical name(s)
Kava-Kava, Kavalactones	*Piper methysticum*

DESCRIPTION

Kava is a large shrub with broad, heart-shaped leaves and is a member of the pepper family. It is native to many islands of the South Pacific, including New Guinea, Fiji, Tahiti, Samoa, and Hawaii. The roots of the plant are used in herbal remedies.

OVERVIEW

Studies support the use of kava for reducing anxiety, although it is not certain how it works. The safe dosage of kava needed to reduce anxiety has not been determined. Side effects appear to increase with large doses.

How is it promoted for use?

Kava is promoted primarily for anxiety, nervous tension, stress, restlessness, and at higher doses, insomnia. Many users say the herb enhances mood and brings on a sense of well being, relaxation and even euphoria. In South Pacific folk medicine, kava has been used to treat uterine inflammations, headaches, colds, rheumatism, and menopausal symptoms. They also drink it to relieve headaches, restore vigor, promote urination, soothe upset stomachs, ease symptoms of asthma and tuberculosis, and to cure fungal infections. Some users believe that kava inhibits gonorrhea. Used as a cream, kava is used to soothe stings and skin inflammations.

Kava has no direct application to cancer treatment, but its ability to ease anxiety may be of interest to people with cancer. There are other effective medications for treating anxiety that patients should discuss with their physician.

What does it involve?

Kava is on the Commission E (Germany's regulatory agency for herbs) list of approved herbs. It is available in tablets, capsules, cream, and powder, which can be made into tea or mixed with other drinks. Daily doses range from 100 to 200 mg of kavalactones (the active ingredient in kava). A safe dosage has not been determined, and, it should not be taken for more than 3 months.

What is the history behind it?

The native people of the South Pacific have used kava socially, ceremonially, and medicinally for generations. A beverage prepared from the kava root is traditionally offered to visiting royalty and dignitaries and served at meetings of village elders. The drink is also often present at social gatherings.

Accounts of kava first came to the West from the English naval officer Captain James Cook, who encountered the plant during a trip to Polynesia from 1772 to 1775. Interest in kava spread quickly. Kava first underwent serious medical investigation in the 1860s and, by the end of the 19th century, kava preparations were available in German pharmacies.

What is the evidence?

Kava has been the focus of dozens of medical studies, many of which support the claims made about the herb's anti-anxiety properties. Kava does indeed appear to ease symptoms of anxiety and stress. In recent studies, patients with varying levels of anxiety took kava extract and reported relief within days or weeks.

Some researchers have found that kava compares favorably to prescription anti-anxiety medications, yet causes fewer side effects and is not addictive. For instance, one study showed that kava does not impair reaction time and may even improve concentration. In comparison, common prescription drugs for anxiety slow reaction time.

Exactly how kava works is still somewhat of a mystery. Some scientists speculate that the active ingredients, kavalactones, soothe a part of the brain called the amygdala, which can be described as the brain's alarm center. Very early research findings indicate that kava may offer some protection against brain damage during stroke, and that the herb may have some antimicrobial effects.

Are there any possible problems or complications?

In rare cases, moderate use of kava can lead to a scaly rash. Heavy use can sometimes lead to metabolic abnormalities including increased levels of liver enzymes. Commission E reports that kava may reduce motor reflexes and judgement when driving or operating heavy machinery. Some evidence suggests that kava should not be taken with anti-anxiety medicines or alcohol which could cause extreme drowsiness. People taking antidepressants or antipsychotic drugs and children under the age of 12 should not take kava.

Other possible side effects include an increase of symptoms of Parkinson's disease, absence of urination, numbness of the mouth, and painful twisting movements of the trunk. Women who are pregnant or breast-feeding should not use kava.

References

Blumenthal M, ed. *The Complete German Commission E Monographs: Therapeutic Guide to Herbal Medicines*. Austin, Tx: American Botanical Council; 1998.

Cerrato PL. Natural tranquilizers? RN. 1998 Dec;61:61-62.

Cupp MJ. Herbal remedies: adverse effects and drug interactions. *Am Fam Physician*. 1999;59:1239-1245.

Fetrow CW, Avila JR. *Professional's Handbook of Complementary and Alternative Medicines*. Springhouse, Pa: Springhouse Corp; 1999.

Heiligenstein E, Guenther G. Over-the-counter psychotropics: a review of melatonin, St. John's wort, valerian, and kava-kava. *J Am Coll Health*. 1998;46:271-276.

Medical Economics. *PDR for Herbal Medicines*. Montvale, NJ: Medical Economics Company; 1998.

Wong AH, Smith M, Boon HS. Herbal remedies in psychiatric practice. *Arch Gen Psychiatry*. 1998;55:1033-1044.

Herbs / Vitamins / Minerals

Larch

Other common name(s)	Scientific/medical name(s)
American Larch, European Larch, Larch Arabinogalactan, Common Larch	*Larix occidentalis, Larix laricina, Larix decidua, Larix europaea*

DESCRIPTION

The larch is a tall, deciduous tree that grows in central Europe, North America, northern Russia, and Siberia. The bark and its resin are used in herbal remedies.

OVERVIEW

There is no scientific evidence that larch bark is effective in treating cancer or any other disease. Limited laboratory evidence suggests that a polysaccharide found in larch may stimulate the immune system, but clinical trials are needed to determine what effect, if any, it may have in humans.

How is it promoted for use?

Proponents believe that larch can be used to treat bronchitis, colds, and other respiratory conditions. The polysaccharide found in larch, called *larch arabinogalactan*, is said to stimulate the immune system and increase the effectiveness of some drugs (including chemotherapy medications). Some claim that the compound also inhibits the spread of cancer to the liver, although there has been no scientific evidence to support these claims.

What does it involve?

Larch is available in the form of ointments, gels, and oils. *Larch arabinogalactan* is available as a fiber supplement in powder form.

What is the history behind it?

The bark of the larch tree has been used in various folk medicine traditions to treat rheumatism, jaundice, skin problems, and as a poultice for wounds. Resins from the bark were used by Native Americans as a chewing gum and to relieve indigestion. *Larch arabinogalactan* was first isolated from the bark of the larch tree in 1992.

What is the evidence?

In one laboratory study, researchers at the University of Minnesota concluded that *Larch arabinogalactan* is a safe source of dietary fiber and may be effective in boosting the immune system. The research was sponsored, however, by the company that owns the patent to the extract. Another laboratory study conducted in Germany found that *arabinogalactan* from *Larix ocidentalis* stimulated the action of natural killer cells (a type of white blood cell). Laboratory studies may show a certain compound holds promise as a beneficial treatment, but further studies are necessary to determine if the results apply to humans.

Are there any possible problems or complications?

The *larix* species is listed in the FDA's Poisonous Plant Database. This is a list of plants that are associated with toxic effects. There have been no definitive conclusions as to its safety or toxicity.

References

Adams J. University of Minnesota researchers uncover immune-boosting fiber. *Minnesota Daily.* January 7, 1999.

Bown D. *Encyclopedia of Herbs & Their Uses.* New York, NY: DK Publishing Inc; 1995.

Hauer J, Anderer FA. Mechanism of stimulation of human natural killer cytotoxicity by arabinogalactan from Larix occidentalis. *Cancer Immunol Immunother.* 1993;36:237-244.

Medical Economics. *PDR for Herbal Medicines.* Montvale, NJ: Medical Economics Company; 1998.

Licorice

Other common name(s)	Scientific/medical name(s)
Sweet Root, Licorice Root	Gan Cao, *Glycyrrhiza glabra,* *Glycyrrhiza uralensis*

DESCRIPTION

Licorice is a perennial plant that grows in southern Europe, Asia, and the Mediterranean. The dried roots and underground stems of the plant are used in herbal remedies.

OVERVIEW

Licorice appears to have some use in the treatment of peptic ulcers; however, it is associated with side effects that can cause serious problems. Licorice can cause a fluid imbalance in the body, involving salt and water metabolism. More research is needed to determine if licorice extract has any role in cancer prevention or treatment.

How is it promoted for use?

Licorice is promoted as an herb that can treat peptic ulcers, eczema, skin infections, cold sores, menopausal symptoms, liver disease, respiratory ailments, inflammatory problems, chronic fatigue syndrome, AIDS, and even cancer. It has also been promoted to relieve symptoms of Addison's disease, lower cholesterol and triglyceride levels, strengthen the immune system, and treat hepatitis.

Many food products are widely available which contain small traces of licorice. Some licorice candy that is sold in the United States is actually flavored with anise and does not contain licorice. Glycyrrhizin (an active ingredient from the plant) is used as a flavoring in candy, gum, cookies, beverages, and cough syrup.

What does it involve?

Licorice is packaged as capsules, tablets, and as a liquid extract. It can be purchased at grocery stores, health food stores, or pharmacies. According to Commission E (Germany's regulatory agency for herbs), the recommended dosage is 200-600 mg for no more than 4 weeks for peptic ulcers.

What is the history behind it?

Licorice extract has been used in Chinese medicine for centuries (see Chinese Herbal Medicine). The Chinese used it as a mild laxative and also to help regulate the heart beat for those with heart problems. Its medicinal properties were also known in ancient Egypt, Greece, and Rome. In 1948, F. E. Revers, MD, first reported in a peer-reviewed article that licorice could be used to treat peptic ulcers.

What is the evidence?

Research suggests that licorice can treat peptic ulcers by increasing the production of prostaglandins (substances present in many tissues that control functions such as blood pressure or smooth muscle control), which is essential to the healing of ulcers.

The value of licorice as a cancer-prevention agent has not been proven. In the early 1990s, one study suggested that licorice could block the cancer-stimulating properties of estrogen due to the effects of its main ingredient, glycyrrhizin, a substance 50 times sweeter than sugar. However, this research has not been repeated.

Licorice has also been reported to have anti-cancer properties in mice by increasing the activity of certain enzymes that detoxify cancer-causing chemicals. However, animal studies may show a certain substance holds promise as a beneficial treatment, but further studies are necessary to determine if the results apply to humans.

Are there any possible problems or complications?

Regular consumption of licorice has been shown to cause headaches, lethargy, water retention, high blood pressure, and muscle weakness. In extremely large amounts, it can cause heart failure. People with high blood pressure, irregular heart beat, or cardiovascular, kidney, or liver diseases should avoid its use unless administered under the supervision of a physician. Women who are pregnant or breast-feeding should not use licorice.

References

Baker ME. Licorice and enzymes other than 11 beta-hydroxy-steroid dehydrogenase: an evolutionary perspective. *Steroids.* 1994;59:136-141.

Blumenthal M, ed. *The Complete German Commission E Monographs: Therapeutic Guide to Herbal Medicines.* Austin, Tx: American Botanical Council; 1998.

Davis EA, Morris DJ. Medicinal uses of licorice through the millennia: good and plenty of it. *Mol Cell Endocrinol.* 1991;78:1–6.

Edwards CR. Lessons from licorice. *N Engl J Med.* 1991;325:1242-1243.

Guide to Medicinal and Aromatic Plants. Licorice Review. Purdue University Web site. Available at: http://www.hort.purdue.edu/newcrop/med-aro/factsheets/LICORICE.html. Accessed May 8, 2000.

Mirsalis JC, Hamilton CM, Schindler JE, Green CE, Dabbs JE. Effects of soya bean flakes and liquorice root extract on enzyme induction and toxicity in B6C3F1 mice. *Food Chem Toxicol.* 1993;31:343-350.

Suzuki F, Schmitt DA, Utsunomiya T, Pollard RB. Stimulation of host resistance against tumors by glycyrrhizin, an active component of licorice roots. *In Vivo.* 1992;6:589-596.

Herbs / Vitamins / Minerals

Marijuana

Other common name(s)	Scientific/medical name(s)
Pot, Grass, Cannabis, Weed, Hemp	*Cannabis sativa*, delta-9-tetrahydrocannabinol (THC)

DESCRIPTION

Cannabis sativa is an annual plant that grows wild throughout the world in warm and tropical climates and is cultivated commercially. Parts of the plant (leaves and buds) have been used in herbal remedies for centuries. Scientists have identified 66 biologically active ingredients, called cannabinoids, in marijuana. The most potent of these is thought to be the chemical delta-9-tetrahydrocannabinol (THC).

OVERVIEW

The cannabinoid drug THC has been approved by the FDA for use in relieving nausea and vomiting, and for helping to increase appetite. Use of the raw marijuana plant, however, is illegal in the United States.

How is it promoted for use?

There is some evidence that THC has the potential to relieve pain, control nausea and vomiting, and stimulate appetite of people with cancer and AIDS. Researchers also believe that THC decreases pressure within the eyes, therefore preventing or reducing the severity of glaucoma.

Some supporters claim that marijuana dilates the respiratory tract (which may ease the severity of asthma attacks), has antibacterial actions, and inhibits tumor growth. Others claim that marijuana can be used to effectively control convulsions and muscle spasms in people who have multiple sclerosis, epilepsy, and spinal cord injuries. There is no scientific evidence to support these claims.

What does it involve?

Delta-9-tetrahydrocannabinol (THC) has been available by prescription (as dronabinol) since 1985 in the form of pills and suppositories. Several pharmaceutical companies are also developing inhalers to deliver therapeutic doses of THC. In raw form, marijuana is most commonly smoked in pipes or homemade cigarettes. It is also eaten directly or mixed with foods. Raw marijuana is illegal in the United States and is not approved by the FDA for medical applications.

What is the history behind it?

Marijuana has been described in Indian and Chinese medical texts for over 3,000 years (see Chinese Herbal Medicine). It was used to treat conditions such as beriberi, constipation, gout, malaria, rheumatism, and absent-mindedness, and also for depression, insomnia, vomiting, tetanus, and coughs. In the middle ages, herbalists used it externally to relieve muscle and joint pain. In the mid-1800s, the plant was mentioned as a treatment for gonorrhea and angina (chest pains related to heart disease). It was also used to treat gastrointestinal pain, cholera, epilepsy, strychnine poisoning, acute bronchitis, whooping cough, and asthma. Marijuana is legal in many parts of Asia and the Middle East but illegal in most Western countries.

In the last few years, marijuana has been the subject of extensive medical research. However, the political and legal controversies surrounding its status as an illegal substance, as well as concerns about the drug's potentially harmful side effects, have hampered the process of scientific inquiry in many countries, including the United States. Despite this, researchers continue to study whether marijuana has genuine medical applications.

What is the evidence?

Much of the research into marijuana has been centered on cannabinoids (the active ingredients in marijuana). Research findings about THC are mixed. One review of studies published between 1975 and 1996 concluded that oral THC is as effective or more effective for reducing nausea associated with chemotherapy than commonly used prescription drugs, and that it may be useful at low doses for appetite stimulation in patients with AIDS. The researchers also found that THC reduces eye pressure in people who have glaucoma. None of the studies, however, showed that THC or other ingredients in marijuana addressed the underlying causes of glaucoma. They reported that marijuana may cause toxic side effects, and the therapeutic benefits of THC should be carefully weighed against its potential risks. They concluded that currently the evidence does not support the use of smoked marijuana as a medication, and that additional research is needed.

Another comprehensive review of marijuana studies found there was not enough persuasive evidence to recommend marijuana as a treatment for nausea. However, a more recent study concluded that specific chemicals in marijuana, or synthetic copies of those chemicals, may prove beneficial to some patients with specific illnesses or symptoms, including nausea.

The most in-depth investigation into the medical use of marijuana was authorized by the US Government in 1997. The Office of National Drug Control Policy commissioned the Institute of Medicine (IOM) to assess the potential health benefits and risks of marijuana. The IOM is considered an independent research body affiliated with the National Academy of Sciences. The IOM issued its final report in 1999 and offered several conclusions regarding marijuana's usefulness.

First, they found that scientific data indicate that cannabinoids, particularly THC, have some potential to relieve pain, control nausea and vomiting, and stimulate appetite. Also, cannabinoids probably affect control of movement and memory, but their effects on the immune system are unclear. They found some of the effects of cannabinoids, such as anxiety reduction, sedation, and euphoria may be beneficial for certain patients and situations and undesirable for others. Based on the numerous studies they reviewed, they also found that smoking marijuana delivers harmful substances and may be an important risk factor in the development of respiratory diseases and certain types of cancers. The IOM stated that because marijuana contains numerous biologically active compounds, it cannot be expected to provide precise effects unless the individual components are isolated.

The National Cancer Institute (NCI) notes that THC may be useful for some cancer patients who have chemotherapy-induced nausea and vomiting that cannot be controlled by other drugs. But THC also causes a high similar to that caused by smoking natural marijuana. The NCI also said that more studies are needed to fully evaluate the potential use of marijuana for people with cancer.

Are there any possible problems or complications?

Smoking or eating raw marijuana can cause a number of effects, including feelings of euphoria, short-term memory loss, difficulty in completing complex tasks, alterations in the perception of time and space, sedation, anxiety, confusion, and inability to concentrate. Other side effects include low blood pressure, tachycardia (fast heart beat), and heart palpitations.

Many researchers agree that marijuana contains known carcinogens (chemicals that can cause cancer). They caution that smoking marijuana may decrease reproductive function as well as increase the risk of respiratory diseases and cancers of the lungs, mouth, and tongue. It may also suppress the body's immune system, and increase the risk of leukemia in children whose mothers smoked marijuana during pregnancy. Women who are pregnant or breast-feeding should not use marijuana.

The symptoms of a marijuana overdose include nausea, vomiting, hacking cough, disturbances to heart rhythms, and numbness in the limbs. Chronic use can also lead to laryngitis, bronchitis, and general apathy.

References

Barsky SH, Roth MD, Kleerup EC, Simmons M, Tashkin DP. Histopathologic and molecular alterations in bronchial epithelium in habitual smokers of marijuana, cocaine, and/or tobacco. *J Natl Cancer Inst.* 1998;90:1198-1205.

DuPont RL. Examining the debate on the use of medical marijuana users. *Proc Assoc Am Physicians.* 1999;111:166-172.

Joy JE, Watson SJ Jr, Benson JA Jr, eds. *Marijuana and Medicine: Assessing the Science Base.* Washington, DC: National Academy Press; 1999.

Kalb C. No green light yet: a long-awaited report supports medical marijuana. So now what? Newsweek Web site. Available at: http://newsweek.com/nw-srv/issue/13_99a/printed/ us/na/na0113_1.htm. Accessed May 8, 2000.

Medical Economics. *PDR for Herbal Medicines.* Montvale, NJ: Medical Economics Company; 1998.

Nahas G, Latour C. The human toxicity of marijuana. *Med J Aust.* 1992;156:495-497.

National Cancer Institute. Marijuana use in supportive care for cancer patients. NCI Cancernet Web site. Available at: http://cancernet.nci.hih.gov. Accessed May 8, 2000.

Schwartz RH, Voth EA, Sheridan MJ. Marijuana to prevent nausea and vomiting in cancer patients: A survey of clinical oncologists. *South Med J.* 1997;90:167-172.

Smigel K. Cancer problems lead list for potential marijuana research studies. *J Natl Cancer Inst.* 1997;89:1255.

Voth EA, Schwartz RH. Medicinal applications of delta-9-tetrahydrocannabinol and marijuana. *Ann Intern Med.* 1997;126:791-798.

Milk Thistle

Other common name(s)	Scientific/medical name(s)
Mary Thistle, Marian Thistle, Holy Thistle, Lady Thistle, Silymarin	*Silybum marianum*

DESCRIPTION

Milk thistle, a plant that belongs to the same family as daisies, grows in Mediterranean regions, Europe, North America, South America, and Australia. The parts used in herbal remedies are the seeds, which contain the antioxidant silymarin. Silymarin (also called milk thistle fruit) is thought to be responsible for milk thistle's therapeutic effects.

OVERVIEW

Laboratory research has shown that silymarin may be a useful agent for treating various liver diseases. Randomized clinical trials are needed to determine if these findings apply to humans, as well as to determine what role silymarin plays in preventing or treating cancer or reducing the side effects of chemotherapy.

How is it promoted for use?

Proponents claim that milk thistle detoxifies and protects the liver and is an effective treatment for hepatitis C, jaundice, and cirrhosis. They also claim it strengthens the spleen and gallbladder, benefits people with diabetes and slows the growth of certain types of cancer cells, including skin cancer, breast cancer, and prostate cancer. Some believe that milk thistle is an antidote for certain varieties of poisonous mushrooms.

Proponents also state that silymarin is a potent antioxidant. Antioxidants are compounds that block the action of activated oxygen molecules, known as free radicals, that can damage cells.

What does it involve?

Milk thistle supplements are available in capsules, tablets, powder, and liquid extract. Powdered milk thistle can be made into a tea. A typical dosage ranges from 200 to 400 mg of silymarin daily.

What is the history behind it?

Milk thistle has been used for generations in Europe as a liver restorative. It has also been used to treat malaria and conditions affecting the uterus.

What is the evidence?

Silymarin has been studied extensively in the laboratory for the treatment of acute and chronic liver disease, and to a lesser extent for some types of cancer. The few clinical studies that have been done have not been published in peer-reviewed medical journals and have come under a great deal of criticism.

Some research indicates that silymarin may be a useful chemical for treating various liver diseases, particularly those caused by excess toxins. Commission E (Germany's regulatory agency for herbs) approved the use of milk thistle fruit (ie, silymarin) as a treatment for toxic liver disease, and as a supportive treatment for chronic inflammatory liver disease and cirrhosis of the liver.

One review of both clinical and laboratory research said that silymarin may be effective for patients with hepatitis, alcoholic liver disease, and cirrhosis. However, the researchers noted that all of the clinical trials were conducted outside of the United States, were difficult to interpret, involved small numbers of patients, and followed inconsistent scientific methods.

Peer-reviewed studies of laboratory mice concluded that silymarin provides substantial protection against skin cancer caused by chemical carcinogens or ultraviolet radiation, possibly because of the drug's potent antioxidant properties. Cell culture studies (using cancer cells grown in the laboratory) found that silymarin reduced growth of breast and prostate cancer cells. Laboratory studies may show that a certain substance holds promise as a beneficial treatment, but further studies are necessary to determine if the results apply to humans.

Are there any possible problems or complications?

Milk thistle is generally considered safe. However, one case study reported that a woman suffered sweating, nausea, abdominal pain, diarrhea, vomiting, and weakness whenever she took milk thistle extract. It is not know for certain whether her reaction was caused by the herb or by another ingredient in her supplements.

Milk thistle extract may act as a mild laxative. Women who are pregnant or breastfeeding should not use this herb.

References

Adverse Drug Reactions Advisory Committee. An adverse reaction to the herbal medication milk thistle. *Med J Aust.* 1999;170:218-219.

Blumenthal M, ed. *The Complete German Commission E Monographs: Therapeutic Guide to Herbal Medicines.* Austin, Tx: American Botanical Council; 1998.

Fetrow CW, Avila JR. *Professional's Handbook of Complementary and Alternative Medicines.* Springhouse, Pa: Springhouse Corp; 1999.

Flora K, Hahn M, Rosen H, Benner K. Milk thistle (Silybum marianum) for the therapy of liver disease. *Am J Gastroenterol.* 1998;93:139-143.

Katiyar SK, Korman NJ, Mukhtar H, Agarwal R. Protective effects of silymarin against photocarcinogenesis in a mouse skin model. *J Natl Cancer Inst.* 1997;89:556-566.

Medical Economics. *PDR for Herbal Medicines.* Montvale, NJ: Medical Economics Company; 1998.

Xiaolin Z, Feyes D, Agarwal R. Anticarcinogenic effect of a flavonoid antioxidant, silymarin, in human breast cancer cells MDA-MB 468: Induction of G1 arrest through an increase in cip1/p21 concomitant with a decrease in kinase activity of cyclin-dependent kinases and associated cyclins. *Clin Cancer Res.* 1998;4:1055-1064.

Xiaolin Z, Grasso AW, Hsing-Jien K, Agarwal R. A flavonoid antioxidant, silymarin, inhibits activation of erbB1 signaling and induces cyclin-dependent kinase inhibitors, G1 arrest, and anticarciniogenic effects in human prostate carcinoma DU145 cells. *Cancer Res.* 1999;59:622-632.

Zi X, Agarwal R. Silibinin decreases prostate-specific antigen with cell growth inhibition via G1 arrest, leading to differentiation of prostate carcinoma cells: Implications for prostate cancer intervention. *Proc Natl Acad Sci U S A.* 1999;96:7490-7495.

Mistletoe

Other common name(s)	Scientific/medical name(s)
All Heal, Bird Lime, Devil's Fuge, Golden Bough	*Viscum album*

DESCRIPTION

Mistletoe is a semi-parasitic plant that grows on several species of trees native to England, Europe, and western Asia. It differs from the mistletoe found in the United States. The parts of the plant used in herbal remedies are its leaves and twigs.

OVERVIEW

A number of laboratory experiments suggest mistletoe may have the potential to treat cancer, but these results have not yet been reflected in clinical trials. Studies are needed to determine if there are any anticancer effects in humans.

How is it promoted for use?

It is claimed that mistletoe stimulates the immune system, helping the body fight more efficiently against cancer and other diseases. Mistletoe extracts are promoted as a remedy for a wide range of cancers, including tumors of the cervix, ovaries, breast, stomach, colon, lung, and also as a treatment for leukemias, sarcomas, and lymphomas. Supporters claim mistletoe extract injected directly into or near a tumor can slow and possibly reverse the growth of cancer cells, even in advanced cases of cancer.

They also claim mistletoe can lower blood pressure, decrease heart rate, relax spasms, and relieve symptoms of arthritis and rheumatism. It is further claimed to have sedative effects, and is promoted to relieve the side effects of chemotherapy and radiation. There is no scientific evidence to support these claims.

What does it involve?

Commission E (Germany's regulatory agency for herbs) has approved mistletoe as palliative therapy for malignant tumors (to help treat symptoms, not cure disease). The herb is prepared as an injectable whole plant extract, and is not used orally. The plant itself is poisonous and not safe to eat.

For people with cancer, mistletoe extracts are injected under the skin near the tumor. Daily injections are often given before and after surgery, chemotherapy, or radiation therapy and may continue for 10 to 14 days. Mistletoe injections promoted to prevent cancer may involve 3 to 7 injections a week over several months to several years.

What is the history behind it?

Mistletoe is surrounded by fascinating myths and legends that date back many centuries. More than 2,000 years ago, the Druids (members of the educated class among the ancient Celts in Europe) used mistletoe in many religious rituals. Their name for mistletoe meant "all healer," because they believed it had magical powers. Today, its name in Brittany, Wales, Scotland and Ireland ("an t'uil") still translates the same. The tradition of kissing under mistletoe dates back to Scandinavian mythology, where, in one tale, the plant became a symbol of love.

The liquid extract from the mistletoe plant has been used as an alternative method to treat cancer for more than 75 years. Modern research of mistletoe began in 1916 with Rudolph Steiner, PhD. Steiner combined spiritual and scientific approaches to medicine and to the treatment of cancer in particular. He believed that cancer formed when regulation of the body's physical or spiritual defenses faltered, and that mistletoe could reestablish that regulatory balance and fight back the tumor. Later researchers carried Steiner's beliefs further, contending that some of the chemicals in mistletoe could stop cancer growth and even kill cancer cells directly while enhancing the body's immune system.

Mistletoe injections are currently among the most widely used unconventional cancer treatments in Europe. Physicians in Switzerland, the Netherlands, and Great Britain commonly prescribe the treatment. In Europe, the most common commercial preparations are sold under the trade names Iscador and Helixor. Only the European species are used for cancer treatment. Mistletoe injections are not available in the United States, except in clinical trials, because the drug is not approved for sale by the FDA.

What is the evidence?

Researchers have completed numerous studies of mistletoe and its effects on cancer. No controlled human clinical studies have shown mistletoe to have any significant antitumor activity. Most of the studies that have found positive results from mistletoe extract in the treatment or prevention of cancer are not considered scientifically dependable. For example, in a review of 11 clinical studies, only one showed that mistletoe extract had no effect. However, that one was the only study in the group that was considered scientifically reliable. Other reviews of recent research have also suggested that mistletoe has no measurable effect on cancer growth.

Mistletoe preparations vary widely depending on how they are prepared (eg, fermented or non-fermented), the particular species from which they are obtained, and the season in which the plant was harvested. Researchers are working to identify the most important components, which are thought to be the lectins (proteins). A number of laboratory experiments suggest that mistletoe extracts may have some potential to combat and kill cancer cells, but these results have yet to be reflected in human trials. Laboratory experiments also hint that mistletoe increases the activity of lymphocytes, which are cells that attack invading organisms.

Are there any possible problems or complications?

Mistletoe is generally considered safe. Possible side effects include temporary redness at the injection site, headaches, fever, and chills. In rare cases, people allergic to mistletoe can develop a severe reaction and potentially life-threatening condition called anaphylactic shock. Some researchers suggest using purified preparations of mistletoe lectins to reduce the occurrence of toxic effects.

Mistletoe should not be eaten because all parts of the plant are poisonous. Consuming mistletoe has been known to cause seizures and death. Other symptoms include blurred vision, nausea and vomiting, stomach pain, diarrhea, irregular heartbeat, confusion, convulsions, disorientation, and drowsiness. Women who are pregnant or breast-feeding should not use this herb.

References

Alternative Medicine: Expanding Medical Horizons. *A Report to the National Institutes of Health on Alternative Medical Systems and Practices in the United States.* Washington, DC: US Government Printing Office; 1994. NIH publication 94-066.

Barrett S, Herbert V. Questionable cancer therapies. Quackwatch Web site. Available at: http://www.quackwatch.com. Accessed October 11, 1999.

Blumenthal M, ed. *The Complete German Commission E Monographs: Therapeutic Guide to Herbal Medicines.* Austin, Tx: American Botanical Council; 1998.

Fetrow CW, Avila JR. *Professional's Handbook of Complementary and Alternative Medicines.* Springhouse, Pa: Springhouse Corp; 1999.

Iscador report. Canadian Breast Cancer Research Initiative Web site. Available at: http://www.breast.cancer.ca. Accessed October 11, 1999.

Medical Economics. *PDR for Herbal Medicines.* Montvale, NJ: Medical Economics Company; 1998.

University of Texas Center for Alternative Medicine Research in Cancer. Mistletoe summary report. University of Texas-Houston Health Science Center Web site. Available at: http://www.sph.uth.tmc.edu/utcam/summary/mistletoe.htm. Accessed May 8, 2000.

US Congress, Office of Technology Assessment. *Unconventional Cancer Treatments.* Washington, DC: US Government Printing Office; 1990. Publication OTA-H-405.

Molybdenum

Other common name(s)	Scientific/medical name(s)
None	Mo

DESCRIPTION

Molybdenum is a scarce mineral that is present in very small quantities in the human body. The mineral is involved in many important biological processes, possibly including development of the nervous system, waste processing in the kidneys, and energy production in cells.

OVERVIEW

Molybdenum is an essential element in human nutrition, but its precise function and interactions with other chemicals are not well understood. Some evidence suggests that too little molybdenum in the diet may be responsible for some health problems. However, more research is needed to determine its role, if any, in preventing cancer and other diseases.

How is it promoted for use?

Proponents claim molybdenum is an antioxidant that prevents cancer by protecting cells from free radicals, the destructive molecules that may damage cells. Some supporters also claim that molybdenum prevents anemia, gout, dental cavities, and sexual impotence; however, there is no scientific evidence to support these claims.

What does it involve?

Diet is the major source of molybdenum for most people. Common sources of molybdenum include legumes, cereals, leafy vegetables, liver, and milk. Humans require very small amounts of molybdenum, which a well-balanced diet usually provides.

Molybdenum is also sold as a supplement in some health food stores and over the Internet. It is usually found in capsule form in combination with other nutrients. A typical dosage is 75 µg daily.

What is the history behind it?

Knowledge of molybdenum dates back to the Middle Ages. Pure molybdenum was first produced in 1893. Serious research into molybdenum's importance in the human body began only within the past decade.

What is the evidence?

Although researchers believe that molybdenum plays an important role in human health, its precise function and interactions with other chemicals are not well known. Some animal research suggests molybdenum supplements reduce the incidence of tumors in the esophagus and stomach of animals, and breast cancer in rats. Animal studies may show that a certain substance holds promise as a beneficial treatment, but further studies are necessary to determine if the results apply to humans.

A large, randomized study was conducted in Linxian, an area of north central China whose residents suffer very high rates of esophageal and stomach cancers. Researchers gave more than 30,000 people one of several different combinations of essential minerals and nutrients. One group received a combination of vita-

min C and molybdenum. The scientists did not find any reductions in cancer mortality rates among those that received molybdenum. Some evidence indicated that soil containing low levels of molybdenum may lead to the formation of chemicals in plants that increase the risk of cancers of the esophagus and stomach, but much more research is needed to determine a connection.

Some evidence suggests that too little molybdenum in the diet may be responsible for some health problems. Deficiencies may occur in areas where the soil contains little or no molybdenum. A study conducted in Japan suggested that low levels of molybdenum in the body were associated with decreased levels of cancer of the esophagus in women, but were also linked to higher levels of cancer of the pancreas. No relationship between molybdenum and cancer was found in men. The investigators cautioned that more research is needed.

Are there any possible problems or complications?

Little is known about the effects of too much or too little molybdenum in the body. Overdoses are extremely rare. Some research indicates that high levels of the mineral can irritate the upper respiratory tract, and cause swelling and deformities of the knees, hands, and feet. High levels may also cause gout.

Molybdenum deficiencies are very rare among humans, therefore most practitioners do not recommend supplements. People who eat diets that are very low in molybdenum may be at higher risk for vision problems, rapid heart rate, and rapid breathing. However, the impact on health may be minimal and cause no symptoms at all.

References

Barceloux DG. Molybdenum. *J Toxicol.* 1999;37:231-237.

Blot WJ, Li JY, Taylor PR, Guo W, Dawsey SM, Li B. The Linxian trials: Mortality rates by vitamin-mineral intervention group. *Am J Clin Nutr.* 1995;62(Suppl):1424S-1426S.

Cassileth B. *The Alternative Medicine Handbook*. New York, NY: W. W. Norton & Co. 1998.

Nakadaira H, Endoh K, Yamamoto M, Katoh K. Distribution of selenium and molybdenum and cancer mortality in Niigata, Japan. *Arch Environ Health*. 1995;50:374-380.

Rajagopalan KV. Molybdenum: An essential trace element in human nutrition. *Annu Rev Nutr*. 1988;8:401-427.

Seaborn CD, Yang SP. Effect of molybdenum supplementation on N-nitroso-N-methylurea-induced mammary carcinogenesis and molybdenum excretion in rats. *Biol Trace Elem Res*. 1993;39:245-256.

Mugwort

Other common name(s)	Scientific/medical name(s)
Ai Ye, Felon Herb, St. John's Plant, Wild Wormwood	*Artemesia vulgaris*

DESCRIPTION

Mugwort is a perennial flowering plant that is a member of the daisy family. It is native to Asia, Europe, and North America. The dried leaves and roots of the plant are used in herbal remedies. Mugwort should not be confused with wormwood or St. John's Wort.

OVERVIEW

There is no scientific evidence that mugwort is effective in treating gastrointestinal problems or any other medical condition, including cancer.

How is it promoted for use?

Mugwort is promoted to treat gastrointestinal disorders such as colic, persistent vomiting, diarrhea, constipation, flatulence, and cramps. The herb has also been promoted as a treatment for a wide range of other conditions, including headaches, nose bleeds, muscle spasm, epilepsy, circulatory problems, menopausal and menstrual complaints, chills, fever, rheumatism, asthma, dermatitis, dysentery, gout, and infertility. Proponents also claim mugwort oil has antibacterial and antifungal properties, and is used to treat worm infestations and snakebites.

Some proponents claim mugwort is a sedative and use it to treat neuroses, hysteria, general irritability, restlessness, insomnia, anxiety, mild depression, anorexia, and opium addiction. Dried mugwort (moxa) is used in moxibustion treatments to treat cancer (see Moxibustion). There is no scientific evidence to support these claims.

What does it involve?

Mugwort is available as dried leaves and roots, extracts, tinctures, teas, and pills. It can be used as a poultice as well. Mugwort is on the Commission E (Germany's regulatory agency for herbs) list of unapproved herbs. This means that it is not recommended for use because it has not been proven to be safe or effective.

What is the history behind it?

Herbalists have prescribed mugwort to treat many different conditions over the years. The Chinese have also used dried mugwort leaves (moxa) in moxibustion for centuries (see Chinese Herbal Medicine). In the middle ages in England, when

Herbs / Vitamins / Minerals

worn on St. John's Eve, mugwort was thought to protect the wearer from evil possession. Young women were told to sew mugwort into a small piece of cloth and place it under their pillows to induce vivid dreams. In the 1830s, Portuguese sailors introduced mugwort to France where it became popular as a cure for blindness and other illnesses. Mugwort was also used as a flavoring in beer.

What is the evidence?

Research on mugwort has focused on its properties related to allergic sensitivities. No research or clinical studies have been done on the alternative use of mugwort. There is no scientific evidence to support any of the claims made for mugwort including its use in moxibustion as a treatment for people with cancer.

Are there any possible problems or complications?

Mugwort is generally considered safe. However, it may increase the effects of anticoagulant medications (drugs that slow blood clotting). People with bleeding abnormalities are advised not to take mugwort. Mugwort pollen is known to cause hay fever in some people. The herb may also cause uterine contractions. Women who are pregnant or breast-feeding should not use this herb.

References

Blumenthal M, ed. The Complete German Commission E Monographs: Therapeutic Guide to Herbal Medicines. Austin, Tx: American Botanical Council; 1998.

Fetrow CW, Avila JR. Professional's Handbook of Complementary and Alternative Medicines. Springhouse, Pa: Springhouse Corp; 1999.

Medical Economics. PDR for Herbal Medicines. Montvale, NJ: Medical Economics Company; 1998.

Oleander Leaf

Other common name(s)	Scientific/medical name(s)
Oleander, Dogbane, Laurier Rose, Rose Bay, Anvirzel™	*Nerium oleander, Oleandri polium, Thevetia peruviana*

DESCRIPTION

Oleander is a poisonous evergreen shrub identified by its fragrant white, rose, or purple flowers, whorled leaves, and long follicles containing seeds. It grows in mild climates or as an indoor plant. The active ingredients are extracted from the leaves.

OVERVIEW

There is no scientific evidence that oleander is effective in treating cancer or any other disease. There have been reports of poisoning and death from ingestion of oleander, oleander leaf tea, and some of its extracts. Even a small amount of oleander can cause fatal respiratory paralysis and cardiac effects. One of the substances in oleander that causes the dangerous effects on the heart is called oleandrin. Because of these dangerous effects, oleander should not be used.

How is it promoted for use?

Even though oleander is poisonous, heavily diluted oleander preparations have been promoted to treat a variety of conditions including muscle cramps, asthma, corns, menstrual pain, epilepsy, paralysis, skin diseases, heart problems, and cancer. It has also been used in folk remedies as an insecticide.

What does it involve?

There is no established therapeutic dose of oleander extract. The oleander leaf is on the Commission E (Germany's regulatory agency for herbs) list of unapproved herbs. This means that it is not recommended for use because it has not been proven to be safe or effective. The raw botanical (herb, flower, or other plant part) can be toxic.

An oleander extract with the trade name of Anvirzel is available, but it has not been approved for study or use by the FDA as an investigational new drug (IND). In March 2000, the FDA requested the company who manufactures Anvirzel to immediately cease distribution and use of materials that promote the product as an IND, including misleading information on their Web site.

What is the history behind it?

Although this plant is poisonous, derivatives from oleander have been used for centuries as herbal medicine. Historical records show that the Mesopotamians, in the 15th century BC, believed in the healing properties of oleander. The Babylonians used a mixture of oleander and licorice to treat hangovers. Pliny, the Elder of ancient Greek, wrote about the appearance, as well as the poisonous and beneficial properties, of oleander. Arab physicians first used oleander as a cancer treatment in the 8th century AD.

Approximately 25 years ago, Huseyin Z. Ozel, MD, a Turkish physician, published medical papers describing his study of oleander. He developed an oleander extract which he patented and trademarked in the United States and Europe as Anvirzel. He had initiated this study because of folk traditions that suggested that an extract from oleander had antileukemic activity.

What is the evidence?

The effectiveness of oleander has not been proven. There have been no controlled studies of oleander or its extract. Although there are claims that Anvirzel improves quality of life, reduces pain, increases energy, and causes cancer regression and remission, there is no scientific evidence to support these claims. Phase I and Phase II clinical trials on Anvirzel are scheduled to begin in the near future.

Are there any possible problems or complications?

The oleander plant is poisonous, and people have died from eating parts of the plant. Death has resulted from heart failure or respiratory paralysis. Some of the symptoms and signs of oleander toxicity are nausea, vomiting, colic, appetite loss, dizziness, drowsiness, hyperkalemia (high potassium levels), rapid heart rate, heart block, dilated pupils, bloody diarrhea, seizures, loss of consciousness, and slow irregular pulse. There have been reports of death occurring after oral and/or rectal administration of the extract from the plant. The FDA has received reports of at least two deaths associated with the use of Anvirzel prior to the filing of the IND. This herb should be avoided, especially by women who are pregnant or breast-feeding.

References

Blumenthal M, ed. *The Complete German Commission E Monographs: Therapeutic Guide to Herbal Medicines.* Austin, Tx: American Botanical Council; 1998.

Clark RF, Selden BS, Curry SC. Digoxin-specific Fab fragments in the treatment of oleander toxicity in a canine model. *Ann Emerg Med.* 1991;20:1073-1077.

Fetrow CW, Avila JR. *Professional's Handbook of Complementary and Alternative Medicines.* Springhouse, Pa: Springhouse Corp; 1999.

Langford SD; Boor PJ. Oleander toxicity: examination of human and animal toxic exposures. *Toxicology.* 1996;109:1-13.

Moss R. *Herbs Against Cancer.* New York, NY: Equinox Press; 1998.

Orthomolecular Medicine

Other common name(s)	Scientific/medical name(s)
None	None

DESCRIPTION / OVERVIEW

Orthomolecular medicine is the use of very high doses of vitamins, minerals, or hormones to prevent and treat a wide variety of conditions. The doses are well above the recommended daily allowance (RDA) and are sometimes used along with special diets and conventional treatment. The concept of orthomolecular medicine dates back to the early 1950s, and Nobel prize winner Linus Pauling, PhD, coined the term in 1968. Proponents believe that taking mega-doses of these nutrients may correct "biochemical abnormalities," and thereby reverse a wide variety of conditions, such as alcoholism, arthritis, asthma, allergies, cancer, depression, epilepsy, heart disease, high blood pressure, hyperactivity, migraine headaches, mental retardation, and schizophrenia. There is no scientific evidence to support these claims. While a balanced diet may be sufficient for people who are healthy, proponents of orthomolecular medicine claim that sick people need far more nutrients than the RDA provides. Consuming large amounts of supplements, however, can be dangerous.

Pau D'Arco

Other common name(s)	Scientific/medical name(s)
Lapachol, Lapacho, Lapacho Morado, Lapacho Colorado, Ipe Roxo, Ipes, Taheebo, Tahuari, Trumpet Bush, Trumpet Tree	*Tabebuia impetiginosa, Tabebuia avellanedae, Tabebuia heptaphylla, Tabebuia ipé*

DESCRIPTION

Pau d'arco is a large tree that grows in the rainforests of Central and South America. There are about 100 species of the tree, which produces large, purple flowers and can grow to 150 feet tall and 6 feet in diameter. The inner bark of the tree is used in herbal remedies.

OVERVIEW

Although some laboratory and animal studies suggest that lapachol, an ingredient in pau d'arco, may have some effects against certain illnesses, no well-designed, controlled studies have shown that this substance is effective against cancer in humans. Pau d'arco also has potentially dangerous side effects.

How is it promoted for use?

Pau d'arco is promoted as a cure for dozens of illnesses and medical conditions, including arthritis, ulcers, diabetes, and cancer. Proponents also claim that when taken internally, it relieves infections, reduces inflammation, promotes digestion, strengthens the immune system, flushes toxins from the body, and protects against cardiovascular disease and high blood pressure. They also use it to treat lupus, osteomyelitis, Parkinson's disease, psoriasis, and to relieve pain. Applied externally, practitioners have used it to treat skin inflammation, fungal infections, hemorrhoids, eczema, and wounds. There is no scientific evidence to support these claims.

What does it involve?

Pau d'arco is available in capsules, tablets, salves, extracts, powder, and teas from health food stores and over the Internet. Recommended dosages vary by manufacturer. When making tea, practitioners say the bark must be boiled for at least 8 minutes to release the active ingredients.

What is the history behind it?

A tea made from pau d'arco is thought to have been a popular herb among the ancient Incas and natives of the South American rain forests, who used it to cure disease and as a tonic to strengthen the body and improve overall health. The native tribes of Brazil used the tree to make bows for hunting. When the Portuguese colonized Brazil, they named the tree pau d'arco, which means "bow stick." The herb remains a popular Brazilian folk remedy.

New interest in pau d'arco arose in the mid-1960s when a Brazilian physician claimed that the substance relieved pain, increased the number of red blood cells, and cured numerous illnesses, including cancer. Since the early 1980s, the herb has been sold in health food stores in the United States, where it is promoted as a treatment for virtually every kind of medical complaint.

What is the evidence?

One of the active ingredients in pau d'arco that has been studied is called lapachol. In laboratory animals, lapachol was found to be effective against malaria and certain kinds of animal tumor cells, such as sarcoma, but did not have an effect against other kinds of cancer, including leukemia and adenocarcinoma. Animal and laboratory studies may show a substance has certain effects, but further studies are necessary to determine if the results apply to humans.

There have only been a few studies on lapachol in humans. A noncontrolled study sponsored by the National Cancer Institute in the early 1970s found no toxic effects on liver or kidney tissue. However, doses high enough to affect tumors posed a serious risk of side effects, such as prevention of blood clotting. Based on these results, approval was not sought for lapachol as a new anticancer drug, research in the area was discontinued, and in Canada, a ban on the substance was recently imposed.

Pau d'arco contains at least 20 other active compounds, including quercetin and other flavonoids, whose effects are not yet known. Unconfirmed tests showed that crude extracts of the tree bark stimulated activity of certain immune system cells (macrophages). The substance also killed lung cancer cells grown in culture and reduced the rate of lung metastases in mice who had undergone surgery to remove the initial tumor. The bark extract also may work to kill bacteria or fungi. Extracted compounds are not the same as the raw bark. Study results of extracts will not necessarily be consistent with studies using the raw bark.

Are there any possible problems or complications?

Pau d'arco has some potentially serious side effects. Some of the chemicals in pau d'arco, such as hydroquinone, are known to be toxic. High doses may cause liver and kidney damage. Even low doses of the pau d'arco can cause vomiting and diarrhea and interfere with blood clotting. This herb should be avoided, especially by women who are pregnant or breast-feeding.

References

American Cancer Society. Questionable methods of cancer management: 'nutritional' therapies. *CA Cancer J Clin.* 1993;43:309-319.

Cassileth BR. Evaluating complementary and alternative therapies for cancer patients. *CA Cancer J Clin.* 1999;49:362-345.

Dinnen RD, Ebisuzaki K. The search for novel anticancer agents: a differentiation-based assay and analysis of a folklore product. *Anticancer Res.* 1997;17:1027-1033.

Fetrow CW, Avila JR. *Professional's Handbook of Complementary and Alternative Medicines.* Springhouse, Pa: Springhouse Corp; 1999.

Montbriand MJ. Past and present herbs used to treat cancer: medicine, magic, or poison? *Oncol Nurs Forum.* 1999;26:49-60.

US Congress, Office of Technology Assessment. *Unconventional Cancer Treatments.* Washington, DC: US Government Printing Office; 1990. Publication OTA-H-405.

PC-SPES

Other common name(s)	Scientific/medical name(s)
None	None

DESCRIPTION

PC-SPES is a formula consisting of a combination of eight herbs which contain a range of plant chemicals including flavonoids, alkanoids, polysaccharides, amino acids, and trace minerals such as selenium, calcium, magnesium, zinc, and copper (see Calcium, Copper, Selenium, and Zinc). The herbs include chrysanthemum, isatis, licorice, Ganoderma lucidum, Panax pseudo-ginseng, Rabdosia rubescens, saw palmetto, and skullcap (see Licorice and Saw Palmetto). "PC" stands for prostate cancer; "SPES" is the Latin word for hope.

OVERVIEW

While some research findings are promising, others show that the formula causes troubling side effects and may interfere with conventional therapies. More research is needed to determine whether PC-SPES is an effective and safe treatment for prostate cancer.

How is it promoted for use?

PC-SPES is promoted primarily as a treatment for prostate cancer. Proponents claim that the herbal preparation may prevent or delay the recurrence of prostate cancer, inhibit the growth of prostate tumors, lengthen the survival time of prostate cancer patients, improve the effectiveness of conventional treatments, and delay the use of chemotherapy. Some also state that PC-SPES stimulates the immune system, prevents benign prostatic hyperplasia (enlargement of the prostate gland), neutralizes blood toxins, suppresses cancer-causing genes, reduces inflammation, and has antioxidant qualities.

What does it involve?

PC-SPES comes in capsules and is taken daily, in varying dosages. It is available in health food stores, from some nutritionists, and directly from manufacturers. One study found that the potency of PC-SPES varies widely from batch to batch, so it can be difficult to know if the formula contains the correct amount of active ingredients.

What is the history behind it?

PC-SPES was developed in the early 1990s by a chemist named Sophie Chen, PhD, who claimed to have developed the formula by integrating modern science and ancient Chinese herbal wisdom (see Chinese Herbal Medicine). By the mid 1990s, the formula became widely promoted in the United States and was named PC-SPES.

What is the evidence?

PC-SPES shows some promise as a treatment for prostate cancer, but more research is needed before firm conclusions can be reached. Some investigators have found that PC-SPES lowers the level of prostate specific antigen (PSA), a protein secreted by cancerous prostate cells. A small study involving use of PC-SPES for at least 3 months in 9 patients with prostate cancer found that 5 of them responded to treatment as measured by an average decline in PSA levels of 62%. A decrease in PSA production often means that a prostate tumor is shrinking, but the study did not show that PC-SPES reduced tumor size or slowed the rate at which tumors spread. The study concluded that PC-SPES may prove to be useful in treating hormonally sensitive prostate cancer; but when used with conventional treatments, it may have mixed results.

Animal and laboratory studies have reported that PC-SPES had positive effects. A recent animal study found that PC-SPES reduced tumor incidence, rate of tumor growth, and metastasis. In one laboratory study, scientists found that PC-SPES appeared to inhibit the growth of certain types of prostate cancer cells, but concluded more research is necessary to evaluate the long-term effects. Animal and laboratory studies may show a certain remedy holds promise as a beneficial treatment, but further studies are necessary to determine if the results apply to humans.

Are there any possible problems or complications?

Side effects associated with the use of PC-SPES can be troubling. A recent laboratory study found that PC-SPES contains compounds that act like estrogen in the body. Such estrogen compounds can cause increased breast size and nipple tenderness in men taking PC-SPES. The estrogenic activity of PC-SPES appears to interfere with male hormones by lowering testosterone levels, which can reduce sex drive (libido). There is also an increased risk of developing blood clots, which are potentially fatal.

References

De La Taille A, Hayek OR, Buttyan R, Bagiella E, Burchardt M, Katz AE. Effects of phytotherapeutic agent, PC-SPES, on prostate cancer: a preliminary investigation on human cell lines and patients. *BJU Int.* 1999;84:845-850.

DiPaola RS, Zhang H, Lambert GH, et al. Clinical and biologic activity of an estrogenic herbal combination (PC-SPES) in prostate cancer. *N Engl J Med.* 1998;339:785-791.

Hsieh T, Chen SS, Wang X, Wu JM. Regulation of androgen receptor (AR) and prostate specific antigen (PSA) expression in the androgen-responsive human prostate LNCaP cells by ethanolic extracts of the Chinese herbal preparation, PC-SPES. *Biochem Mol Biol Int.* 1997;42:535-544.

Tiwari RK, Geliebter J, Garikapaty VP, Yedavelli SP, Chen S, Mittelman A. Anti-tumor effects of PC-SPES, an herbal formulation in prostate cancer. *Int J Oncol.* 1999;14:713-719.

Peppermint

Other common name(s)	Scientific/medical name(s)
Peppermint Oil, Mint, Balm Mint, Brandy Mint, Green Mint	*Mentha piperitae*

DESCRIPTION

Peppermint is a plant native to Europe, which is now cultivated widely in the United States and Canada. The oil from the leaves and flowering tops of the plant is used in herbal remedies.

OVERVIEW

There is no scientific evidence that peppermint oil is effective in treating side effects related to chemotherapy and radiation; however, there is some evidence that it may be effective in controlling nausea after surgery. There is mixed evidence about its effectiveness in treating symptoms of irritable bowel syndrome, such as stomach cramps.

How is it promoted for use?

Proponents claim peppermint oil improves digestion and relieves many gastrointestinal ailments, including gas, indigestion, cramps, diarrhea, and symptoms of irritable bowel syndrome and food poisoning. Some state it has a soothing effect and reduces anxiety.

Sprays and inhalants containing peppermint oil are promoted to relieve sore throats, toothaches, colds, coughs, laryngitis, bronchitis and nasal congestion, and inflammation of the mouth and throat. Some claim salves made from menthol (one of the major active ingredients in peppermint) ease muscle pain and soreness associated with injuries, arthritis, rheumatism, and neuralgia. Menthol vapors are also believed to relieve respiratory and sinus congestion.

Aromatherapists claim peppermint scent alone increases concentration, stimulates the mind and body, decreases inflammation, improves digestion, and relieves stomach pain (see Aromatherapy).

What does it involve?

Peppermint oil is the most frequently used form of the plant. The pure oil, or a liquid extract containing the oil, can be taken directly or swallowed in capsules. Peppermint oil is on the Commission E (Germany's regulatory agency for herbs) list of approved herbs. Common dosages are 1 to 2 capsules 3 times a day for irritable bowel syndrome; 1 tablespoon of leaves in a cup of boiling water for tea, 2 or 3 times a day; 3 to 4 drops in hot water for inhalation; 1% to 5% essential oil for nasal ointments; and 5% to 20% essential oil for other ointments applied to the skin.

Peppermint is also available as sprays and inhalants for treating ailments of the throat, mouth, and respiratory tract, and the leaves are sometimes brewed as a tea. Many well-known commercial products also contain menthol (the active ingredient in peppermint), which is rubbed directly on the skin or whose fumes are inhaled. Peppermint is often used to flavor pharmaceuticals, toothpaste, mouthwashes, cosmetics, and candy.

What is the history behind it?

Peppermint may have been used as a digestive aid thousands of years ago in ancient Egypt. More recently, peppermint has been a classic folk remedy for stomach cancer, nausea, vomiting, morning sickness, respiratory infections, and menstrual problems. Preparations containing menthol have a long history as a treatment for muscle soreness and pain, itching, sunburn, and to clear nasal congestion.

What is the evidence?

There are many anecdotal reports that support the use of peppermint as a treatment for various digestive and respiratory complaints. However, there is not enough scientific evidence to conclude that peppermint lives up to all the claims made by proponents, including its use as a treatment for stomach cancer or any other type of cancer.

Although there is no scientific evidence that peppermint oil is effective in treating side effects related to chemotherapy and radiation, it was found to be useful in controlling nausea after surgery. A randomized clinical trial in England found that patients who had received peppermint oil before surgery experienced less nausea after their operations than those who did not receive it.

There is debate about whether peppermint oil is effective in treating irritable bowel syndrome. Both a major scientific journal, as well as a major review article, reported that the evidence for this use is contradictory, and the effectiveness of peppermint oil has not been clearly established. A randomized clinical trial in Germany found that a preparation consisting of peppermint oil and caraway oil was effective for treating an upset stomach. Some preliminary evidence suggests that instilling peppermint oil into the colon during a barium enema (and perhaps colonoscopy) may reduce spasms and decrease the need for intravenous antispasm medications; however, more well-controlled studies are needed to make definite conclusions.

Are there any possible problems or complications?

Peppermint is considered safe but may cause irritation when applied to the skin. Because peppermint may increase symptoms associated with esophageal reflux disease and hiatal hernia, people with these conditions are advised to avoid the herb. People with gall stones or liver damage should also use caution when using peppermint. Products containing peppermint oil should not be applied to faces of infants or small children.

References

Blumenthal M, ed. *The Complete German Commission E Monographs: Therapeutic Guide to Herbal Medicines.* Austin, Tx: American Botanical Council; 1998.

Fetrow CW, Avila JR. *Professional's Handbook of Complementary and Alternative Medicines.* Springhouse, Pa: Springhouse Corp; 1999.

Kingham JGC. Peppermint oil and colon spasm. *Lancet.* 1995;346:986.

Madisch A, Heydenreich CJ, Wieland V, Hufnagel R, Hotz J. Treatment of functional dyspepsia with a fixed peppermint oil and caraway oil combination preparation as compared to cisapride. A multicenter, reference-controlled double-blind equivalence study. *Arzneimittelforschung.* 1999;49:925-932.

Medical Economics. *PDR for Herbal Medicines.* Montvale, NJ: Medical Economics Company; 1998.

Pittler MH, Ernst E. Peppermint oil for irritable bowel syndrome: a critical review and metaanalysis. *Am J Gastroenterol.* 1998;93:1131-1135.

Tate S. Peppermint oil: a treatment for postoperative nausea. *J Adv Nurs.* 1997;26:543-549.

Phytochemicals

Other common name(s)	Scientific/medical name(s)
Antioxidants, Flavonoids, Carotenoids, Sulfides, Polyphenols	None

DESCRIPTION

The term "phytochemicals" refers to a wide variety of compounds produced by plants. They are found in fruits, vegetables, beans, grains, and other plants. Scientists have identified thousands of phytochemicals, although only a small fraction have been studied closely. Some of the more commonly known phytochemicals include beta carotene, ascorbic acid (vitamin C), folic acid, and vitamin E (see Beta Carotene, Folic Acid, Vitamin C, Vitamin E).

OVERVIEW

Some phytochemicals have either antioxidant or hormone-like actions. Eating fruits, vegetables, and grains reduces cancer risk, and researchers are looking for specific compounds in these foods that may account for the beneficial effects in humans. There is no evidence that taking phytochemical supplements is as beneficial as consuming the fruits, vegetables, beans, and grains from which they are taken.

How is it promoted for use?

Phytochemicals are promoted for the prevention and treatment of numerous health conditions, including cancer, heart disease, diabetes, and high blood pressure. There is some evidence that phytochemicals may help prevent the formation of potential cancer-causing substances (carcinogens), block the action of carcinogens on their target organs or tissue, or act on cells to suppress cancer development. Some scientists estimate that people can reduce their risk of cancer by 30% to 40% simply by eating more fruits, vegetables, and other plant sources that contain phytochemicals.

There are several major groups of phytochemicals. One group, the polyphenols, includes a subgroup of chemicals called flavonoids. Flavonoids are plant chemicals found in a broad range of fruits, grains, and vegetables. The flavonoids found in soy beans, soy products, garbanzo beans, chickpeas, licorice, and tea, may mimic the actions of the female hormone estrogen (see Green Tea, Licorice, and Soy). Estrogen-like substances from these plant sources are called phytoestrogens. Flavonoids are being studied to determine whether they can prevent chronic diseases such as cancer and heart disease.

Antioxidants make up another broad category of phytochemicals. They are commonly found in vegetables such as broccoli, brussels sprouts, cabbage, and cauliflower (see Broccoli). These phytochemicals are thought to eliminate harmful molecules in the body known as free radicals, which can damage a cell's DNA and are thought to trigger some forms of cancer and other diseases.

Carotenoids, which give carrots, yams, cantaloupe, butternut squash, and apricots their orange color, are also promoted as anticancer agents. Tomatoes, red peppers, and red grapefruit contain lycopene which proponents claim is a powerful antioxidant (see Lycopene). The phytochemicals lutein and zeaxanthin, found in spinach, kale, and turnip greens, may reduce the risk of lung cancer. According to some nutritionists, grapes, eggplant, red cabbage, and radishes all contain anthocyanins–phytochemicals that protect against cancer and heart disease (see Grapes). Ellagic acid, found in raspberries, blackberries, cranberries, strawberries, and walnuts, also is said to have anticancer effects (see Ellagic Acid).

Another group of phytochemicals, called sulfides, are found in garlic and onions (see Garlic). Sulfides, according to supporters, stimulate enzymes that inhibit the growth of bacteria and may reduce the risk of stomach cancer, lower blood pressure, and strengthen the immune system.

What does it involve?

Phytochemicals are present in virtually all of the fruits, vegetables, legumes (beans and peas), and grains we eat, so it is quite easy for most people to include them in their diet. For instance, a carrot contains more than 100 phytochemicals. According to one estimate, more than 4,000 phytochemicals are catalogued, but only about 150 have been studied in detail.

Some of the better-known phytochemicals, such as vitamin A, vitamin E, beta carotene, and lycopene, are also available as supplements. However, most nutrition researchers believe that single supplements are not as beneficial as the foods from which they are derived.

What is the history behind it?

Only a few years ago, the term "phytochemical" was barely known. But physicians, nutritionists, and other health care practitioners have long advocated a low-fat diet that includes a variety of fruits, vegetables, legumes, and whole grains. Historically, cultures that consume such a diet experience lower rates of certain cancers and heart disease.

What is the evidence?

It has become a widely accepted notion that a diet rich in fruits, vegetables, legumes, and grains reduces the risk of cancer, heart disease, and other illnesses. But only recently have researchers begun to seriously try to determine the effects of specific phytochemicals contained in those foods.

Much of the evidence so far has come from observations of cultures whose diets consist mainly of plant sources, and which appear to experience noticeably lower rates of certain types of cancer and heart disease. For instance, the relatively low rates of breast and endometrial cancers in some Asian cultures is credited at least partially to dietary habits. These cancers are much more common in the United States, possibly because the typical American diet consists of a high proportion of fat and a low proportion of fruits, vegetables, legumes, and grains. Further evidence shows that the risk of breast cancer increases among Asian women who move to the United States, which may be the result of a shift to a diet that is high in fat and low in fruits and vegetables.

Because of the number of phytochemicals and the complexity of the chemical processes they are involved in, researchers face the challenging task of trying to determine which phytochemicals in foods are truly beneficial to health, which may fight cancer and other diseases, and which may even be harmful.

Researchers have conducted many laboratory and clinical studies examining the relationship between cancer risk and eating fruits and vegetables, legumes, and grains. Much of the evidence indicates that a higher consumption of these foods is associated with a reduced risk of some cancers and other illnesses. Some of the associations between individual phytochemicals and cancer risk are very compelling and make a very strong case for additional investigation. To date, none of the findings are conclusive, and knowledge about which of the numerous phytochemicals in fruits and vegetables actively help the body fight disease remains to be determined.

Researchers have also shown much interest in phytochemical supplements. Studies so far indicate that the value of most phytochemicals decreases when they are obtained through supplements and not through diet.

Until conclusive research findings emerge, health care professionals advise a balanced diet with emphasis on fruits, vegetables, legumes, and whole grains. According to ACS dietary guidelines, at least 5 servings of fruits and vegetables per day are recommended. Experts also stress that diet, regardless of how healthy, may reduce the risk of cancer and other diseases, but other crucial factors, such as genetics and the environment, clearly play a role as well.

Are there any possible problems or complications?

Phytochemical supplements should not be taken with benzodiazepine-type drugs, such as valium or other sedatives. Some phytochemical supplements may actually be toxic when taken in large doses.

There are some concerns that much of the fruits and vegetables grown in the United States are contaminated by pesticides, but most experts agree that the benefits of a diet rich in fruits and vegetables far outweigh any risks.

References

Barrett S. Antioxidants and other phytochemicals: current scientific perspective. Quackwatch Web site. Available at: http://www.quackwatch.com. Accessed May 8, 2000.

Craig WJ. Health-promoting properties of common herbs. *Am J Clin Nutr.* 1999;70:491S-499S.

Setchell KDR, Cassidy A. Dietary isoflavones: biological effects and relevance to human health. *J Nutr.* 1999;129:758S-767S.

Ziegler RG, Colavito EA, Hartge P, et al. Importance of alpha-carotene, beta-carotene, and other phytochemicals in the etiology of lung cancer. *J Natl Cancer Inst.* 1996;88:612-615.

Ziegler RG, Mayne ST, Swanson CA. Nutrition and lung cancer. *Cancer Causes Control.* 1996;7:157-177.

Pokeweed

Other common name(s)	Scientific/medical name(s)
Common Pokeweed, Pokeroot, Poke Salad, Pokeberry, Poke, Virginia Poke, Inkberry, Cancer Root, Crowberry, Bear's Grape, American Nightshade, Pigeon Berry	*Phytolacca americana*

DESCRIPTION

Pokeweed is a shrub that is native to eastern North America, and cultivated throughout the world. It can grow to a height of more than 10 feet. The berries and dried roots, which are the most potent sections of the plant, are used in herbal remedies.

OVERVIEW

Some research has shown that a protein contained in pokeweed, called pokeweed antiviral protein, has antitumor effects in mice and laboratory studies. Clinical trials have not yet been done to determine if these effects apply to humans. All parts of the mature plant contain chemically active substances such as phytolaccine, formic acid, tannin, and resin acid, and all parts are at least mildly poisonous when eaten.

How is it promoted for use?

Proponents claim that pokeweed can be used internally to treat a number of conditions, including rheumatoid arthritis, tonsillitis, mumps, swollen glands, chronic excess mucus, bronchitis, mastitis, and constipation. They also say that the herb is an effective treatment for fungal infections, joint inflammation, hemorrhoids, breast abscesses, ulcers, and bad breath. Herbalists also claim that external application of a preparation made from the plant relieves itching, inflammation, and skin diseases. There is no scientific evidence to support these claims.

Some supporters believe that the plant has anticancer and antiviral properties, protects cells against HIV, and may prevent the virus from replicating. Current studies are investigating the possible benefits of pokeweed as an anticancer agent in osteosarcomas and certain kinds of leukemia.

What does it involve?

Pokeweed supplements are available as liquid extracts, tinctures, powders, and poultices. There is no standard dose for pokeweed. Pokeweed berries are one of the ingredients in the Hoxsey formula (see Hoxsey Formula). For research purposes, scientists have learned to make pokeweed protein because pokeweed antiviral protein (PAP) is difficult to remove from the plant.

What is the history behind it?

Young pokeweed shoots, which contain very low levels of toxins, were used as food by Native Americans. They also used pokeweed in herbal remedies as a heart stimulant and to treat cancer, rheumatism, itching, and syphilis. European settlers adopted the therapeutic use of pokeweed, which went on to become a common folk medicine.

Juice from the berries was once used to make ink and dye and is still used by the food industry to manufacture red food coloring. Farmers and dairymen use an alcohol extract or tincture of pokeweed to reduce swelling of cows' udders. Followers of President James Polk wore pokeweed twigs during their candidate's election campaign, mistakenly believing that the plant was named for him.

What is the evidence?

Research has shown that pokeweed contains a compound that appears to enhance the immune system and has some anticancer effects in animals. According to one animal study, a protein contained in pokeweed called PAP demonstrated anticancer effects in rodents. Another study found that PAP combined with an immunotherapy drug (TP-3) holds some promise as a potential treatment for advanced osteosarcomas and some soft tissue sarcomas. Animal and laboratory studies may show a certain compound holds promise as a beneficial treatment, but further studies are necessary to determine if the results apply to humans.

Are there any possible problems or complications?

All parts of the pokeweed are poisonous, particularly the berries, roots, and seeds. Cooking the plant reduces its toxicity. The effects of eating the uncooked plant can include nausea, vomiting, diarrhea, abdominal cramps, headaches, blurred vision, confusion, dermatitis, dizziness, and weakness. Pokeweed may be fatal in children.

Pokeweed should not be used by people who are taking anti-depressants, Antabuse®, oral contraceptives, or fertility drugs. The plant may cause menstrual cycle irregularities and may also stimulate contractions of the uterus. Women who are pregnant or breastfeeding should not use pokeweed.

References

Anderson PM, Meyers DE, Hasz KC, et al. In vitro and in vivo cytotoxicity of an anti-osteosarcoma immunotoxin containing pokeweed antiviral protein. *Cancer Res.* 1995;55:1321-1327.

Bown D. *Encyclopedia of Herbs & Their Uses.* New York, NY: DK Publishing Inc; 1995.

Ek O, Waurzyniak B, Myers DE, Uckun FM. Antitumor activity of TP3(anti-p80)-pokeweed antiviral protein immunotoxin in hamster cheek pouch and severe combined immunodeficient mouse xenograft models of human osteosarcoma. *Clin Cancer Res.* 1998;4:1641-1647.

Herbs / Vitamins / Minerals

Fetrow CW, Avila JR. *Professional's Handbook of Complementary and Alternative Medicines*. Springhouse, PA: Springhouse Corp; 1999.

Medical Economics. *PDR for Herbal Medicines*. Montvale, NJ: Medical Economics Company; 1998.

Petersdorf RG, Adams RD, Braunwald E, et al. Eds. *Harrison's Principles of Internal Medicine*. 14th ed. New York, NY: McGraw-Hill; 1998.

Potassium

Other common name(s)	Scientific/medical name(s)
None	K, K+

DESCRIPTION

Potassium is an essential mineral found in most foods. Along with sodium and calcium, potassium helps regulate major body functions, including normal heart rhythm, blood pressure, water balance in the body, pH balance (acidity and alkalinity), digestion, nerve impulses, and muscle contractions. The body cannot manufacture potassium on its own and must obtain it from foods including apricots, potatoes, bananas, oranges, pineapples, green leafy vegetables, whole grains, beans, and lean meat.

OVERVIEW

Potassium is a mineral that is essential to normal body functioning. Most people get all the potassium they need in their diet. There is no scientific evidence that potassium supplements can prevent or treat cancer in humans. Excess potassium in the body can be toxic.

How is it promoted for use?
Some alternative medical practitioners maintain that low levels of potassium in the body may be linked to cancer, heart disease, high blood pressure, osteoporosis, depression, and schizophrenia. Some proponents claim that a diet high in sodium (salt) and low in potassium promotes tumor growth by changing the normal pH and water balance in human cells.

What does it involve?
There is no RDA for potassium, but the Estimated Minimum Daily Requirement is 2 g. Because most foods contain potassium, people usually get plenty of potassium from their normal food intake. The kidneys control blood levels of potassium and eliminate excess in the urine.

Supplements may be needed only by those who have low levels of potassium in their bloodstream, a condition known as hypokalemia. The causes of hypokalemia can include digestive disorders that result in diarrhea and vomiting, some types of diuretics (drugs that remove water from the body through urine), overuse of laxatives, diabetes, certain kidney diseases, and excessive sweating.

What is the history behind it?
In the 1930s, Max Gerson began developing a controversial dietary treatment for cancer known as the Gerson Diet Therapy (see Gerson Therapy). The cornerstone of his diet was the

use of potassium supplements in combination with low sodium claimed to restore proper salt-and-water balance within human cells and help stop tumor growth. However, this theory has not been supported by clinical or experimental data.

What is the evidence?

Some animal and human studies have indicated that a diet high in potassium and low in sodium might help prevent high blood pressure in some people. However, similar studies of the effects of a high-potassium diet on cancer have not shown a positive link between potassium intake and the prevention or development of cancer.

Some population studies have found that in a number of countries, where there are high-potassium diets, there are lower cancer rates, and in areas where there are low-potassium diets there are higher cancer rates. These types of studies, however, do not prove a direct connection, because there may be many other factors involved.

One researcher has suggested a link between an increased risk of cancer and low-potassium and high-sodium levels in cells. However, there is no scientific evidence that shows that changes in dietary potassium have any impact on potassium concentrations inside cancer cells. Potassium concentration in the body is actually regulated by the kidneys. Further studies are needed to determine the effects of a high-potassium/low-sodium diet on the prevention or formation of cancer.

Are there any possible problems or complications?

People with symptoms of hypokalemia (low potassium levels in their blood) should consult their physician before taking potassium supplements. These symptoms include tiredness, sleepiness, dizziness, muscle fatigue, and, in more serious cases, abnormal heartbeat or muscle paralysis.

Taking excessive potassium supplements can cause potassium to build up in the blood, resulting in a condition known as hyperkalemia. The symptoms of hyperkalemia include muscle numbness and tingling, abnormalities in heart rhythm, muscle paralysis, and possibly even heart failure. Severe kidney failure and Addison's disease (a hormone deficiency) may also cause hyperkalemia.

References

Cassileth B. *The Alternative Medicine Handbook.* New York, NY: W. W. Norton & Co; 1998.

Grimm RH Jr, Neaton JD, Elmer PJ, et al. The influence of oral potassium chloride on blood pressure in hypertensive men on a low-sodium diet. *N Eng J Med.* 1990;322:569-574.

Jacobs MM. Potassium inhibition of DMH-induced small intestinal tumors in rats. *Nutr Cancer.* 1990;14:95-101.

Jansson B. Potassium, sodium, and cancer: a review. *J Environ Pathol Toxicol Oncol.* 1996;15:65-73.

Negri E, La Vecchia C, Franceschi S, et al. Intake of selected micronutrients and the risk of breast cancer. *Int J Cancer.* 1996;65:140-144.

Tobian L. Dietary sodium chloride and potassium have effects on the pathophysiology of hypertension in humans and animals. *Am J Clin Nutr.* 1997;65:606S-611S.

Van Leer EM, Seidel JC, Kromhout D. Dietary calcium, potassium, magnesium and blood pressure in the Netherlands. *Int J Epidemiol.* 1995;24:1117-1123.

US Pharmacopeia Quality Review. USP Web site. Available at: http://www.usp.org. Accessed May 9, 2000.

Psyllium

Other common name(s)	Scientific/medical name(s)
Psyllium Seed Husk, Isphagula, Isapgol	*Planatago psyllium, Plantago ovata, Plantago isphagula*

DESCRIPTION

Psyllium comes from the crushed seeds of the Plantago ovata plant, an herb native to parts of Asia, Mediterranean regions of Europe, and North Africa. It is now cultivated extensively in India and Pakistan as well as in the southwestern United States. The seed husks are used in herbal remedies.

OVERVIEW

Psyllium has been used for many years to treat constipation and it may also be effective in reducing cholesterol. Although psyllium and other fiber supplements are useful in treating constipation, fruits and vegetables are considered to be more effective in lowering cancer risk. Psyllium should be taken with an adequate amount of water to avoid choking and obstruction of the esophagus, throat, and intestines.

How is it promoted for use?

The psyllium seed husk is used primarily as a fiber supplement to promote bowel movements and ease constipation. Fiber is the indigestible material in plant foods, also known as roughage. High fiber diets help the digestive tract function properly. Psyllium absorbs water and expands as it travels through the digestive tract, which is why it is referred to as a bulk-forming laxative. Psyllium is also sometimes used to treat side effects of conventional cancer treatment, such as diarrhea, and constipation.

What does it involve?

Psyllium seed husk is approved by Commission E (Germany's regulatory agency for herbs) for chronic constipation. It is also supported by the FDA which has issued a food-specific positive health claim for oats that includes psyllium fiber.

Psyllium is available in powder, tablet, and capsule form. In any form, it must be taken with adequate amounts of water (1 or 2 glasses per 3.5 g). Commission E recommends 4-20 g/day of the drug as needed. Psyllium is also available as the most common ingredient contained in laxatives that are used by over 4 million Americans a day. These laxatives are available over the counter and by prescription.

What is the history behind it?

Psyllium seed husk has been used as a laxative for generations. The leaves of the plant have been used in many folk medicine traditions to treat a variety of conditions, such as blisters, bleeding, abrasions, sprains, insect bites, stings, burns, poison ivy, throat irritation, gout, inflammation of mucous membranes and skin, and as a wash for sore eyes, dysentery, urinary tract disorders, chronic diarrhea, and coughs.

What is the evidence?

Psyllium has been found to be effective in treating constipation and research suggests that it may also help reduce cholesterol. It is well known that a diet high in fiber helps the digestive tract perform most efficiently. An inadequate amount of fiber in the diet can lead to constipation, hemorrhoids and diverticulitis. Fiber supplements such as psyllium have been proven to be effective for easing constipation, but most nutritionists agree that the best source of fiber is from the diet. Good sources of fiber are beans, vegetables, whole grains, and fruits.

Dietary fiber is thought by some nutritionists to help reduce the risk of colorectal cancer, although it is not yet known whether the protective factor is fiber itself or other components of the plant. Conflicting results from studies of dietary fiber and colorectal cancer risk have caused some confusion among the general public and some health professionals. Studies clearly show that a diet high in fruits and vegetables can lower colorectal cancer risk, as well as the risk of several other diseases. A recent study found that fiber may not be the beneficial ingredient in fruits and vegetables. The study does confirm the benefits of eating fruits and vegetables, but suggests that other substances in these foods may be responsible for their protective effect.

Are there any possible problems or complications?

The use of psyllium is generally safe. However, excessive amounts can cause abdominal distention, diarrhea, gas, and gastrointestinal obstruction. Not drinking enough water with psyllium can cause choking and obstruction of the esophagus, throat, and intestines. Some people are allergic to the plant, as well as to the psyllium powder.

Psyllium may delay the absorption of some medications taken at the same time. Diabetics who are insulin-dependent may need to reduce insulin dosage while taking psyllium products. Patients with a history of intestinal obstruction, fecal impaction, narrowing of the gastrointestinal tract, and those who have difficulty controlling diabetes should avoid psyllium.

References

Anderson JW, Allgood LD, Turner J, Oeltgen PR, Daggy BP. Effects of psyllium on glucose and serum lipid responses in men with type 2 diabetes and hypercholesterolemia. *Am J Clin Nutr.* 1999;70:466-473.

Blumenthal M, ed. *The Complete German Commission E Monographs: Therapeutic Guide to Herbal Medicines.* Austin, Tx: American Botanical Council; 1998.

Fetrow CW, Avila JR. *Professional's Handbook of Complementary and Alternative Medicines.* Springhouse, Pa: Springhouse Corp; 1999.

Fuchs CS, Giovannucci EL, Colditz GA, et al. Dietary fiber and the risk of colorectal cancer and adenoma in women. *N Engl J Med.* 1999;340:169-176.

Ganji V, Kies CV. Psyllium husk fiber supplementation to the diets rich in soybean or coconut oil: hypocholesterolemic effect in healthy humans. *Int J Food Sci Nutr.* 1996;47:103-110.

Medical Economics. *PDR for Herbal Medicines.* Montvale, NJ: Medical Economics Company; 1998.

Roberts-Andersen J, Mehta, T, Wilson RB. Reduction of DMH-induced colon tumors in rats fed psyllium husk or cellulose. *Nutr Cancer.* 1987;10:129-136.

Pycnogenol

Other common name(s)	Scientific/medical name(s)
Pinebark Extract, Pycnogenol™	None

DESCRIPTION

The name pycnogenol is used in several ways. Pycnogenol often refers to a trademarked compound extracted from the bark of the European coastal pine tree (Pinus maritima) that contains naturally occurring chemicals called proanthocyanidins. Pycnogenol is also the name of a variety of compounds that contain proanthocyanidins taken from a variety of natural sources, such as grape seeds (see Grapes) and plants, which contain a high concentration of these chemicals.

OVERVIEW

Although interest in pycnogenol is growing among medical researchers, there is little data from clinical trials to support the health claims made for any form of pycnogenol.

How is it promoted for use?

Proponents claim that pycnogenol is one of the most powerful antioxidants. Antioxidants are compounds that block the action of activated oxygen molecules, known as free radicals, that can damage cells. Supporters believe that pycnogenol protects against arthritis, complications from diabetes, cancer, heart disease, and circulatory problems such as swelling and varicose veins. Other reported benefits include helping to improve memory, reducing the effects of stress, improv]ing flexibility in joints, and reducing inflammation. Some claim that Pycnogenol supplements are much more effective in eliminating free radicals than vitamins E and C (see Vitamin C and E). There is no scientific evidence to support these claims.

What does it involve?

Pycnogenol is available as tablets and capsules. Practitioners use 25-300 mg/day for up to 3 weeks. They suggest a maintenance dose of 40-800 mg/day.

What is the history behind it?

In 1951, French researcher Dr. Jacques Masquelier extracted proanthocyanidins from the bark of the European coastal pine tree. He patented the process and named the compound Pycnogenol.

In 1970, proanthocyanidins were also extracted from grape seeds. The compound found in grape seeds and plants is referred to as either proanthocyanidins or pycnogenol. However, it differs somewhat from the Pycnogenol developed by Dr. Masquelier.

What is the evidence?

There is not enough data from clinical trials to support the health claims made for any form of pycnogenol, although interest in proanthocyanidins among medical researchers is growing. There are anecdotal reports that pycnogenol is effective in treating circulatory disorders. The results of one animal study suggest that pycnogenol from a pine tree bark extract may protect against lung cancer. A small human study found that a single high dose of pycnogenol in the form of a bioflavonoid mixture was effective in reducing platelet aggregation in smokers for over 6 days.

More research is needed to determine if pycnogenol may have any benefit for people with cancer or any other disease.

References

Fetrow CW, Avila JR. *Professional's Handbook of Complementary and Alternative Medicines.* Springhouse, Pa: Springhouse Corp; 1999.

Huynh HT, Teel RW. Effects of intragastrically administered Pycnogenol on NNK metabolism in F344 rats. *Anticancer Res.* 1999;19:2095-2099.

Putter M, Grotemeyer KH, Wurthwein G, et al. Inhibition of smoking-induced platelet aggregation by aspirin and pycnogenol. *Thromb Res.* 1999;95:155-161.

Tyler VE. Pycnogel fights cancer and the diseases of aging. *Prevention.* 1998;50:93.

Rabdosia Rubescens

Other common name(s)	Scientific/medical name(s)
None	None

DESCRIPTION / OVERVIEW

Rabdosia rubescens is a Chinese herb promoted as a treatment for cancer of the esophagus. It is also one of the eight herbs used in PC-SPES, an herbal formula promoted as a treatment for prostate cancer (see PC-SPES). There is no scientific evidence to support the claims for Rabdosia rubescens.

Red Clover

Other common name(s)	Scientific/medical name(s)
Purple Clover, Trefoil, Wild Clover	*Trifolium pratense*

DESCRIPTION

Red clover is a native plant of Europe, central Asia, and northern Africa. It now grows in many other parts of the world. The flower head is the part of the plant used in herbal remedies.

OVERVIEW

There is no scientific evidence that red clover is effective in treating or preventing cancer, menopausal symptoms, or any other medical conditions. It may also increase the risk of excessive bleeding in some people.

How is it promoted for use?

Proponents claim that red clover is useful for relieving menopausal symptoms because it contains chemicals that are similar to the hormone estrogen. They also claim that the herb suppresses coughs (particularly whooping cough), speeds wound healing, eases chronic skin conditions such as psoriasis, and is an anticoagulant (a compound that slows blood clotting). People who take prescription anticoagulant medication may be able to reduce their dosage by taking red clover supplements, according to some practitioners.

Other supporters claim that red clover is effective for treating cancers of the breast, ovaries, and lymphatic system. A few claim that the herb acts as an antibiotic, an appetite suppressant, and a relaxant; however, there is no scientific evidence to support these claims.

What does it involve?

Red clover supplements are available as tablets, capsules, or in liquid extract form. Dried red clover can be brewed into a tea. Practitioners generally use a daily dosage of about 4 g of dried red clover, or 1.5-3.0 ml of liquid extract. The liquid extract can be rubbed directly on skin or applied with a compress.

What is the history behind it?

For centuries, red clover has been grown in pastures to feed cattle and other grazing animals. The herb is an ingredient in the Hoxsey formula, Jason Winters' tea, and Essiac tea, which are common herbal remedies (see Hoxsey Herbal Treatment and Essiac).

What is the evidence?

Scientists have identified estrogen-like substances called isoflavonoids and anticoagulant chemicals called coumarins in red clover. However, the therapeutic claims made for the herb have not been verified in humans through randomized clinical trials.

One laboratory study found that red clover contains substances similar to the hormones estrogen and progesterone. Most studies suggest that long-term use (10 years or more) of estrogen replacement therapy after menopause may increase the risk of breast and endometrial cancers. Scientists have been seeking alternatives to estrogen that do not increase the risk of cancer.

In a small clinical study, researchers concluded that a diet supplemented with red clover sprouts and other plants that contain estrogen-like substances may reduce the severity of menopause. However, this conclusion needs to be confirmed in other studies before red clover can be routinely recommended.

Are there any possible problems or complications?

Not enough is known about the herb to determine its safety. Patients with bleeding problems or who take anticoagulant medications should avoid red clover because it may increase the risk of serious bleeding. Women with a history of estrogen receptor-positive cancers, or who are pregnant or breast-feeding should not use this herb.

References

Bown D. *Encyclopedia of Herbs & Their Uses.* New York, NY: DK Publishing Inc; 1995.

Fetrow CW, Avila JR. *Professional's Handbook of Complementary and Alternative Medicines.* Springhouse, Pa: Springhouse Corp; 1999.

Medical Economics. *PDR for Herbal Medicines.* Montvale, NJ: Medical Economics Company; 1998.

Wilcox G, Wahlqvist ML, Burger HG, Medley G. Oestrogenic effects of plant foods in postmenopausal women. *BMJ.* 1990;301:905-906.

Zava DT, Dollbaum CM, Blen M. Estrogen and progestin bioactivity of foods, herbs, and spices. *Proc Soc Exp Biol Med.* 1998:217:369-378.

Saw Palmetto

Other common name(s)	Scientific/medical name(s)
None	*Serenoa repens*

DESCRIPTION

Saw palmetto is a low-growing palm tree found in the West Indies and in coastal regions of the southeastern United States. The tree grows 6 to 10 feet in height and has a crown of large leaves. The berries are used in herbal remedies.

OVERVIEW

There is some scientific evidence that saw palmetto relieves symptoms associated with benign prostatic hyperplasia (BPH), such as difficult and frequent urination. However, saw palmetto is not an effective treatment for prostate cancer.

How is it promoted for use?

Saw palmetto is not effective as a treatment for prostate cancer, but may aid in relieving some of the symptoms of BPH (an enlarged prostate gland), which include difficult and frequent urination. Chemicals in saw palmetto berries are believed to interfere with the action of prostate hormones that stimulate cell growth.

Saw palmetto is also promoted as a treatment for prostatitis (inflamed prostate gland). Some proponents claim it also increases sex drive and fertility, and can be used to treat low thyroid function, although there is no scientific evidence to support these claims.

What does it involve?

Saw palmetto supplements are available as capsules, tablets, extracts, and tea. There is no standard dosage. In some clinical studies for the treatment of BPH, patients received 320 mg/day, divided into 2 doses.

What is the history behind it?

Native Americans ate the berries of the saw palmetto believing they served as a tonic that nourished the body, stimulated appetite, and promoted weight gain. They also used the herb to treat problems of the urinary tract and genital systems, such as difficulty urinating or frequent nighttime urination. Saw palmetto supplements are very popular in Europe, especially Germany, where physicians often prescribe them for patients with BPH.

What is the evidence?

Some research has found that saw palmetto extract may reduce symptoms of BPH. In 1998, the *Journal of the American Medical Association* published a review of 18 scientific studies on saw palmetto conducted over the last 30 years which involved more than 3,000 patients. The report concluded that the extract improved urinary symptoms, such as frequent nighttime urination and problems with urine flow. The improvements from using palmetto extract were similar to those seen in men who took the prescription drug finasteride for BPH. Saw palmetto also caused fewer and milder side effects than finasteride. Finasteride appears to reduce the size of the prostate, but it is still not clear whether saw palmetto causes the prostate to shrink.

Most of the studies using saw palmetto have included small numbers of patients, lasted an average of only 9 weeks, and varied in their design. Also, different dosages and forms of saw palmetto were used, which makes it difficult to establish a standard preparation. More research is needed to determine saw palmetto's long-term effectiveness and ability to prevent complications from BPH.

It is important to note that BPH is not cancer, and there is no published scientific evidence that saw palmetto has any value in the treatment of prostate cancer.

Are there any possible problems or complications?

The long-term effects and safety of saw palmetto are unknown. Side effects are not common, but may include headache, nausea, vomiting, upset stomach, dizziness, constipation or diarrhea, difficulty sleeping, fatigue, and in rare instances, heart pain. Men who have symptoms of BPH, which include difficult, frequent, or urgent urination, should see a physician as soon as possible, rather than treating themselves with saw palmetto. Similar symptoms can also result from prostate cancer, and self-treatment with saw palmetto may delay diagnosis and treatment of cancer.

It is not known if saw palmetto interferes with the measurement of prostate-specific antigen (PSA), which is a protein made by prostate cells used to determine the presence and extent of prostate cancer. Researchers have not yet thoroughly studied the effects of saw palmetto on blood PSA levels or determined whether saw palmetto interferes with accuracy of the PSA test. Since saw palmetto affects testosterone metabolism in the same way as finasteride, some physicians recommend that men also have a baseline PSA test and digital rectal exam before starting treatment with saw palmetto.

References

Fetrow CW, Avila JR. *Professional's Handbook of Complementary and Alternative Medicines.* Springhouse, Pa: Springhouse Corp; 1999.

Medical Economics. *PDR for Herbal Medicines.* Montvale, NJ: Medical Economics Company; 1998.

University of Texas Center for Alternative Medicine Research in Cancer. Saw palmetto summary. Available at: http://www.sph.uth.tmc.edu/utcam/summary/sawpalmetto.htm. Accessed October 29, 1999.

Wilt TJ, Ishani A, Stark G, MacDonald R, Lau J, Mulrow C. Saw palmetto extracts for treatment of benign prostatic hyperplasia. A systematic review. *JAMA.* 1998;280:1604-1609.

Herbs / Vitamins / Minerals

Selenium

Other common name(s)	Scientific/medical name(s)
None	Se

DESCRIPTION

Selenium is an essential mineral nutrient for both humans and animals. It is found in soil all over the world in varying amounts. Plants and small living organisms convert selenium to organic compounds, including selenomethione, which is the major source of selenium in foods.

OVERVIEW

Selenium shows promise as a nutrient that may prevent the development and progression of cancer; however, more research is needed. A small amount of selenium is all the human body needs. Large amounts in supplement form can be toxic.

How is it promoted for use?

Selenium is said to help preserve elasticity in body tissues, slow the aging process, improve the flow of oxygen to the heart, and help prevent abnormal blood clotting. Researchers think selenium is an antioxidant, a compound that blocks the action of activated oxygen molecules, known as free radicals, that can damage cells. Selenium may stimulate the formation of antibodies (proteins that help fight invading microorganisms) in response to vaccines. Selenium may also play a role in normal growth, development, and fertility.

Selenium is claimed to protect the body against cancer by causing cancer cells to die before they have a chance to grow and spread, a process known as apoptosis; however, this has not yet been proven.

What does it involve?

The best nutritional sources of selenium are seafood, liver, kidney, whole grains, cereals, and Brazil nuts. Selenium is also present in drinking water in very low levels. Selenium in food and water is easily absorbed by the human body and used where needed. A very small amount of selenium is good for the body, but too much can be toxic and have a negative effect on the immune system. The recommended intake of selenium is 5.5 µg per day for adults.

Since a normal diet provides about 50 to 150 µg/day, supplements are usually not needed. However, some research suggests that supplements may help prevent certain types of cancer, but the amount of the supplements should not exceed 400 µg/day taken on a regular basis. Supplements are available in drug and health food stores.

What is the history behind it?

Selenium was first discovered as an element in 1817 by Jons Berzelius, but it was not until the 1960s that selenium began to be associated with cancer prevention. Researchers hypothesized that selenium's antioxidant properties could inhibit tumor growth and boost the immune system. Animal research into the relationship between selenium and cancer began in the 1960s, and one human trial followed in the 1980s.

What is the evidence?

Both animal and human studies suggest that selenium may play a role in lowering a person's risk of developing cancer, and reducing death rates from cancer in those who already have the disease. However, a recent report by the National

Herbs / Vitamins / Minerals

Academy of Sciences (NAS) concluded that there is not enough evidence that taking high doses of antioxidants can prevent chronic diseases.

Epidemiological studies indicate that in areas of the world where selenium levels in the soil are high, mortality rates from cancer are significantly lower when compared with death rates in areas where the selenium levels are low. This finding is true for deaths from cancers of the lung, esophagus, bladder, breast, colon and rectum, pancreas, ovary, and cervix, and for total cancer deaths. However, a recent report by the National Academy of Sciences (NAS) concluded that there is not enough evidence that taking high doses of antioxidants can prevent chronic diseases.

There was one long-term controlled study of people with a history of skin cancer that began in 1983. The supplement had no effect on the patients' skin cancer; however, it was found that patients given a selenium supplement of 200 µg/day had significantly fewer cancers of the lung, colon and rectum, and prostate, and fewer deaths from lung cancer than those who did not receive it.

Animal studies have also shown a protective effect from selenium against the development of various cancers; however, observational studies in humans have had mixed results. Some have shown a cancer-protective benefit of selenium, while others have found no association between selenium and cancer. It is too early to conclude positively that selenium can prevent the development and progression of cancer until more long-term controlled human studies are conducted.

Are there any possible problems or complications?

Taking selenium supplements can be toxic to the human body if the supplements raise selenium levels beyond what the body can tolerate. No one knows for sure what that level is, however. The signs of selenium poisoning include deformed nails, vomiting, fatigue, numbness and loss of control in the arms and legs, as well as loss of hair, teeth, and nails. Massive overdoses can result in

death. In rare cases, eating vegetables grown in areas where selenium levels in the soil are high, such as the western United States, may also cause selenium poisoning.

On the other hand, a deficiency of selenium resulting from eating a poor diet over a long time or eating vegetables grown in selenium-poor soil can cause heart disease, muscle pain, and premature aging.

According to the US Department of Health and Human Services, one compound of selenium, selenium sulfide (a chemical compound used in antidandruff shampoos), might cause cancer if taken internally and therefore should not be ingested. Using antidandruff shampoos is considered safe because skin does not absorb selenium sulfide.

References

ADAM Pediatric Encyclopedia. Selenium in diet. HealthScout Web site. Available at: http://www.healthscout.com. Accessed May 8, 2000.

Cassileth B. *The Alternative Medicine Handbook.* New York, NY: W. W. Norton & Co; 1998.

Clark CC, Combs GF Jr, Turnbull BW, et al. Effects of selenium supplementation for cancer prevention in patients with carcinoma of the skin. *JAMA.* 1996;276:1957-1963.

Combs GF Jr, Gray WP. Chemopreventive agents: selenium. *Pharmacol Ther.* 1998;79:179-192.

Food and Nutrition Board, Institute of Medicine. Dietary Reference Intakes for Vitamin C, Vitamin E, Selenium, and Carotenoids. Washington, DC: National Academy Press; 2000. Also available at: http://books.nap.edu. Accessed April 25, 2000.

Ip C. Lessons from basic research in selenium and cancer prevention. *J Nutr.* 1998;128:1845-1854.

Patterson BH, Levander OA. Naturally occurring selenium compounds in cancer chemoprevention trials: A workshop summary. *Cancer Epidemiol Biomarkers Prev.* 1997;6:63-69.

University of Texas Center for Alternative Medicine Research in Cancer. Selenium summary. University of Texas-Houston Health Science Center Web site. Available at: http://www.sph.uth.tmc.edu/utcam/summary/selenium.htm. Accessed May 8, 2000.

Herbs / Vitamins / Minerals

Siberian Ginseng

Other common name(s)	Scientific/medical name(s)
None	*Eleutherococcus senticosus*

DESCRIPTION

Siberian ginseng is an herb that grows in Siberia, China, Korea, and Japan. The dried root and other underground parts of the plant are used in herbal remedies. Siberian ginseng should not be confused with Asian ginseng or American ginseng, which belong to a different family of herbs.

OVERVIEW

There is no scientific evidence that Siberian ginseng is effective in treating cancer or reducing the side effects of chemotherapy or radiation therapy. There have been no studies of its safety or long-term effects.

How is it promoted for use?

Proponents of Siberian ginseng claim that it stimulates the immune system, increases energy, improves concentration and memory, quickens recovery from illness, and heightens mental acuity, and physical prowess. Some practitioners claim that the herb regulates blood pressure, reduces inflammation, has a restorative effect on many organs, lowers blood sugar levels, and enables chemotherapy drugs to penetrate cancer cells more easily. There is no scientific evidence to support these claims.

What does it involve?

Siberian ginseng is on the Commission E (Germany's regulatory agency for herbs) list of approved herbs, and the supplements are available in tablets and liquid extracts. The powdered or cut root can be brewed as a tea. An average dose is 2-3 g/day. Typically, Siberian ginseng is taken regularly for 6 to 8 weeks, followed by a 1 or 2 week break before resuming.

What is the history behind it?

Siberian ginseng has been used in traditional Chinese medicine for 2,000 years to treat rheumatism, weak liver and kidneys, low energy levels, and to prevent respiratory tract infections, colds and the flu. Athletes from the former Soviet Union used Siberian ginseng to enhance athletic performance during competitions.

Herbalists have long prescribed Siberian ginseng for menopausal complaints, weakness in elderly people, physical and mental stress, insomnia caused by anxiety, and even to treat cancer and reduce the toxic effects of chemotherapy and radiation therapy. After the Chernobyl nuclear reactor disaster, Russian and Ukrainian citizens reportedly received the herb to counter the effects of radiation poisoning.

What is the evidence?

Few animal studies of Siberian ginseng have been published in peer-reviewed medical journals. There is no evidence that demonstrates the herb's effectiveness against cancer, and there is little evidence that supplements enhance athletic ability. One clinical study in the United States concluded that Siberian ginseng did not improve performance during aerobic exercise.

Health risks associated with Siberian ginseng have not been established, although side effects seem to be rare. A few cases of diarrhea and insomnia have been reported. People with high blood pressure should avoid the supplements. There have been no studies of Siberian ginseng's long-term effects.

References

Bown D. *Encyclopedia of Herbs & Their Uses.* New York, NY: DK Publishing Inc; 1995.

Blumenthal M, ed. *The Complete German Commission E Monographs: Therapeutic Guide to Herbal Medicines.* Austin, Tx: American Botanical Council; 1998.

Dowling EA, Redondo DR, Branch JD, et al. Effect of Eleutherococcus senticosus on submaximal and maximal exercise performance. *Med Sci Sports Exerc.* 1996;28:482-489.

Medical Economics. *PDR for Herbal Medicines.* Montvale, NJ: Medical Economics Company; 1998.

Six Flavor Tea

Other common name(s)	Scientific/medical name(s)
Liu Wei Di Huang, Gold Book Tea, Jin Gui Shen Qi	None

DESCRIPTION / OVERVIEW

Six Flavor Tea is a Chinese herbal tonic that is promoted to enhance conventional treatment of small-cell lung cancer (see Chinese Herbal Medicine). However, it is primarily sold as a treatment for kidney deficiencies, which practitioners claim can cause a buildup of disease-causing toxins. They contend Six Flavor Tea can also treat weakness or pain in the lower back, insomnia, night sweats, dizziness, tinnitus, impotence, and high blood pressure. There is no scientific evidence to support any of these claims.

St. John's Wort

<table>
<tr><td>

Other common name(s)
Goatweed, Amber, Klamath Weed,
Tipton Weed, Kira®, Tension Tamer®,
Hypercalm®

</td><td>

Scientific/medical name(s)
Hypericum perforatum

</td></tr>
</table>

DESCRIPTION
St. John's wort is a shrub-like perennial plant with bright yellow flowers that is native to Europe, western Asia, and northern Africa. It is also cultivated in the United States and other parts of the world. The parts of the plant used in herbal remedies are taken from the flowering tops.

OVERVIEW
St. John's wort has been shown to be effective in treating mild to moderate depression, with fewer side effects than standard antidepressants (ie, tricyclics). There is no data about its effectiveness in treating severe depression or how well it compares with newer antidepressants. More research is needed to compare extracts and different extract formulas with standard antidepressants. It also has the potential to interfere with a number of prescription drugs.

How is it promoted for use?
St. John's wort is widely used in Europe to treat depression, anxiety, and sleep disorders. In Germany, doctors prescribe it more often than Prozac®, which is a popular antidepressant drug. Hypericin is the most commonly studied active ingredient in St. John's wort.

The herb is also promoted to treat bronchial inflammation, burns, wounds, bedwetting, stomach problems, hemorrhoids, hypothyroidism, insect bites and stings, skin diseases, insomnia, migraines, kidney disorders, and scabies. There is no scientific evidence to support these further claims.

What does it involve?
Commission E (Germany's regulatory agency for herbs) has approved St. John's wort for the treatment of depression and anxiety, as well as for burns and skin lesions. It is available by prescription only in Germany; however, it can be purchased in drug and health food stores in the United States. An average daily dosage is 300 mg (.3% hypericin) of standardized extract preparation 3 times/day for 4 to 6 weeks.

There is a wide range of potency and purity of the different extracts that are available. Researchers have found that most brands of St. John's wort contain lower potency than is listed on the label. In some cases, the potency is less than half the promised amount–even as low as 20%. Standardized products contain .3% hypericin.

What is the history behind it?
Use of St. John's wort dates back many centuries, and is surrounded with much folklore. Greeks used it to fight fevers and evil spirits. The scientific name comes from the Greek words hyper (over) and eikon (ghost). In pre-Christian rituals in England, the plant was used to protect a house from evil spirits and to banish witches. It was thought that a person would be protected from death during the following year by putting a piece of the plant under a pillow on St. John's Eve, then

the Saint would appear in a dream and give his blessing. The plant's common name reflects the fact that the flowers typically bloom around the birthday of St. John the Baptist (June 24).

St. John's wort has also been used as a folk remedy for centuries to treat everything from wounds, headaches, gout, and kidney problems to nervous disorders. Native American Indians used several species of St. John's wort to treat diarrhea, wounds, and snakebites.

In the United States, the plant was not well known until after the 1900s. In 1959, the plant was first studied for its ability to fight bacteria. Extracts of St. John's wort have become extremely popular in the United States. People spent an estimated $400 million on products containing St. John's wort in 1998.

What is the evidence?

Clinical trials have shown that hypericin is effective in treating mild to moderate depression, with fewer side effects than standard antidepressants (ie, tricyclics). There is no data about its effectiveness in treating severe cases of depression or about how it compares to newer antidepressants such as Prozac® (ie, selective serotonin reuptake inhibitors). Its long-term effectiveness is also unknown, and it may not work with all types of depression. Researchers are uncertain about how the hypericin in St. John's wort works to relieve depression. Some think that the active ingredient may even be another compound in the herb.

One review that analyzed 23 randomized clinical trials concluded that hypericin was more effective than a placebo (an inactive substance) for the treatment of mild to moderately severe depression, and was found to be as effective as standard antidepressants. A more recent review of controlled, double-blinded studies reached a similar conclusion. However, they reported that there were problems with the way the studies were designed and analyzed. For example, many of the studies used low doses of tricyclic antidepressants. The authors stated that additional well-designed studies are needed before concluding that St. John's wort is an effective antidepressant.

The National Institutes of Health—in cooperation with the Office of Alternative Medicine, the National Institute of Mental Health, and the Office of Dietary Supplements–has launched a multicenter clinical trial using hypericin (St. John's wort) in the treatment of patients with major depression. A total of 336 patients will be followed over a period of 2 to 6 months at two clinical sites in the United States. The study will compare the effects of hypericin, a placebo, and a newer antidepressant.

Are there any possible problems or complications?

Information on the long-term effects or usage of St. John's wort is not currently known. Side effects are not common, but include gastrointestinal discomfort, fatigue, dry mouth, dizziness, skin rash, and hypersensitivity to sunlight. St. John's wort should not be used with alcohol, narcotics, amphetamines, anticoagulants, antibiotics, or cold and flu medicines such as pseudoephedrine. It should not be used with other antidepressants because it could cause serotonin syndrome–a potentially fatal complication involving changes in thoughts, behavior, and autonomic and central nervous system functioning caused by an increase in serotonin activity. People with severe depression or manic depression and women who are pregnant or breastfeeding should not use St. John's wort.

In response to a report in the medical journal Lancet, the FDA issued a public health alert on St. John's wort on February 10, 2000. The herb may interfere with a number of prescription drugs such as warfarin, indinavir, cyclosporine, digoxin, oral contraceptives, and antiretrovial medications (used for HIV). People taking any prescription medications, or other herbal preparations, should consult their physicians before taking St. John's wort.

References

Barrett S. St. John's wort. Quackwatch Web site. Available at: http://www.quackwatch.com. Accessed May 8, 2000.

Blumenthal M, ed. *The Complete German Commission E Monographs: Therapeutic Guide to Herbal Medicines.* Austin, Tx: American Botanical Council; 1998.

Center for Drug Evaluation and Research, Public Health Advisory: Risk of drug interactions with St. John's Wort and Indinavir and other drugs. FDA Web site. Available at: http://www.fda.gov/cder/drug/advisory/stjwort.htm. Accessed February 10, 2000.

Fetrow CW, Avila JR. *Professional's Handbook of Complementary and Alternative Medicines.* Springhouse, Pa: Springhouse Corp; 1999.

Kim HL, Streltzer J, Goebert D. St. John's wort for depression: a meta-analysis of well-defined clinical trials. *J Nerv Ment Dis.* 1999;187:532-538.

Linde K, Ramirez G, Mulrow CD, et al. St John's wort for depression–an overview and meta-analysis of randomised clinical trials. *BMJ.* 1996;313:253-258.

Medical Economics. *PDR for Herbal Medicines.* Montvale, NJ: Medical Economics Company; 1998.

Piscitelli SC, Burstein AH, Chaitt D, Alfaro RM, Falloon J. Indinavir concentrations and St. John's wort. *Lancet.* 2000;355:547-548.

National Center for Complementary and Alternative Medicine. Public Alert on St. John's Wort. National Institute of Mental Health Web site. Available at: http://nccam.nih.gov/nccam/mainmenu/one.html. Accessed March 2, 2000.

Ruschitzka F, Meier PJ, Turina M, Luscher TF, Noll G. Acute heart transplant rejection due to Saint John's wort. *Lancet.* 2000;355:548-549.

Vorbach EU, Arnoldt KH, Hubner WD. Efficacy and tolerability of St. John's wort extract LI 160 versus imipramine in patients with severe depressive episodes according to ICD-10. *Pharmacopsychiatry.* 1997;30:81-85.

Strychnos nux-vomica

Other common name(s)	Scientific/medical name(s)
Poison nut, strychnos seed, Quaker buttons	*Strychnos nux-vomica*

DESCRIPTION

Strychnos nux-vomica *is the name of an evergreen tree native to southeast Asia, especially India and Myanmar. Its dried seeds and bark (called nux vomica) are used in herbal remedies. The seeds contain organic substances, strychnine and brucine, that act as stimulants in the human body.*

OVERVIEW

There is no scientific evidence that Strychnos nux-vomica is effective in treating the side effects of conventional cancer treatment or any other conditions. The chemicals in the seeds are poisonous and may cause convulsions and death.

How is it promoted for use?

In herbal medicine, *Strychnos nux-vomica* is recommended for upset stomach, vomiting, abdominal pain, constipation, intestinal irritation, hangovers, heartburn, insomnia, certain heart diseases, circulatory problems, eye diseases, depression, migraine headaches, nervous conditions, problems related to menopause, and respiratory diseases in the elderly. In folk medicine, it is used as a healing tonic and appetite stimulant. There is no evidence to support these claims.

What does it involve?
The seeds of the *Strychnos nux-vomica* tree are removed from the ripened berries of the tree and dried in the sun. Various herbal preparations are made from the dried seeds, including tablets, liquid extracts, and tinctures. Some practitioners use single dosages that range from .02 g to 1 g. The maximum daily dosage should not exceed 2 g.

What is the history behind it?
Native tribes in Central and South America have used this remedy for centuries as a medicine to inhibit muscle contractions and as a poison for the tips of arrows. Some physicians used *Strychnos nux-vomica* in the treatment of stomach cancer in the late 19th century. It was given to patients to induce vomiting, which helped relieve the patient's discomfort.

Today it is used almost exclusively in homeopathy as an herbal remedy for the various conditions listed above (see Homeopathy). It is also used by industry as an active ingredient in pest control products.

What is the evidence?
Strychnos nux-vomica has not been proven to be effective for the treatment of any illness. Since the herb contains strychnine, which is poisonous to humans, conventional medical practitioners do not recommend it as a medicine. Some research has shown that the level of toxicity of nux vomica preparations may depend greatly on how the seeds are processed.

The herbal remedy is on the Commission E (Germany's regulatory agency for herbs) list of unapproved herbs. This means that it is not recommended for use because it has not been proven to be safe or effective.

Are there any possible problems or complications?

The strychnine in nux vomica is a poison that, in doses of 5 mg or more (equal to 30 to 50 mg of the herb formulation), may cause anxiety, restlessness, painful convulsions of the body, breathing difficulties, and even death resulting from suffocation or exhaustion. In addition, long-term intake of strychnine can cause liver damage. This herb should be avoided, especially by women who are pregnant or breast-feeding.

References

Blumenthal M, ed. *The Complete German Commission E Monographs: Therapeutic Guide to Herbal Medicines.* Austin, Tx: American Botanical Council; 1998.

Cai BC, Wang TS, Kurokawa M, Shiraki K, Hattori M. Cytotoxicities of alkaloids from processed and unprocessed seeds of Strychnos nux-vomica. *Chung Kuo Yao Li Hsueh Pao* 1998;19:425-428.

Medical Economics. *PDR for Herbal Medicines.* Montvale, NJ: Medical Economics Company; 1998.

Tea Tree Oil

Other common name(s)	Scientific/medical name(s)
Australian Tea Tree Oil, Melaleuca Oil	*Melaleuca alternifolia*

DESCRIPTION

Tea tree oil is a concentrated plant oil that is distilled through a steam process from the leaves of a large myrtle tree native to Australian coastal areas known as Melaleuca alternifolia *(or tea tree). The oil is used as an herbal remedy.*

OVERVIEW

Tea tree oil has been used in Australia for many years to treat skin infections. It holds promise today as an alternative to antibiotics that are resistant to certain bacteria; however, there is no evidence that it boosts the immune system. Tea tree oil is toxic when swallowed and it should never be taken internally.

How is it promoted for use?

Some proponents believe tea tree oil may be an antibiotic and antiseptic that is effective in combating germs. It has been used to treat cuts, minor burns, athlete's foot, and insect bites. Some claim it can treat bacterial and fungal skin infections, wound infections, gum infections, acne, head lice, eczema, vaginal candidiasis (a yeast infection), colds, pneumonia, and other respiratory illnesses.

While no one claims tea tree oil can prevent or treat cancer, some proponents claim the oil can boost the immune system. In addition, household cleaners that contain tea tree oil have been promoted as alternatives to products that contain possible cancer-causing chemicals, such as formaldehyde. One herbalist claims that tea tree oil can be used as a "lymphatic recharge" for a "sluggish" lymphatic system. There is no scientific evidence to support these claims.

What does it involve?

Tea tree oil can be dissolved in water or used in full strength. It is available as an ointment, cream, lotion, and soap. Tea tree oil is often sold in dark glass bottles with a dropper on the cap to prevent light from affecting its potency. When used to treat infections and skin conditions, the oil can be applied directly to the skin in full strength or diluted form using cotton swabs. The oil can also be found in deodorants, shampoos, soaps, antiseptic first-aid creams, and household cleaning products.

It should never be taken internally. For colds and other respiratory illnesses, the oil is added to a vaporizer so that the fumes can be inhaled to kill germs in the nose and throat. Drops of the oil can be added to bath water to treat skin diseases. The oil is sometimes mixed in water as a mouthwash to prevent gum infections.

What is the history behind it?

The Aborigines in Australia were the first to discover the healing properties of tea tree oil thousands of years ago. They treated cuts, burns, and skin infections by crushing the leaves of the tree in mudpacks and applying the packs to the injured skin. In the 1770s, the British explorer Captain Cook observed the native Aborigines brewing tea from the leaves and then he brewed tea of his own to give to his men to prevent scurvy. He coined the name tea tree.

In the 1920s, Australian physicians began to use the oil to sterilize wounds and prevent infections after surgery. They found it to be more effective than carbolic acid, the antiseptic most used at that time. Average Australians began to use the oil as a common household remedy for skin conditions and fungus infections. During World War II, tea tree oil was included in the first-aid kits given to all Australian soldiers and sailors.

After the discovery of penicillin and other antibiotics in the late 1940s, tea tree oil went out of favor as an antibiotic until the 1980s when it was discovered that some forms of staphylococcal bacteria were resistant to certain antibiotics, such as methicillin and vancomycin. Today, there is renewed interest in tea tree oil as an alternative to these antibiotics.

What is the evidence?

Recent laboratory experiments suggest that tea tree oil holds promise as an antibiotic when spread on top of the skin to treat staph bacteria that are resistant to methicillin and vancomycin and other infectious agents. Laboratory studies may show a certain substance holds promise as a beneficial treatment, but further studies are necessary to determine if the results apply to humans. There is also no clinical evidence for the effectiveness of tea tree oil for treating skin problems and infections.

Are there any possible problems or complications?

Tea tree oil is toxic when swallowed. As a result, it can cause drowsiness, poor muscle coordination, vomiting, diarrhea, and stomach upset. In rare cases, some people develop allergic reactions, such as inflammation of the skin. There is some evidence that the oil should not be used on burns. The oil is not recommended for children. Women who are pregnant or breast-feeding should not use this oil.

References

Carson CF, Riley TV. Antimicrobial activity of the major components of the essential oil of Melaleuca alternifolia. *J Appl Bacteriol.* 1995;78:264-269.

Faoagali J, George N, Leditschke JF. Does tea tree oil have a place in the topical treatment of burns? *Burns.* 1997;23:349-351.

Fetrow CW, Avila JR. *Professional's Handbook of Complementary and Alternative Medicines.* Springhouse, Pa: Springhouse Corp; 1999.

Rubel DM, Freeman S, Southwell IA. Tea tree allergy: what is the offending agent? Report of three cases of tea tree allergy and review of the literature. *Australas J Dermatol.* 1998;39:244-247.

Thuja

Other common name(s)	Scientific/medical name(s)
Eastern White Cedar, Yellow Cedar, Tree of Life, Arborvitae, Hackmatack, Swamp Cedar	*Thuja occidentalis*

DESCRIPTION

Thuja is an eastern white cedar tree. It is an evergreen in the cypress family that is native to eastern North America. The tree is also grown in Europe as an ornamental plant. The parts used in herbal remedies are the leaves, branches, and needles, which contain the oil thujone (see Wormwood).

OVERVIEW

There is no scientific evidence that thuja or its extract is safe or effective. Taken internally, this herb can cause serious side effects, and may be toxic in large doses.

How is it promoted for use?

Thuja is promoted as a treatment for many medical conditions, including cancer. Some proponents claim that thuja decreases the toxic effects of chemotherapy and radiation therapy.

Herbalists prescribe thuja to treat coughs and other respiratory ailments (including strep throat and respiratory distress related to congestive heart failure), and viral and bacterial infections. They also use it as a diuretic (to increase urination) and an astringent, to purify the blood, reduce inflammation, and cleanse the body of toxins. Thuja is sometimes used together with antibiotics to treat bacterial skin infections and herpes sores. It has even been used by practitioners to stimulate abortions. Thuja ointment is applied to the skin for ailments such as psoriasis, eczema, vaginal infections, warts, muscular aches, and rheumatism. There is no scientific evidence to support any of these claims.

What does it involve?

Liquid extracts, tinctures, and tea made from thuja are taken internally. There is no standardized dose. Thuja ointment is applied directly to the skin. Thuja oil and capsules are available in health food stores and over the Internet.

What is the history behind it?

Native Americans of the eastern United States and Canada used thuja for generations to treat menstrual problems, headaches, and heart ailments (see Native American Healing). Loggers drank tea made from white cedar twigs to relieve rheumatism. During the 17th century, some people called the eastern white cedar the "tree of life," because they believed that its sap had healing powers. In the late 1800s, the US Pharmacopoeia listed thuja as a treatment to stimulate the uterus and as a diuretic (to increase urine flow).

What is the evidence?

There is no scientific evidence that thuja is effective in treating cancer or any other disease. The medical literature contains no studies on the effects of thuja in humans, and there is very little scientific data to verify that the herb has any therapeutic value. Many supporters base their claims on limited laboratory experiments or anecdotal reports. One laboratory study conducted in

Germany found that a polysaccharide from thuja enhanced the immune system's ability to fight off invading organisms, such as HIV. Laboratory studies may show a certain substance holds promise as a beneficial treatment, but further studies are necessary to determine if the results apply to humans.

Are there any possible problems or complications?

Taken internally, in large doses, thuja is potentially toxic, although the amount that constitutes a high dose has not been determined. Some people who have consumed thuja reportedly experienced asthma attacks, gastrointestinal irritation, excess stimulation of the nervous system, and spontaneous abortion.

People with seizure disorders or gastrointestinal problems (such as ulcers or gastritis) should avoid thuja. Women who are pregnant or breast-feeding should not use this herbal treatment. In fact, because so little is known about thuja, it is not recommended for any use.

References

Fetrow CW, Avila JR. *Professional's Handbook of Complementary and Alternative Medicines.* Springhouse, Pa: Springhouse Corp; 1999.

Medical Economics. *PDR for Herbal Medicines.* Montvale, NJ: Medical Economics Company; 1998.

Offergeld R, Reinecker C, Gumz E, et al. Mitogenic activity of high molecular polysaccharide fractions isolated from the cuppressaceae Thuja occidentalis L. Enhanced cytokine-production by thyapolysaccharide, g-fraction (TPSg). *Leukemia.* 1992; 3:189S-191S.

Turmeric

Other common name(s)	Scientific/medical name(s)
Indian Saffron, Indian Valerian, Jiang Huang, Radix, Red Valerian	*Curcuma longa*

DESCRIPTION

Turmeric is a spice grown in India and other tropical regions of Asia. It has a long history of use in herbal remedies, particularly in China, India, and Indonesia. The root of the plant contains the active ingredient, curcumin.

OVERVIEW

Turmeric is a common food flavoring and coloring in Asian cuisine. Animal and laboratory studies have found that curcumin (the active ingredient in turmeric) demonstrated some anti-cancer effects. However, clinical research is needed to determine curcumin's role in cancer prevention and treatment in humans.

Herbs / Vitamins / Minerals

How is it promoted for use?

Some researchers believe turmeric may prevent and slow the growth of a number of cancers, particularly tumors of the esophagus, mouth, intestines, stomach, breast and skin, although there is no evidence from human studies to support these claims. One researcher states that curcumin, the active ingredient in turmeric, inhibited the formation of cancer-causing enzymes in rodents, although this has not been tested in humans. Some researchers have speculated that curcumin, after it enters the body, changes into tetrahydrocurcumin, which may be a potent antioxidant. An antioxidant is a compound that blocks the action of activated oxygen molecules, known as free radicals, that can damage cells.

Turmeric is promoted primarily as an anti-inflammatory herbal remedy that is said to produce far fewer side effects than conventional pain relievers. Some practitioners prescribe turmeric to relieve inflammation caused by arthritis, muscle sprains, swelling, and pain caused by injuries or surgical incisions. It is also promoted as a treatment for rheumatism and as an antiseptic for cleaning wounds. Some proponents claim turmeric interferes with the actions of some viruses, including hepatitis and HIV.

Supporters also claim that turmeric protects against liver diseases, stimulates the gall bladder and circulatory systems, reduces cholesterol levels, dissolves blood clots, helps stop external and internal bleeding, and relieves painful menstruation and angina (chest pains usually associated with heart disease). It is also used as a remedy for digestive problems such as irritable bowel syndrome, colitis, Crohn's disease, and illnesses caused by the parasite *Giardia* and by the *Salmonella* toxin. There is no scientific evidence to support any of these claims.

What does it involve?

Turmeric root is on the Commission E (Germany's regulatory agency for herbs) list of approved herbs, and it is available in powdered form in most grocery stores. It can also be made into a tea or purchased as a tincture or tablets. An ointment made from turmeric can be applied to the skin. Although there is no standardized dose for turmeric, some practitioners recommend taking a teaspoon with each meal.

What is the history behind it?

The use of turmeric was described in traditional Chinese and Indian medicine as early as the 7th century AD (see Chinese Herbal Medicine). In various Asian folk medicine traditions, turmeric has been used to treat a long list of conditions, including diarrhea, fever, bronchitis, colds, parasitic worms, leprosy, and bladder and kidney inflammations. Herbalists have applied turmeric salve to bruises, leech bites, festering eye infections, mouth inflammations, skin conditions, and infected wounds. Some people inhale fumes of burning turmeric to relieve chronic coughs. Turmeric mixed with hot water and sugar is considered by some herbalists to be a remedy for colds.

In India and Malaysia, there is a custom of pasting turmeric onto the skin, a practice now under study for the possibility that it may prevent skin cancer. The bright red forehead mark worn by some Hindu women is created by mixing turmeric with lime juice. Chefs frequently add turmeric to their creations because of its rich flavor and deep yellow color. The seasoning is an important ingredient in Indian curries. It is also used to add color to foods such as butter, margarine, cheese and mustard, to tint cotton, silk, paper, wood and cosmetics, as a food preservative, and to make pickles.

What is the evidence?

Researchers have studied turmeric extensively to determine if it is an effective antioxidant and anti-inflammatory agent, and whether it holds any promise as a cancer drug. However, all of the evidence so far comes from laboratory or animal studies. Animal and laboratory studies may show a certain substance holds promise as a beneficial treatment, but further studies are necessary to determine if the results apply to humans.

According to a review article published by researchers from the Ohio State University in Columbus, curcumin demonstrated anticancer effects at virtually all stages of tumor development in rodents and showed potential to kill cancer cells and prevent normal cells from becoming cancerous. This was particularly true for cancers of the breast, intestines, colon, stomach, and skin in rodents; however, this was not tested in humans.

A French laboratory study concluded that curcumin appeared to be a potent inhibitor of cancer development. Several additional laboratory studies also concluded that curcumin might prevent and slow the growth of some types of tumor cells. Two animal studies conducted in India found that curcumin slowed the growth and spread of cancer in mice. Controlled clinical trials are needed to determine what, if any, medical benefits turmeric offers to humans.

Are there any possible problems or complications?

When used as a spice in foods, turmeric is considered safe. More research is needed to establish the safety of turmeric when used in herbal remedies. Little is known about the potential risks of taking the larger quantities used to treat illnesses. An overdose may result in stomach pain. Contact dermatitis (skin allergy) and stomach ulcers have been reported after long-term use.

People taking anticoagulant medications, drugs that suppress the immune system, or non-steroidal pain relievers (such as Ibuprofen) should avoid turmeric. Persons with bleeding disorders, obstructions of the bile duct, or a history of ulcers, also should avoid turmeric. Women who are pregnant or breast-feeding should not use this herb.

References

Blumenthal M, ed. *The Complete German Commission E Monographs: Therapeutic Guide to Herbal Medicines.* Austin, Tx: American Botanical Council; 1998.

Bown D. *Encyclopedia of Herbs & Their Uses.* New York, NY: DK Publishing Inc; 1995.

Deshpande SS, Ingle AD, Maru GB. Inhibitory effects of curcumin-free aqueous turmeric extract on benzo[a]pyrene-induced forestomach papillomas in mice. *Cancer Lett.* 1997; 118:79-85.

Hastak K, Lubri N, Jakhi SD, More C, John A, Ghaisas SD, Bhide SV. Effect of turmeric oil and turmeric oleoresin on cytogenetic damage in patients suffering from oral submucous fibrosis. *Cancer Lett.* 1997:116:265-269.

Fetrow CW, Avila JR. *Professional's Handbook of Complementary and Alternative Medicines.* Springhouse, Pa: Springhouse Corp; 1999.

Medical Economics. *PDR for Herbal Medicines.* Montvale, NJ: Medical Economics Company; 1998:786-787.

Nagabhushan M, Bhide SV. Curcumin as an inhibitor of cancer. *J Am Coll Nutr.* 1992;11:192-198.

Simon A, Allais DP, Duroux JL, et al. Inhibitory effect of curcuminoids on MCF-7 cell proliferation and structure-activity relationships. *Cancer Lett.* 1998;129:111-116.

Stoner GD, Mukhtar H. Polyphenols as cancer chemopreventive agents. *J Cell Biochem.* 1995;22:169-180.

Valerian

Other common name(s)	Scientific/medical name(s)
Valerian Tea, Valerian Root, Valerian Extract	*Valeriana officinalis*

DESCRIPTION

Valerian is a flowering plant native to Europe, Asia, and the Americas. In herbal remedies, the plant's foul-smelling root is chopped up and made into a tea or extract that is used primarily as a sedative.

OVERVIEW

Valerian is an herb used for anxiety and insomnia. Although some research suggests that it is effective, the results have been conflicting, and the methods have been flawed. More research is needed to make definite conclusions about its effectiveness.

How is it promoted for use?

Herbal practitioners claim that valerian root or extract can lessen anxiety and nervous tension, aid sleep, help people quit smoking, ease congestion, and relieve muscle spasms. There are no claims that valerian is useful for treating or preventing cancer.

What does it involve?

Valerian root is on the Commission E (Germany's regulatory agency for herbs) list of approved herbs. Supplements are available in tablets, capsules, or tinctures, and it can also be brewed as a tea. To ease sleep and combat insomnia, the usual dosage of valerian extract in tablet form is 300-900 mg to be taken an hour before bedtime. For stress and anxiety, the recommended dosage is 50-100 mg taken 2 to 3 times/day.

What is the history behind it?

For thousands of years, the Chinese, Greeks, Romans, and Indians have used valerian as a mild sedative. The origin of the word "pew" is said to come from the foul odor of the valerian root, which a first century AD Roman physician, Dioscorides, called "phu." In the mid-1800s in the United States, the Shakers began growing valerian and other herbs to market to physicians and pharmacists in America and Europe. Valerian is often used to flavor foods and beverages such as root beer.

What is the evidence?

At least three controlled human studies have been conducted in the United States comparing valerian with a placebo (an inactive substance). These studies showed that those who took valerian experienced less insomnia and had improved quality of sleep. One randomized clinical trial conducted in Germany compared a combination of valerian and St. John's wort to diazepam (an antianxiety drug) in 100 people with anxiety symptoms and found significantly greater symptom improvement in those who took the herbs (see St. John's Wort). While promising, these studies are limited by small sample sizes and short follow-up periods.

On the basis of animal studies and several clinical trials in Europe, German health officials have approved valerian as a sleep aid and mild sedative. Expert advisors to the US Pharmacopeial Convention have concluded that the scientific evidence is insufficient and too conflicting to recommend valerian for the treatment of insomnia. More research is needed to determine the effectiveness of valerian.

Are there any possible problems or complications?

Valerian is considered to be relatively safe. However, some people may experience restlessness and heart palpitations, especially with long-term use of valerian as a sedative. Long-term or excessive use is not recommended due to the potential side effects, which include headaches, blurred vision, heart palpitations, excitability, hypersensitivity reactions, insomnia, and nausea.

Valerian should not be taken with alcohol, certain antihistamines, muscle relaxants, psychotropic drugs, sedatives, barbiturates, or narcotics. People with liver or kidney disease should seek their physician's advice before taking valerian. In very high doses, the herb may weaken the heartbeat and cause paralysis. Women who are pregnant or breastfeeding should not take valerian.

References

Barrett B, Kiefer D, Rabago D. Assessing the risks and benefits of herbal medicine: an overview of scientific evidence. *Altern Ther Health Med.* 1999;5:40-49.

Blumenthal M, ed. *The Complete German Commission E Monographs: Therapeutic Guide to Herbal Medicines.* Austin, Tx: American Botanical Council; 1998.

Fetrow CW, Avila JR. *Professional's Handbook of Complementary and Alternative Medicines.* Springhouse, Pa: Springhouse Corp; 1999.

Garges HP. Cardiac complications and delirium associated with valerian root withdrawal. *JAMA.* 1998;280:1566-1567.

Miller L. Herbal medicinals: selected clinical considerations focusing on know or potential drug-herb interactions. *Arch Intern Med.* 1998;158:2200-2211.

O'Hara M, Kiefer D, Farrell K, Kemper K. A review of 12 commonly used medicinal herbs. *Arch Fam Med.* 1998;7:523-536.

Venus Flytrap

Other common name(s)	Scientific/medical name(s)
Carnivora®, Plumbagin	*Dionaea muscipula*

DESCRIPTION

The Venus flytrap is a perennial plant that traps and eats insects. It is found in low-lying wetlands of the southeastern United States. Some believe that the primary active ingredient in the Venus flytrap is plumbagin. Carnivora is a commercially available liquid that is extracted from the plant.

OVERVIEW

There is no scientific evidence that the extract from the Venus flytrap plant is effective in treating skin cancer or any other type of cancer. Some side effects have been reported with its use.

How is it promoted for use?

Proponents claim that Carnivora has immune stimulant and anticancer properties. Some even claim that Carnivora applied directly to some skin cancer lesions could substitute for radiation therapy and chemotherapy. One practitioner claims that Carnivora can lead to the total reversal of skin and other forms of cancer. Supporters also claim that Carnivora is effective for treating colitis, Crohn's disease, rheumatoid arthritis, multiple sclerosis, neurodermatitis, chronic fatigue syndrome, HIV, and certain types of herpes. There is no scientific evidence to support any of these claims.

What does it involve?

Proponents suggest that full-strength or diluted, Carnivora can be placed under the tongue or mixed with water to make a drink. Carnivora can also be injected into the skin, inhaled through a vaporizer, or applied directly to the skin. There is no standardized dose for the drug. One practitioner gives patients 30 drops of Carnivora mixed with water or tea 5 times/day, or applies the extract directly to skin lesions. Carnivora contains 30% alcohol.

What is the history behind it?

In the 1970s, a German physician began testing liquids pressed from the Venus flytrap to determine if they would digest abnormal proteins found in cancer cells. Several years later he patented Carnivora. In a 1985 study, he claimed that out of 210 people with various types of cancer, 56% experienced either remission or stabilization of their tumors. He published the findings in a little-known German medical journal, and the results were never verified. Carnivora is not approved by the FDA, and physicians in this country cannot legally prescribe the drug.

What is the evidence?

There is no scientific evidence to support any of the claims made for Carnivora. It is also not clear whether plumbagin is actually the active ingredient in the Venus flytrap plant.

Most of the studies that have been done were conducted by the physician who patented the drug, and who also has a large financial stake in a clinic that administers the drug and in the manufacturing company.

An animal study conducted in India to study the effects of plumbagin from the Indian medicinal plant Plumbago rosea combined with radiation therapy was inconclusive. A second animal study in India found that plumbagin demonstrated a small degree of antitumor activity. The results of several other studies from India were positive but inconclusive. A laboratory study in Japan indicated that plumbagin had some effect against intestinal tumors. Animal and laboratory studies may show a certain substance holds promise as a beneficial treatment, but further studies are necessary to determine if the results apply to humans.

Are there any possible problems or complications?

Carnivora does not appear to be toxic, but not enough is known about the active ingredients for scientists to ensure that it is safe. Reported side effects from Carnivora injections include nausea and vomiting. Relying on this treatment alone, and avoiding conventional medical care, may have serious health consequences.

References

Devi PU, Rao BS, Solomon FE. Effect of plumbagin on the radiation-induced cytogenetic and cell cycle changes in mouse Ehrlich ascites carcinoma in vivo. Indian J Exp Biol. 1998;36:891-895.

Kini DP, Pandey S, Shenoy BD, et al. Antitumor and antifertility activities of plumbagin-controlled release formulations. Indian J Exp Biol. 1997;35:374-379.

Sugie S, Okamoto K, Rahman KM, et al. Inhibitory effects of plumbagin and juglone on azoxymethane-induced intestinal carcinogenesis in rats. Cancer Lett. 1998;127:177-183.

Vitae Elixxir

Other common name(s)	Scientific/medical name(s)
None	None

DESCRIPTION / OVERVIEW

Vitae Elixxir is an herbal and mineral mixture that is promoted as a treatment for arthritis, multiple sclerosis, lymphomas, leukemias, and multiple myeloma. There is no scientific evidence to support these claims. The ingredients of the formula are not well documented and people have reported that it has an unpleasant taste. It is taken orally by drops mixed with food and drink. Proponents also recommend mixing Vitae Elixxir with DMSO to make a foot bath for people with advanced cancer who cannot tolerate taking the preparation orally; however, it has not been proven to be effective (see DMSO).

Vitamin A

Other common name(s)	Scientific/medical name(s)
None	Retinol

DESCRIPTION

Vitamin A is a fat-soluble nutrient that is essential to growth and development. It is obtained in the diet from animal sources, and is also derived from beta carotene in plant foods (see Beta Carotene). Beta carotene is converted to Vitamin A in the small intestine and stored in the liver until needed by the body. Vitamin A and closely related molecules are also known as retinoids.

OVERVIEW

Vitamin A has not been proven to be effective in preventing cancer in humans. However, clinical studies are currently being done to examine the role of vitamin A and other retinoids in cancer prevention and treatment. High doses of vitamin A are toxic, and long-term use of high dose supplements may increase the risk of lung cancer among people at high risk, such as smokers.

How is it promoted for use?

Vitamin A is essential for normal growth, bone development, reproduction, vision, the maintenance of healthy skin and mucous membranes (which line the nose and mouth), and protection against infections in the respiratory, digestive, and urinary tracts. It enters the body directly as vitamin A from animal sources, such as liver, fish-liver oils, and dairy products, and indirectly as beta carotene, which the body converts to retinol, from many fruits and vegetables, including carrots, broccoli, spinach, squash, peaches, and apricots.

Some research suggests that vitamin A and some other retinoids have the ability to modify cancer cells and prevent normal cells from becoming cancerous. This is currently under investigation. Some proponents say that vitamin A supplements prevent cancer; however, most scientific studies do not support this claim.

What does it involve?

Vitamin A is a fat-soluble vitamin, which means that it is absorbed from dietary fats in the intestine and stored in the liver until needed by the body. It does not need to be consumed every day. The best way to get this vitamin is to eat a well-balanced diet. People who eat a balanced diet of fruits, vegetables, dairy products, and animal fats usually obtain enough vitamin A for good health, although supplements are available. The RDA of vitamin A is 4,000 IU (2.4 mg) per day for women and 5,000 IU (3 mg) per day for men.

What is the history behind it?

A popular theory in the 1920s was that vitamin A could be used to fight infections, such as respiratory infections and measles. At least 30 studies were done, with mixed results. In 1926, a Japanese researcher proposed a possible relationship between vitamin A deficiency and the development of cancer. Within the past 20 years, vitamin A has been extensively studied as an anticancer nutrient in laboratory, animal, and human population studies.

What is the evidence?

Studies on vitamin A are often hard to interpret because they have been done using different methods and different levels and combinations of retinoids. Results have been mixed, and there have been no consistent findings showing a decreased risk of cancers of the lung, stomach, intestines, skin, breast, cervix, bladder, or prostate due to vitamin A in the diet.

The use of vitamin A supplements has also not been proven to be effective in reducing can-

cer risk in humans. It appears that the combination of antioxidants in fruits, vegetables, legumes, and grains, rather than individual vitamins is more likely to be beneficial (see Phytochemicals). A clinical trial studied the effects of vitamin A and beta-carotene supplements on lung cancer and cardiovascular disease, researchers found that supplements did not benefit the patients studied and may have increased the incidence of lung cancer and cardiovascular disease in cigarette smokers and asbestos workers. Because of the evidence of possible harm to the study participants, the researchers ended the study early.

Some animal studies have found that vitamin A and other retinoids may enhance the immune system, slow tumor growth, decrease the size of tumors, and increase the effectiveness of some cancer treatments. Some laboratory, animal, and human studies have found that certain retinoids may also inhibit cancer development. Retinoids have shown significant activity in the reversal of cervical, mouth, throat, and skin premalignancies. However, further clinical research is needed. Several large clinical trials involving retinoids are currently being conducted.

Retinoids are not currently used as a cancer therapy, except in one notable case. A relatively rare type of leukemia, promyelocytic leukemia, often responds to a combination of retinoic acid (a retinoid) and chemotherapy.

Are there any possible problems or complications?

High doses of vitamin A supplements can cause nausea, tiredness, headaches, itchiness, scaling of the skin, diarrhea, and loss of appetite. High doses of vitamin A supplements should be avoided because they can cause bone pain, hair loss, irregular menstruation in women, birth defects if taken during pregnancy, as well as temporary or permanent liver damage.

A deficiency of vitamin A, which is rare in developed countries, can cause a lowered resistance to infection, poor night vision or even blindness, poor growth in children, weak bones and teeth, inflamed eyes, diarrhea, and poor appetite.

References

de Klerk NH, Musk AW, Ambrosini GL, et al. Vitamin A and cancer prevention II: comparison of the effects of retinol and beta-carotene. *Int J Cancer*. 1998;75:362-367.

Kushi LH, Fee RM, Sellers TA, Zheng W, Folsom AR. Intake of vitamins A, C, and E and postmenopausal breast cancer. The Iowa Women's Health Study. *Am J Epidemiol*. 1996;144:165-174.

Omenn GS, Goodman GE, Thornquist MD, et al. Effects of a combination of beta carotene and vitamin A on lung cancer and cardiovascular disease. *N Eng J Med*. 1996;334:1150-1155.

Vainio H, Rautalahti M. An international evaluation of the cancer preventive potential of vitamin A. *Cancer Epidemiol Biomarkers Prev*. 1999;8:107-109.

Vitamin A summary. Canadian Breast Cancer Research Initiative Web site. Available at: http://www.breast.cancer.ca. Accessed October 11, 1999.

Vitamin B Complex

Other common name(s)	Scientific/medical name(s)
B Vitamins, Vitamin B_1, Vitamin B_2, Vitamin B_3, Vitamin B_5, Vitamin B_6, Vitamin B_7, Vitamin B_9, Vitamin B_{12}	Thiamine, Riboflavin, Niacin, Pantothenic Acid, Pyridoxine, Biotin, Folic Acid, Cobalamin

DESCRIPTION

B vitamins are essential nutrients for growth, development, and a variety of other bodily functions. They play a major role in the activities of enzymes (proteins) that regulate chemical reactions in the body. B vitamins are found in a variety of plant and animal food sources.

OVERVIEW

There is not enough scientific evidence to determine what amount of B vitamins are needed to reduce the risk of cancer or other diseases. Vitamin B_9 may have some protective effect against colon cancer, but more studies are needed (see Folic Acid). There is no evidence that B vitamins are an effective treatment for people who already have cancer.

How is it promoted for use?

Scientists know that B vitamins influence several important bodily functions. Vitamin B_1 (thiamine) regulates enzymes that influence the functions of the muscles, nerves, and heart. Vitamin B_2 (riboflavin) influences the production of energy in cells and health of the skin and mucous membranes of the digestive and respiratory systems. Vitamin B_3 (niacin) also has a role in production of energy in cells and in maintaining health of the skin, nervous system, and digestive system. Vitamin B_5 (pantothenic acid) influences normal growth and development. Vitamin B_6 (pyridoxine) has an effect on protein, carbohydrate, and fat metabolism, and on maintaining health of red blood cells, skin, the nervous system, and digestive system. Vitamin B_7, $_H$ (biotin) helps break down protein, fatty acids, and carbohydrates. Vitamin B_9 (folic acid) influences growth, reproduction, blood-cell produc-

Herbs / Vitamins / Minerals

tion, and the nervous system. Vitamin B_{12} (cobalamin) plays a role in growth, development, the production of blood cells, the functions of the nervous system, and how the body uses folic acid and carbohydrates.

Some alternative medical practitioners claim that deficiencies in B vitamins weaken the immune system and make the body vulnerable to cancer. They recommend high doses of B vitamins as treatments for people with cancer. However, current scientific evidence has not found any effect of B vitamin supplements on the growth and spread of cancer. Many scientific studies in progress, are studying the relationships between vitamin intake and risk of developing certain cancers.

What does it involve?

Nutritionists maintain that a balanced diet that includes plenty of fresh fruits and vegetables is sufficient to provide the body with all the B vitamins it needs. Only small amounts of these vitamins are needed to fulfill the RDA. The RDA of vitamin B_9 (folic acid) is 400 µg a day. The National Academy of Science (NAS) recommends that adults over the age of 50 receive B vitamin supplements, or foods enriched with these vitamins, in order to prevent deficiency, which is common in this age group.

Vitamins B_1 and B_2 are found in cereals and whole grains. B_1 is also found in potatoes, pork, seafood, liver, and kidney beans. B_2 is found in enriched bread, dairy products, liver, and green leafy vegetables. Vitamin B_3 is found in liver, fish, chicken, lean red meat, nuts, whole grains, and dried beans. Vitamin B_5 is found in almost all foods. Fish, liver, pork, chicken, potatoes, wheat germ, bananas, and dried beans are good sources of vitamin B_6. Vitamin B_7, H is manufactured by intestinal bacteria and is also present in peanuts, liver, egg yolks, bananas, mushrooms, watermelon, and grapefruit. Green leafy vegetables, liver, citrus fruits, mushrooms, nuts, peas, dried beans, and wheat bread contain vitamin B_9.

Supplements that contain several of the B vitamins, usually in combination with other nutrients, are sold in grocery stores, health food stores, and over the Internet in pill form. Dosages vary by manufacturer.

What is the history behind it?

B vitamins have been studied for decades to determine how they affect the human body. In 1998, the NAS said that except for folate, recommended intakes of the B vitamins have not changed much since the last recommendations were made in 1989 and in Canada in 1990.

Research on their possible role in preventing cancer, if any, is relatively new and merits more investigation.

What is the evidence?

In 1998, the NAS released a report that said there has been much research over the past two decades that has focused on the roles that B vitamins may have in reducing the risk of cardiovascular disease, cancers, and various psychiatric conditions. There is some evidence showing that increased intake of vitamin B_9 (folic acid) may lower colorectal cancer risk, but the evidence is not conclusive. The study also reported that vitamin B_6 may reduce elevated levels of homocysteine (an amino acid) in the blood. Decreased levels of homocysteine have been linked with decreased risk of heart disease. However, other studies have not shown a positive benefit from B_6 in relation to vascular and heart disease. Some studies have also shown a possible link between intake of certain B vitamins and cancers of the breast and prostate. While these results are preliminary and not conclusive, they deserve further study.

Based on the NAS report, it is still unclear what intake levels are needed to reduce the risk of these diseases or whether an increase in B vitamin intake will produce any positive effect.

Supplements containing B vitamins are generally considered safe but should not be taken in large doses. Some possible side effects include gouty arthritis, hyperglycemia, and skin problems. Overdoses can lead to heart and liver problems. High doses of folate supplements can interfere with at least one chemotherapy drug, methotrexate.

Women who are pregnant and breastfeeding require more folic acid than others. All women of childbearing age may be urged by their physicians to increase their intake of folic acid to help prevent certain birth defects in their children.

B vitamin deficiency can cause anemia, tiredness, loss of appetite, abdominal pain, depression, numbness and tingling in the arms and legs, muscle cramps, respiratory infections, hair loss, eczema, poor growth in children, and birth defects in the fetuses of pregnant women.

References

Food and Nutrition Board, Institute of Medicine. *Dietary Reference Intakes for Thiamin, Riboflavin, Niacin, Vitamin B6, Folate, Vitamin B12, Pantothenic Acid, Biotin, and Choline.* Washington, DC: National Academy Press; 1998.

Key TJ, Silcocks PB, Davey GK, Appleby PN, Bishop DT. A case-control study of diet and prostate cancer. *Br J Cancer.* 1997;76:678-687.

Wu K, Helzlsouer KJ, Comstock GW, Hoffman SC, Nadeau MR, Selhub J. A prospective study on folate, B12, and pyridoxal 5'-phosphate (B6) and breast cancer. *Cancer Epidemiol Biomarkers Prev.* 1999;8:209-217.

Vitamin C

Other common name(s)	Scientific/medical name(s)
None	Ascorbic Acid, Ascorbate

DESCRIPTION

Vitamin C is an essential vitamin the human body needs to function well. It is a water-soluble vitamin that must be obtained from the diet. Vitamin C is found in abundance in citrus fruits, such as oranges, grapefruit, and lemons, and in green leafy vegetables, potatoes, strawberries, bell peppers, and cantaloupe.

OVERVIEW

Many studies have shown a connection between eating foods rich in vitamin C, such as fruits and vegetables, and a reduced risk of cancer. Studies of supplement use and cancer have found mixed results that make it difficult to determine the role of supplements and their effect on cancer risk. High doses of vitamin C can cause a number of side effects.

How is it promoted for use?

Vitamin C is an antioxidant, a compound that blocks the action of activated oxygen molecules, known as free radicals, that can damage cells. Vitamin C is thought by some to enhance the immune system by stimulating the activities of natural killer cells (a type of white blood cell) and anticancer agents. Some claim that the vitamin can prevent a variety of cancers from developing, including lung, prostate, bladder, breast, cervical, intestinal, esophageal, stomach, pancreatic, and salivary gland cancers, as well as leukemia and non-Hodgkin's lymphoma. Vitamin C is also said to prevent tumors from spreading, help the body heal after cancer surgery, enhance the effects of certain anticancer drugs, and reduce the toxic effects of other drugs used in chemotherapy. These claims are currently under investigation.

There is controversy over whether the reduction in cancer risk provided by eating fruits and vegetables that contain vitamin C together with many other nutrients can also be gained from vitamin C supplements.

Vitamin C may help control high blood pressure according to a recent study published in the *Lancet*. Some practitioners recommend high doses of vitamin C supplements to protect against and treat colds, although this has not been proven.

What does it involve?

Vitamin C is water-soluble, which means that the body uses what it needs and eliminates the rest. The RDA of vitamin C for women is 75 mg/day and for men is 90 mg/day. These recommendations were revised by the Food and Nutrition Board of the National Academy of Sciences (NAS) in April 2000. Experts at the National Cancer Institute (NCI) have argued that the RDA should be increased to 100-200 mg/day, to be obtained from fruits and vegetables whenever possible. The recent NAS report set the upper limit from both food and supplements at 2,000 mg/day.

Vitamin C supplements are available in powder or chewable pill form at grocery stores, health food stores, drug stores, and over the Internet. Recommended dosages vary by manufacturer.

What is the history behind it?

First identified in 1928 by Nobel Prize winner Albert Szent-Gyorgyi, vitamin C has been studied ever since for its nutritional and disease-preventing role. In 1970, two-time Nobel Prize winner Linus Pauling advocated large doses of vitamin C (1,000 mg/day or more) to prevent colds and reduce their severity.

Then in 1979, in a book called *Vitamin C and Cancer,* Pauling claimed that high doses of vitamin C could also be effective against cancer. His claim was based on a 1976 study he did with a Scottish physician in which 100 patients with advanced cancer were given 10,000 mg of vitamin C. The study concluded that the patients treated with vitamin C survived 3 to 4 times longer than patients not given the supplements. The Pauling study has been criticized by the NCI for being poorly designed, and subsequent studies done at the Mayo Clinic found that advanced cancer patients given the same dosage of vitamin C did not survive any longer than those not given the supplement. However, the Mayo Clinic trials have also been criticized for not fully addressing all the issues related to the effects of vitamin C, which still left questions about its effectiveness in the treatment of cancer.

What is the evidence?

Many scientific studies of the protective effects of vitamin C have shown that consuming a diet high in fruits and vegetables (containing vitamin C) significantly reduces the risk of developing cancers of the pancreas, esophagus, larynx, mouth, stomach, colon and rectum, breast, cervix, and lungs. Many of these studies show that a high intake of vitamin C from dietary sources has about a twofold protective effect when compared to a low intake of the vitamin.

However, observational studies and recent experimental trials of vitamin C supplements have not shown the same strong protective effects against formation of cancer. Apparently, vitamin C is most beneficial when consumed naturally in fruits and vegetables because of the other active ingredients in the food.

The 2000 NAS report stated that there is not enough evidence to support claims that taking high doses of antioxidants (such as vitamins C and E, selenium, and beta carotene) can prevent chronic diseases. Some scientists believe that taking high doses of antioxidant vitamins may actually interfere with the effectiveness of radiation and some chemotherapy drugs. No studies have yet been done in humans to test this theory. However, a recent review suggests that a combination of antioxidant vitamin supplements together with diet and lifestyle changes may actually improve the effectiveness of standard and experimental cancer therapies. More research is needed to evaluate the effects.

Are there any possible problems or complications?

The vitamin C supplements are generally considered safe unless doses are higher than 2,000 mg/day. Doses over this amount can cause headaches, diarrhea, nausea, heartburn, stomach cramps, and possibly kidney stones. Many physicians routinely recommend that people with cancer avoid gram-size doses of vitamin C during treatment. People with cancer should consult their physicians before taking vitamin C or other vitamin supplements.

References

Alternative Medicine: Expanding Medical Horizons. *A Report to the National Institutes of Health on Alternative Medical Systems and Practices in the United States.* Washington, DC: US Government Printing Office; 1994. NIH publication 94-066.

Barrett S, Herbert V. Questionable cancer therapies. Quackwatch Web site. Available at: http://www.quackwatch.com. Accessed October 12, 1999.

Byers T, Guerrero N. Epidemiologic evidence for vitamin C and vitamin E in cancer prevention. *Am J Clin Nutr.* 1995;62:1385S-1392S.

Duffy SJ, Gokce N, Holbrook M, et al. Treatment of hypertension with ascorbic acid. *Lancet.* 1999;354:2048-2049.

Food and Nutrition Board, Institute of Medicine. *Dietary Reference Intakes for Vitamin C, Vitamin E, Selenium, and Carotenoids.* Washington, DC: National Academy Press; 2000. Also available at: http//books.nap.edu. Accessed April 25, 2000.

Hwang MY. How much vitamin C do you need? *JAMA.* 1999;281:1415.

Labriola D, Livingston R. Possible interactions between dietary antioxidants and chemotherapy. *Oncology.* 1999;13:1003-1008.

Levine M, Rumsey SC, Daruwala R, Park JB, Wang Y. Criteria and recommendations for vitamin C intake. *JAMA.* 1999;281:1415-1423.

Kushi LH, Fee RM, Sellers TA, Zheng W, Folsom AR. Intake of vitamins A, C, and E and postmenopausal breast cancer. The Iowa Women's Health Study. *Am J Epidemiol.* 1996;144:165-174.

Patterson RE, White E, Kristal AR, Neuhouser ML, Potter JD. Vitamin supplements and cancer risk: the epidemiologic evidence. *Cancer Causes Control.* 1997;8:786-802.

Prasad KN, Kumar A, Kochupillai V, Cole WC. High doses of multiple antioxidant vitamins: essential ingredients in improving the efficacy of standard cancer therapy. *J Am Coll Nutr.* 1999;18:13-25.

University of Texas Center for Alternative Medicine Research in Cancer. Research in process. University of Texas-Houston Health Science Center Web site. Available at: http://www.sph.uth.tmc.edu/utcam/resact.htm. Accessed May 8, 2000.

US Congress, Office of Technology Assessment. *Unconventional Cancer Treatments.* Washington, DC: US Government Printing Office; 1990. Publication OTA-H-405.

Vitamin C summary. Canadian Breast Cancer Research Initiative Web site. Available at: http://www.breast.cancer. Accessed October 11, 1999.

Vitamin E

Other common name(s)	Scientific/medical name(s)
None	Alpha-Tocopherol, Tocopherols, Tocotrienols

DESCRIPTION

Vitamin E is an essential nutrient the human body needs to function normally. The term vitamin E actually represents a group of substances that includes alpha-tocopherol, which is the most important of the group to the body. This vitamin helps build normal cells and form red blood cells. The main sources of vitamin E in the diet are vegetable oils (especially safflower oil, sunflower oil, and cottonseed oil), green leafy vegetables, nuts, cereals, meats, egg yolks, wheat germ, and whole wheat products.

OVERVIEW

There is some evidence of the protective effects of vitamin E against prostate and colorectal cancer; however, more research is needed to confirm its role. There is no evidence that vitamin E significantly affects the growth of cancers that have already formed. High doses of vitamin E supplements can cause certain side effects.

How is it promoted for use?

Vitamin E is an antioxidant, a compound that blocks the action of activated oxygen molecules, known as free radicals, that can damage cells. Some proponents claim vitamin E plays a role in protecting the body against cancer by bolstering the immune system. Some physicians believe the vitamin can also increase the effectiveness of some drugs used in chemotherapy, such as doxorubicin and 5-fluorouracil (5-FU), and reduce some of the side effects of radiation therapy. However, others believe high doses of vitamin E might interfere with the effectiveness of radiation therapy and chemotherapy. These claims are currently under investigation.

Proponents claim that vitamin E supplements protect against heart attacks by preventing a buildup of harmful cholesterol in the blood. However, a recent study published in the *New England Journal of Medicine* found that the supplements had no effect on heart disease. There are also claims that vitamin E eases the inflammation associated with arthritis, speeds the healing of wounds in people who have suffered burns or have had surgery, and slows the progress of Parkinson's and Alzheimer's disease. Vitamin E is also used to protect against the effects of pollution and overexposure to the sun and to lessen the risk of developing cataracts. There is no scientific evidence to support these claims.

What does it involve?

A balanced diet normally provides adequate amounts of vitamin E for the body's needs, especially a diet low in fat and high in green leafy vegetables and fiber from grains and cereals. The RDA of vitamin E for adults is 15 mg/day from food. This recommendation was revised by the National Academy of Science (NAS) in April 2000. They also set the upper limit of intake from supplements at 1,000 mg/day.

Supplements are not usually necessary unless the body has a deficiency of vitamin E, which can lead to a destruction of red blood cells and result in anemia, with symptoms such as tiredness and shortness of breath.

What is the history behind it?

Since the 1940s, researchers and others have suspected that vitamin E might prevent heart disease. More recently, researchers have observed that people who have cancer often also have low levels of vitamin E in their blood. However, no one knows for sure if low levels of vitamin E can increase your chances of getting cancer or if cancer causes a decrease of vitamin E to occur in the blood.

What is the evidence?

Most of the evidence for the preventive effects of antioxidants such as vitamin E comes from animal studies and human observational studies. The largest controlled study of antioxidant vitamins and cancer was conducted in 1994 by the National Cancer Institute (NCI) in the United States and the National Public Health Institute of Finland. The study was designed to find out if antioxidant vitamins in higher doses than the RDA (eg, 50 mg) could reduce the incidence of lung cancer and other cancers and illnesses among 29,000 male smokers. The study found no beneficial effect of vitamin E supplements on lung cancer incidence and mixed results for other cancers. The study did find lower rates of prostate and colorectal cancer among those who received vitamin E, but higher rates of bladder, stomach, and other cancers.

In 1997, a review of epidemiological research reported some protective effects of vitamin E against several cancers. They found that in randomized clinical trials, there were modest protective effects of vitamin E against prostate and colon cancer. However, there have been methodological problems in measuring the association of supplement use and cancer risk. For example, one study found people who take supplements are more likely to exercise regularly, eat four or more servings of fruits and vegetables per day, and eat a low-fat diet.

The 2000 NAS report stated that there is not enough evidence to support claims that taking high doses of antioxidants (such as vitamins C and E, selenium, and beta carotene) can prevent chronic diseases. Some scientists believe that taking high doses of antioxidant vitamins may actually interfere with the effectiveness of radiation and some chemotherapy drugs. No studies have yet been done in humans to test this theory. However, one animal study found that vitamin E actually increased the effectiveness of the chemotherapy drug 5-FU against colon cancer in mice. Animal and laboratory studies may show a certain substance holds promise as a beneficial treatment, but further studies are necessary to determine if the results apply to humans.

Are there any possible problems or complications?

Vitamin E supplements found in multivitamins are generally considered safe as long as the levels are consistent with the RDA. However, excessive doses of vitamin E supplements taken over a long time can cause nausea, vomiting, stomach pain, and diarrhea. High doses of supplements may also slow the way the body absorbs vitamins A, D, and K and result in deficiencies of these vitamins. Megadoses of vitamin E supplements are not advised for people who are taking blood-thinning drugs, such as warfarin, because the supplements might counteract the effects of the drugs. People with cancer should consult their physician before taking vitamin E or other vitamin supplements.

References

Alpha-Tocopherol, Beta Carotene Cancer Prevention Study Group. The effect of vitamin E and beta carotene on the incidence of lung cancer and other cancers in male smokers. *N Eng J Med.* 1994;330:1029-1035.

Chinery R, Brockman JA, Peeler MO, Shyr Y, Beauchamp RD, Coffey RJ. Antioxidants enhance the cytotoxicity of chemotherapeutic agents in colorectal cancer: a p53-independent induction of p21WAF1/CIP1 via C/EBPbeta. *Nat Med.* 1997;3:1233-1241.

Food and Nutrition Board, Institute of Medicine. *Dietary Reference Intakes for Vitamin C, Vitamin E, Selenium, and Carotenoids.* Washington, DC: National Academy Press; 2000. Also available at: http//books.nap.edu. Accessed April 25, 2000.

Health & Living. ABC News Web site. Available at: http://abcnews.go.com/sections/living/DailyNews/vitamine1028.html. Accessed May 8, 2000.

Kimmick GG, Bell RA, Bostick RM. Vitamin E and breast cancer: a review. *Nutr Cancer.* 1997;27:109-117.

Olson KB, Pienta KJ. Vitamins A and E: further clues for prostate cancer prevention. *J Natl Cancer Inst.* 1998;90:414-415.

Oncolink Cancer News. The University of Pennsylvania Web site. Available at: http://www.oncolink.upenn.edu/cancer_news/1994/antiox.html. Accessed August 13, 1999.

Patterson RE, Neuhouser ML, White E, Hunt JR, Kristal AR. Cancer-related behavior of vitamin supplement users. *Cancer Epidemiol Biomarkers Prev.* 1998;7:79-81.

Patterson RE, White E, Kristal AR, Neuhouser ML, Potter JD. Vitamin supplements and cancer risk: the epidemiologic evidence. *Cancer Causes Control.* 1997;8:786-802.

Yusuf S, Dagenais G, Pogue J, Bosch J, Sleight P. Vitamin E supplementation and cardiovascular events in high-risk patients. The Heart Outcomes Prevention Evaluation Study Investigators. *N Engl J Med.* 2000;342:154-160.

Vitamin K

Other common name(s)	Scientific/medical name(s)
Vitamin K, Vitamin K_1, Vitamin K_2, Vitamin K_2, Vitamin K_3	Phylloquinone, Phytonadione, Menaquinone, Menadione

DESCRIPTION

Vitamin K is an essential nutrient the liver needs to form substances that promote blood clotting and prevent abnormal bleeding. There are three forms of vitamin K. Vitamin K_1 (phylloquinone or phytonadione) is a natural nutrient found in green leafy vegetables, such as lettuce, cabbage, broccoli, and turnip greens. It is also found in cereals, dairy products, some fruits, liver, and pork. Vitamin K_2 (menaquinone) is a natural product of bacteria that reside in the lower intestinal tract. Vitamin K_3 (menadione) is a potent synthetic form of vitamin K.

OVERVIEW

Vitamin K is necessary for normal blood clotting. The human body obtains vitamin K from certain foods and bacteria that normally live in the intestines. There is no scientific evidence supporting the use of vitamin K supplements in cancer treatment or prevention.

How is it promoted for use?

Vitamin K is known primarily as a blood-clotting nutrient. However, some alternative medical practitioners claim that vitamin K_3 is also an anticancer agent. Others claim that high doses of both vitamin C and vitamin K_3 supplements can inhibit tumor growth when taken together, however this has not been scientifically proven.

What does it involve?

Most people get all the vitamin K they need from natural sources. The RDA is 60 μg/day for women and 80 μg/day for men. Dietary sources of vitamin K, such as green leafy vegetables, provide the body with about half of the normal supply of the vitamin, while intestinal bacteria produce the rest.

Only those who have symptoms of a vitamin K deficiency may need to take supplements. The signs of a deficiency include abnormal or excessive bleeding, such as frequent nosebleeds, abnormally bleeding gums, or blood in the urine or stool. People who experience these symptoms should consult a physician because these signs may also signify other, more serious, problems. A deficiency may result from extended treatment with antibiotics (killing the bacteria that produce vitamin K) for several weeks or certain liver or intestinal disorders.

Newborn infants lack the bacteria in their intestines to produce vitamin K and are at risk of uncontrolled bleeding. Newborns are usually given vitamin K supplements, either by injection or by mouth, while in the hospital. Babies who received the supplements in the hospital do not need supplements after they leave.

Vitamin K is also promoted for topical use in some cosmetic or herbal creams to lighten the redness from broken capillaries, and to treat skin irritation (burns and sunburns) and scarring. Applications are usually recommended for several weeks.

What is the history behind it?

In 1935, a Danish scientist discovered that vitamin K was essential to blood clotting and named it for the Danish word for clotting, koagulation. Since then, laboratory and animal studies have been conducted to see if vitamin K plays a role in preventing the development or spread of cancer, but there is no convincing evidence that it does. However, in the 1990s, researchers began to suggest a possible link between childhood cancers, especially leukemia, and injections of vitamin K supplements in newborns. Subsequent studies were done in the late 1990s to investigate this link.

What is the evidence?

There is overwhelming scientific evidence that vitamin K is necessary for blood clotting. The intestinal bacteria that produce vitamin K in children and adults are not present at birth. To avoid a deficiency of this vitamin that might lead to impaired blood clotting and excessive bleeding, most pediatricians recommend that an injection of vitamin K be given to newborns. Studies published in the early 1990s suggested a link between childhood cancer (ie, acute lymphoblastic leukemia) and injections of vitamin K supplements in newborn babies. Most supplement studies did not find any association between vitamin K injections and childhood cancer. Some researchers have recommended the oral administration of vitamin K; however, the effectiveness of this method of administration has not been proven and is not currently licensed.

In addition, an animal study done in 1998 at the University of Pittsburgh found that a novel form of vitamin K (a synthetic version) known as compound 5 might be able to stop the spread of liver cancer and possibly other cancers by causing cancer cells to die. While this preliminary study shows promise, much further research is required to determine if this compound might have an anticancer effect in humans.

There have been some studies examining whether menadione (vitamin K_3) can help overcome resistance to certain types of chemotherapy drugs. Results in animal and cell cultures are mixed, but there is no evidence of any significant effects in humans yet. There is no evidence that vitamin K_3 is an active anticancer agent in human patients when used alone. More research is needed on menadione and related compounds to determine if they may have any positive effects for people with cancer.

Are there any possible problems or complications?

Natural vitamin K is considered safe as a normal part of a daily diet. Supplements of the vitamin are not usually needed unless recommended by a physician. Research showing a possible link between the development of leukemia in children who were given injections of vitamin K supplements shortly after birth has led to a recommendation that newborns be given only oral supplements.

References

Ansell P, Bull D, Roman E. Childhood leukaemia and intramuscular vitamin K: findings from a case-control study. *BMJ*. 1996;313:204-205.

Ni R, Nishikawa Y, Carr BI. Cell growth inhibition by a novel vitamin K is associated with induction of protein tyrosine phosphorylation. *J Biol Chem.* 1998;273:9906-9911.

McKinney PA, Juszczak E, Findlay E, Smith K. Case-control study of childhood leukaemia and cancer in Scotland: findings for neonatal intramuscular vitamin K. *BMJ.* 1998;316:173-177.

Parker L, Cole M, Craft AW, Hey EN. Neonatal vitamin K administration and childhood cancer in the north of England: retrospective case-control study. *BMJ.* 1998;316:189-193.

Passmore SJ, Draper G, Brownbill P, Kroll M. Ecological studies of relation between hospital policies on neonatal vitamin K administration and subsequent occurrence of childhood cancer. *BMJ.* 1998;316:184-189.

Passmore SJ, Draper G, Brownbill P, Kroll M. Case-control studies of relation between childhood cancer and neonatal vitamin K administration. *BMJ.* 1998;316:178-184.

Sata N, Klonowski-Stumpe H, Han B, Haussinger D, Niederau C. Menadione induces both necrosis and apoptosis in rat pancreatic acinar AR4-2J cells. *Free Radic Biol Med.* 1997;23:844-850.

Tetef M, Margolin K, Ahn C, et al. Mitomycin C and menadione for the treatment of advanced gastrointestinal cancers: a phase II trial. *J Cancer Res Clin Oncol.* 1995;121:103-106.

von Kries R. Oral versus intramuscular phytomenadione: safety and efficacy compared. *Drug Saf.* 1999;21:1-6.

von Kries R, Hachmeister A, Gobel U. Can 3 oral 2 mg doses of vitamin K effectively prevent late vitamin K deficiency bleeding? *Eur J Pediatr.* 1999;158 Suppl 3:S183-S186.

Xu CJ, Zhang Y, Wang J, Zhang TM. Menadione reduced doxorubicin resistance in Ehrlich ascites carcinoma cells in vitro. *Chung Kuo Yao Li Hsueh Pao.* 1998;19:273-276.

Wild Yam

Other common name(s)	Scientific/medical name(s)
Wild Mexican Yam, Chinese Yam, Colic Root, Rheumatism Root	*Dioscorea villosa, Dioscorea opposita*

DESCRIPTION
Wild yam is native to North America. The roots and other underground parts of wild yams are used in herbal remedies. The plants described here are different from yams and sweet potatoes sold as food.

OVERVIEW
Although creams containing wild yam extracts are becoming popular among women as an alternative to hormone replacement therapy (HRT), there is no scientific evidence that they are safe or effective. Neither estrogen nor progesterone are found in wild yams.

How is it promoted for use?
The wild Mexican yam and the Chinese yam are the two types of yams promoted for therapeutic use. Proponents claim that a cream made from the wild Mexican yam contains natural progesterone (a hormone that plays a vital role in women's health) and is therefore effective in treating premenstrual and menopausal symptoms. They say that using the cream as an alternative to HRT will significantly lower the risk of

breast and endometrial cancer although there is no scientific evidence to support this claim. Cream marketers also claim that their product helps women lose weight, increases energy and stamina, and enhances sex drive.

Supporters claim that the wild Mexican Yam, when taken internally, eases arthritis pain, the symptoms of morning sickness, painful menstruation, bronchitis, asthma, whooping cough, and cramps, and relieves gastrointestinal ailments such as Crohn's disease, colitis, and chronic diarrhea.

The Chinese yam is claimed to stimulate appetite and to be a remedy for chronic diarrhea, asthma, uncontrollable or frequent urination, diabetes, and emotional instability. Used externally, proponents claim the Chinese yam can speed the healing of boils and abscesses. Herbalists also use it to treat colic (see Homeopathy).

What does it involve?
Creams made from wild yams are rubbed directly onto the skin and are available from health food stores. In homeopathic medicine, the wild yam from the *Dioscorea villosa* plant is used fresh or dried and put in liquid extracts. The Chinese yam can also be used fresh or baked with flour or clay. Wild yam cream and wild Mexican yam capsules are available in herbal shops and over the Internet. Dosages vary by manufacturer.

What is the history behind it?
In East Indian traditional medicine, yams are used for sexual and hormonal problems. Chinese herbalists have long used the herb for rheumatism and digestive and urinary complaints (see Chinese Herbal Medicine). Yams have also been used in American folk medicine to treat coughs and to induce sweating and vomiting.

What is the evidence?
Contrary to claims, the wild Mexican yam cannot supply the body with progesterone. The plant contains the chemical diosgenin, which can be converted into progesterone through a lengthy process in the laboratory. The body cannot convert diosgenin into progesterone itself. Some of the chemicals in the plant resemble estrogen, another hormone that is important in female physiology, but their effects on the body are very different from those of progesterone. There are drugs manufactured from diosgenin that are used to treat asthma, arthritis, eczema, and to control fertility.

There is no scientific evidence showing that the wild yam has any effect on the symptoms of menopause or premenstrual syndrome.

Are there any possible problems or complications?

Large doses of wild yam may cause nausea, vomiting, and diarrhea. This treatment should not be used as a replacement for HRT. Women who are pregnant or breastfeeding should not use wild yams.

References
Bown D. *Encyclopedia of Herbs & Their Uses.* New York, NY: DK Publishing Inc; 1995.

Foster S, Duke JA. *A Field Guide to Medicinal Plants: Eastern and Central North America.* Boston, MA: Houghton Mifflin; 1990.

Fugh-Berman, A. Wild yam cream, diosgenin, and natural progesterone: What can they really do for you? *National Women's Health Network, The Network News.* January 1, 1999.

Gorski T. Wild yam cream threatens women's health. Quackwatch Web site. Available at: http://www.quackwatch.com. Accessed May 8, 2000.

Marini R. Yamscam. HealthScout Web site. Available at: http://www.healthscout.com. Accessed August 9, 1999.

Herbs / Vitamins / Minerals

Wormwood

Other common name(s)	Scientific/medical name(s)
Absinthe, Absinthium	*Artemisia absinthium*

DESCRIPTION

Wormwood is a shrubby perennial plant whose upper shoots and leaves are used in herbal remedies. It is native to Europe, northern Africa, and western Asia.

OVERVIEW

There is no scientific evidence that wormwood is effective in treating the side effects of conventional cancer treatment or any other conditions. The plant contains a volatile oil with a high level of thujone, the active component of wormwood oil, which can cause convulsions (see Thuja). In fact, it may be considered harmful when taken internally because there are reports that it can cause serious problems to the liver, as well as neurological symptoms, such as convulsions, numbness of legs and arms, loss of intellect, delirium, and paralysis.

How is it promoted for use?

Wormwood is promoted as a sedative and anti-inflammatory. There are also claims that it can treat loss of appetite, stomach disorders, liver and gallbladder complaints. In folk medicine it is used for a wide range of stomach disorders, fever and irregular menstruation. It is also used to destroy intestinal worms. Externally, it is applied to poorly healing wounds, ulcers, skin blotches, and insect bites. It is also used in Moxibustion treatments for cancer (see Moxibustion). There is no scientific evidence to support these claims.

What does it involve?

Wormwood combinations are taken in small doses for a short period of time. It is taken in liquid form either in water (tincture), or as a tea preparation, as well as in capsules. Wormwood is also applied externally. Although pure wormwood is not available, "thujone-free" wormwood extract has been approved by the FDA for use in foods and as flavoring in alcoholic beverages such as vermouth.

What is the history behind it?

Traditional Chinese medicine has used a related herb, sweet wormwood, *Artemisia annua*, also known as qinghao, for over 2,000 years for the treatment of such diverse complaints as hemorrhoids and fever (see Chinese Herbal Medicine). *Artemisia absinthium* was used by Hippocrates, and the earliest references to wormwood in Western civilization can be found in the Bible. Extract of wormwood was also used in ancient Egypt. The herb is mentioned often in first-century Greek and Roman writings, and reportedly was placed in the sandals of Roman soldiers to help soothe their sore feet. Its ingestion to exterminate tapeworms dates back to the Middle Ages.

In 1797, Henri Pernod developed absinthe, an alcoholic drink, containing essential oil of wormwood. Absinthe became very popular in both Europe and the United States in the 19th century. It was eventually banned in various countries in the early 20th century due to its addictive qualities (found in thujone). Even though absinthe liqueurs are illegal in some countries today, they can still be found in France, Spain, and Italy.

What is the evidence?

No studies have shown any evidence to support the use of wormwood for the treatment of cancer or the side effects of conventional cancer treatment. There is also not enough evidence to support the numerous other indications for which wormwood is recommended. *Artemisia annua* and some of its derivatives have been shown to be effective in the treatment of malaria. In fact, drugs derived from artemisinin, the active ingredient in sweet wormwood, may be registered soon in Europe for the treatment of malaria.

Are there any possible problems or complications?

Due to the thujone content, taking large doses of wormwood internally can lead to vomiting, stomach and intestinal cramps, headaches, dizziness, and disturbances of the central nervous system. Wormwood can also lead to liver failure. The *New England Journal of Medicine* reported that a man who ordered essential oil of wormwood over the Internet, thinking he had purchased absinthe, suffered acute liver failure after ingesting the volatile oil. Wormwood may also lower the seizure threshold, and offset the beneficial effects from known anti-convulsants such as phenobarbital.

The ingestion of thujone, the active ingredient in oil of wormwood and absinthe, can lead to absinthism, a syndrome of hallucinations, sleeplessness, tremors, convulsions, and paralysis associated with long-term use of the liqueur absinthe. This herb should be avoided, especially by women who are pregnant or breast-feeding.

References

Arnold WN. Vincent van Gogh and the thujone connection. *JAMA*. 1998;260:3042-3044.

Blumenthal M, ed. *The Complete German Commission E Monographs: Therapeutic Guide to Herbal Medicines*. Austin, Tx: American Botanical Council; 1998.

Bown D. *Encyclopedia of Herbs & Their Uses*. New York, NY: DK Publishing Inc; 1995.

Fetrow CW, Avila JR. *Professional's Handbook of Complimentary and Alternative Medicines*. Springhouse, PA: Springhouse Corp; 1999.

Medical Economics. *PDR for Herbal Medicines*. Montvale, NJ: Medical Economics Company; 1998.

Miller LG. Selected clinical considerations focusing on known or potential drug-herb interactions. *Arch Intern Med*. 1998;158:2200-2209.

Rediscovering wormwood: qinghaosu for malaria. *Lancet* 1992;339:649-651.

Spencer JW, Jacobs JJ. *Complementary/Alternative Medicine: An Evidence-Based Approach*. St. Louis, MO: Mosby, Inc; 1999.

Van Agtmael MA, Eggelte TA, van Boxtel CJ. Artemisinin drugs in the treatment of malaria: from medicinal herb to registered medication. *Trends Pharmacol Sci*. 1999;20:199-205.

Weisbord SD, Soule JB, Kimmel PL. Poison on line: acute renal failure caused by oil of wormwood purchased through the internet. *N Engl J Med*. 1997;337:825-827.

Yohimbine

Other common name(s)
Yohimbe, Yohimbe Bark, Yohimbine Hydrochloride, Actibine®, Aphrodyne®, Yocon®, Yohimex®, Yomax®

Scientific/medical name(s)
Pausinystalia yohimbine, Corynanthe yohimbine

DESCRIPTION
Yohimbe is an evergreen tree that grows in the jungles of Africa. It can reach a height of 90 feet. The dried bark is used in herbal remedies, and a yohimbine drug, derived from the bark, is approved by the FDA.

OVERVIEW
Yohimbe bark has been used as an aphrodisiac (sexual stimulant) for many years, and yohimbine has recently been studied as a potential treatment for erectile dysfunction (male impotence). Clinical trials of yohimbine have found contradictory results regarding its effectiveness. Yohimbe bark has been declared an unsafe herb in Germany because of such complications as increased heart rate and blood pressure, and even kidney failure.

How is it promoted for use?
Yohimbine hydrochloride is the most important component of yohimbe bark and it is available as a FDA-approved drug for the treatment of impotence. The evidence about its effectiveness is mixed. Yohimbine is also promoted as an aphrodisiac. Chemicals in the bark of the tree are said by proponents to improve blood flow to the penis. Yohimbine has also been promoted to treat exhaustion, drug overdose (from clonidine), and a form of low blood pressure that occurs when standing.

What does it involve?
Yohimbine is available in tablets, capsules, and liquid extracts. Purity of the prescription form of yohimbine is strictly regulated by the FDA. In contrast, the yohimbe bark extracts and yohimbine sold in health food stores and the Internet contains varying amounts of yohimbine as well as other ingredients. Researchers from the FDA analyzed a number of commercial yohimbe bark products available over-the-counter and found that they contained only 7% or less of actual yohimbine compared to what was in the authentic yohimbe bark. The US Department of Agriculture lists the yohimbine bark used in herbal remedies as an unsafe herb. Yohimbe bark is on the Commission E (Germany's regulatory agency for herbs) list of unapproved herbs. This means that it is not recommended for use because it has not been proven to be safe or effective.

The drug yohimbine hydrochloride is regulated and available only as a prescription and approved for the treatment of impotence. The standard recommended dosage is 5.4 mg taken 3 times/day for not more than 10 weeks.

What is the history behind it?
In Africa, yohimbe has been used for generations as an aphrodisiac, a hallucinogenic, an antiseptic, and to treat impotence. It was also used by warriors as a stimulant before battle. In the 1890s, medicinal use of yohimbe appeared in Europe.

What is the evidence?
Clinical trials have found contradictory results

Herbs / Vitamins / Minerals

regarding the effectiveness of yohimbine for treating impotence. One small uncontrolled study found that yohimbine did not result in any improvement for patients with organic erectile dysfunction (impotence caused by a physical problem). However, the American Urological Association guidelines on treatment of organic erectile dysfunction state that evidence clearly shows that yohimbine is better than a placebo (an inactive substance or treatment). A recent randomized clinical trial found that yohimbine may be a useful treatment for nonorganic erectile dysfunction (impotence not related to a physical problem). Another randomized clinical study found that yohimbine was no better than a placebo as an initial treatment for mixed-type impotence. No studies have been done to compare yohimbine to other treatments for impotence.

In a review of previous clinical research, the authors concluded that yohimbine is a reasonable option for the treatment of impotence and that the benefits of the drug seem to outweigh its risks. Another clinical review concluded that yohimbine has a modest effect on psychogenic impotence (caused by psychological factors), but not on organic erectile dysfunction. It is apparent that more research needs to be done to clarify the role of yohimbine in the treatment of impotence. These studies were done using the drug yohimbine hydrochloride. Extracted chemicals are not the same as the raw plant. Study results of extracts will not necessarily be consistent with studies using the raw plant.

Are there any possible problems or complications?

Yohimbine and yohimbe bark may increase heart rate and raise blood pressure at dosages from 20 to 30 mg/day. People with high blood pressure, heart, kidney or liver disease, or who take antidepressants, should avoid the drug. Yohimbine has been associated with psychotic episodes. Other side effects include difficulty breathing, chest pain and palpitations, anxiety, queasiness, insomnia, and vomiting. The less common side effects that do not usually require medical attention include dizziness, headache, flushing, nausea, nervousness, sweating, and tremors.

Yohimbine should not be used by elderly people or women who are pregnant or breastfeeding.

References

Betz JM, White KD, der Marderosian AH. Gas chromatographic determination of yohimbine in commercial yohimbe products. *J AOAC Int.* 1995;78:1189-1194.

Blumenthal M, ed. *The Complete German Commission E Monographs: Therapeutic Guide to Herbal Medicines.* Austin, Tx: American Botanical Council; 1998.

Bown D. *Encyclopedia of Herbs & Their Uses.* New York, NY: DK Publishing Inc; 1995.

Brinker NDF. *Herb Contraindications and Drug Interactions, Second Edition.* Sandy, Ore: Eclectic Medical Publications; 1998.

Cassileth B. *The Alternative Medicine Handbook.* New York, NY: W. W. Norton & Co; 1998.

Ernst E, Pittler MH. Yohimbine for erectile dysfunction: A systemic review and meta-analysis of randomized clinical trials. *J Urol.* 1998;159:433-436.

Fetrow CW, Avila JR. *Professional's Handbook of Complementary and Alternative Medicines.* Springhouse, Pa: Springhouse Corp; 1999.

Kunelius P, Hakkinen J, Lukkarinen O. Is high-dose yohimbine hydrochloride effective in the treatment of mixed-type impotence? A prospective, randomized, controlled double-blind crossover study. *Urology.* 1997;49:441-444.

Medical Economics. *Physicians' Desk Reference.* Montvale, NJ: Medical Economics Company; 1999.

Medical Library. Yohimbine. WebMDHealth Web site. Available at: http://www.my.webnd.com/content/asset/cp_drug_291. Accessed March 6, 2000.

Medicine Center. Yohimbine. Mayo Clinic Web site. Available at: http://mayohealth.org/usp/html/202639.htm. Accessed March 6, 2000.

Pittler MH, Ernst E. Trials have shown yohimbine is effective for erectile dysfunction. *BMJ.* 1998;317:478.

Teloken C, Rhoden EL, Sogari P, et al. Therapeutic effects of high dose yohimbine hydrochloride on organic erectile dysfunction. *J Urol.* 1998;159:122-124.

Vogt HJ, Brandl P, Kockott G, et al. Double-blind, placebo-controlled safety and efficacy trial with yohimbine hydrochloride in the treatment of nonorganic erectile dysfunction. *Int J Impot Res.* 1997;9:155-161.

Wagner G, Saenz de Tejada I. Update on male erectile dysfunction. *BMJ.* 1998;316:678-682.

Zinc

Other common name(s)	Scientific/medical name(s)
Zinc Gluconate, Zinc Sulfate	Zn, Zn++

DESCRIPTION

Zinc is a trace mineral that plays a key role in many bodily processes, including the building of DNA and RNA, energy production, cell metabolism, and regulation of the immune system. It is found in seafood, meats, nuts, eggs, cheese, grains, and other food sources.

OVERVIEW

Some studies have found that zinc supplements may help reduce cancer risk in animals, but this has not been proven in humans. Research that has examined patterns of zinc intake in humans has found a correlation between increased risk of some cancers and low zinc levels or low dietary zinc intake. However, no randomized clinical trials have been done to show the effectiveness of zinc supplements in cancer prevention or treatment. High doses of zinc can lead to some serious side effects.

How is it promoted for use?

Some people claim zinc protects against certain types of cancer, reduces the size of enlarged prostate glands, strengthens the immune system, decreases asthma and allergy symptoms, speeds wound healing, and fortifies the skin. Some also claim that zinc is an antioxidant, a compound that blocks the action of activated oxygen molecules, known as free radicals, that can damage cells. There is no scientific evidence to support these claims.

There are also claims that zinc reduces the severity and duration of the common cold. There is some evidence suggesting that this may be true.

What does it involve?

Zinc is obtained through a number of dietary sources, such as lean meat, seafood, soybeans, nuts, pumpkin and sunflower seeds, eggs, cheese, and wheat bran. The RDA of zinc is 15 mg/day for most adults and 30 mg/day for pregnant women. Zinc gluconate lozenges are available in most drug stores and pharmacies. Zinc spray or ointment is sometimes applied to wounds to accelerate healing.

What is the history behind it?

Zinc has been found in metals that date back to 1400 BC. In the 13th century, metallic zinc was produced in India. In 1500, zinc was recognized as an element by Andreas Marggraf in Germany. In the 1700s, zinc factories were developed in Europe. Medical researchers began serious investigations of zinc in the early 1970s.

What is the evidence?

Some researchers have focused on examining zinc levels in the body associated with cancer and other diseases. A few studies found that zinc levels in serum and/or inside white blood cells were frequently lower in patients with head and neck cancer or childhood leukemia. Low zinc levels were also linked to increased size of head or neck tumors, more advanced stage of disease, and a greater number of unplanned hospitalizations. Another study found a connection between zinc intake (from both food and supplements) and a lower risk of melanoma (the most serious form of skin cancer) and precancerous lesions of the mouth. Protective effects have also been associated with zinc supplements and prostate cancer risk.

Several studies have found that zinc supplements may make laboratory animals less susceptible to chemical carcinogens, but studies of humans have not been done to evaluate the impact of such supplements in cancer risk. There is no clinical evidence to support the use of zinc supplements to affect the growth or spread of cancer.

A randomized clinical trial in Italy involving patients with head and neck cancer found that zinc sulfate tablets reversed the loss of taste caused by radiation therapy. The results suggest that zinc sulfate supplements could become an important component in the supportive care of these patients.

Two randomized, double-blind placebo studies found that zinc gluconate in a glycine base reduced the length of cold symptoms. In a review of eight recent clinical trials, researchers concluded that zinc reduces the duration and severity of the common cold. One study published in the *Journal of the American Medical Association*, however, found that zinc gluconate lozenges were not effective in treating cold symptoms in children and adolescents, and that further study is needed to determine what, if any, role zinc plays in affecting cold symptoms.

Are there any possible problems or complications?

An overdose of zinc can lead to a weakened immune system, vomiting, headache, and fatigue. Very high exposure to zinc (which occurs in some industries) may contribute to the development of prostate cancer.

References

Godfrey JC, Conant Sloane B, Smith DS, Turco JH, Mercer N, Godfrey NJ. Zinc gluconate and the common cold: a controlled clinical study. *J Int Med Res*. 1992;20:234-246.

Godfrey JC, Godfrey NJ, Godfrey Novick S. Zinc for treating the common cold: review of all clinical trials since 1984. *Altern Therapies*. 1996;2:63-72.

Gupta PC, Hebert JR, Vhonsle RB, et al. Influence of dietary factors on oral precancerous lesions in a population-based case-control study in Kerala, India. *Cancer*. 1999;85:1885-1893.

Kirkpatrick CS, White E, Lee JA. Case-control study of malignant melanoma in Washington State. II. Diet, alcohol, and obesity. *Am J Epidemiol*. 1994;139:869-880.

Kristal AR, Stanford JL, Cohen JH, Wicklund K, Patterson RE. Vitamin and mineral supplement use is associated with reduced risk of prostate cancer. *Cancer Epidemiol Biomarkers Prev*. 1999;8:887-892.

Macknin ML, Piedmonte M, Calendine C, Janosky J, Wald E. Zinc gluconatge lozenges for treating the common cold in children: A randomized controlled trial. *JAMA*. 1998;279:1962-1967.

Mossad SB. Treatment of the common cold. *BMJ*. 1998;317:33-36.

Mossad SB, Macknin ML, Medendorp SV, Mason P. Zinc gluconate lozenges for treating the common cold. A randomized, double-blind, placebo-controlled study. *Ann Intern Med*. 1996; 125:81-88.

Phillips MJ, Ackerley CA, Superina RA, et al. Excess zinc associated with severe progressive cholestasis in Cree and Ojibwa-Cree children. *Lancet*. 1996;347:866-868.

Prasad AS, Beck FW, Doerr TD, et al. Nutritional and zinc status of head and neck cancer patients: An interpretive review. *J Amer Coll Nutr*. 1998;17:409-418.

Ripamonti C, Zecca E, Brunelli C, Fulfaro F, et al. A randomized, controlled clinical trial to evaluate the effects of zinc sulfate on cancer patients with taste alterations caused by head and neck irradiation. *Cancer*. 1998;15:1938-1945.

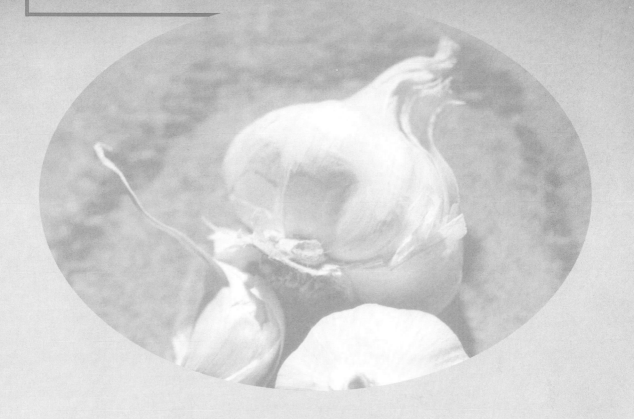

Chapter 8

Diet and Nutrition Methods

This category includes dietary approaches

and special nutritional programs related

to prevention and treatment of disease.

Acidophilus

Other common name(s)	Scientific/medical name(s)
Lactic Acid Bacteria	Lactobacillus acidophilus (L. acidophilus)

DESCRIPTION

Acidophilus is a type of bacterium commonly found in the normal gastrointestinal (GI) tract of mammals, mainly in the small intestine. It is also found in many dairy products, especially yogurt.

OVERVIEW

There have been no studies with humans on the role of L. acidophilus in preventing or treating human cancers. Animal studies on L. acidophilus reducing the occurrence of cancer have shown varying results.

How is it promoted for use?

Acidophilus may be recommended to prevent or treat uncomplicated diarrhea and vaginal infections, lower cholesterol, promote lactose digestion in lactose-sensitive people, and help prevent disease-causing bacteria and yeast from growing.

Acidophilus is promoted to help lower the incidence of cancer by reducing the carcinogens in the diet and by directly killing tumor cells. Other anticancer claims include a reduction in the cholesterol levels that tumor cells need to grow and in the production of B vitamins and vitamin K which are supposed to help the immune system fight off cancer (see Vitamin B Complex and Vitamin K). There is no scientific evidence to support these claims.

What does it involve?

When taking acidophilus, the dosage usually refers to the number of live bacteria. Most sources suggest 1 to 10 billion bacteria as a recommended dose. This amount is available in tablets, capsules, and powder form. Average dosage suggestions vary from 1 to 3 times per day; however, some scientists warn that concentrations of the bacteria in supplemental form

vary widely from one manufacturer to another. Yogurt with "live cultures" and milk supplemented with L. acidophilus bacteria are another source.

What is the history behind it?

Interest in the health benefits of acidophilus began in the late 1800s when it was proposed that the long-life span of the Balkan people was due to their ingestion of fermented milk products. It was later found that these milk products were rich in L. acidophilus. Since then, the exact role of L. acidophilus in the GI tract in human health has been a controversial subject, with little or no clear results.

What is the evidence?

Studies on the ability of L. acidophilus to prevent cancer from occurring have been contradictory. In recent animal studies, animals with diets supplemented with L. acidophilus were less susceptible to DNA damage in the colon after treatment with known carcinogens. These results suggest that L. acidophilus may prevent the occurrence of colon cancer. However, other studies have shown that diets with L. acidophilus had no effect on the formation of breast or skin cancers. In either case, randomized clinical trials have not been done. Animal studies may show a certain substance holds promise as a beneficial treatment, but further studies are necessary to determine if the results apply to humans.

L. acidophilus also has been investigated as possessing direct anti-tumor properties. In two separate studies with human cancer cells grown in the laboratory, milk that was fermented by *L. acidophilus* was able to slow or prevent the growth of cancer cells. One study used a breast cancer cell and the other used colon cancer cells. However, neither animal nor human studies on the effect of *L. acidophilus* on established tumors in the body have been reported. More research is needed to determine what role, if any, acidophilus may play in cancer treatment and prevention.

A recent review of research on the effects of *L. acidophilus* and other closely related bacteria found that it lowered cholesterol in some, but not all, studies. They reported that a related bacterium *(Lactobacillus GG)* may shorten the duration of diarrhea due to viral or bacterial infections, but other health effects of these types of bacteria are not clear.

Are there any possible problems or complications?

In rare cases, acidophilus can cause serious infections that are difficult to treat with antibiotics. People with compromised immune systems, such as those with AIDS, should use acidophilus with caution.

The lack of standardization makes it difficult to determine the quality of acidophilus products. Because acidophilus must contain live cultures in order to be considered effective, proper packaging and storage is essential. Many of these products do not contain adequate levels of the active organisms or may contain other bacteria that are not beneficial.

References

Baricault L, Denariaz G, Houri JJ, Bouley C, Sapin C, Trugnan G. Use of HT-29, a cultured human colon cancer cell line, to study the effect of fermented milks on colon cancer cell growth and differentiation. *Carcinogenesis*. 1995;16:245-252.

Biffi A, Coradini D, Larsen R, Riva L, Di Fronzo G. Antiproliferative effect of fermented milk on the growth of a human breast cancer cell line. *Nutr Cancer*. 1997;28:93-99.

de Roos NM, Katan MB. Effects of probiotic bacteria on diarrhea, lipid metabolism, and carcinogenesis: a review of papers published between 1988 and 1998. *Am J Clin Nutr*. 2000;71:405-411.

Fetrow, CV and Avila, JR. *Professional's Handbook of Complementary and Alternative Medicines*. Springhouse, Pa: Springhouse Corp; 1999.

Hove H, Norgaard H, Mortensen PB. Lactic acid bacteria and the human gastrointestinal tract. *Eur J Clin Nut*. 1999;53:339-350.

Lidbeck A, Nord CE, Gustafsson JA, Rafter J. Lactobacilli, anticarcinogenic activities and human intestinal microflora. *Eur J Cancer Prev*. 1992;1:341-353.

Pool-Zobel BL, Neudecker C, Domizlaff I, et al. Lactobacillus- and bifidobacterium-mediated antigenotoxicity in the colon of rats. *Nutr Cancer*. 1996;26:365-380.

Rao CV, Sanders ME, Indranie C, Simi B, Reddy BS. Prevention of colonic preneoplastic lesions by the probiotic Lactobacillus acidophilus NCFMTM in F344 rats. *Int J Oncol*. 1999;14:939-944.

Rice LJ, Chai YJ, Conti CJ, Willis RA, Locniskar MF. The effect of dietary fermented milk products and lactic acid bacteria on the initiation and promotion stages of mammary carcinogenesis. *Nutr Cancer*. 1995;24:99-109.

Amino Acids

Other common name(s)	Scientific/medical name(s)
None	Arginine, Alanine, Aspartic Acid, Asparagine, Cysteine, Glycine, Glutamine, Glutamic Acid, Histidine, Isoleucine, Leucine, Lysine, Methionine, Phenylalanine, Serine, Threonine, Tryptophan, Tyrosine, Valine

DESCRIPTION

Amino acids are a group of 20 different chemical compounds that are the basic building blocks of all the proteins in the human body. Proteins are needed for human growth and development. Twelve of the amino acids, called nonessential amino acids, can be produced in the human body by metabolism of other substances. Eight of the amino acids, called essential amino acids, cannot be produced by the human body and must be obtained from dietary sources.

OVERVIEW

Amino acids are necessary for human growth and development. However, their effects on cancer are not well studied and not completely known. Some amino acid supplements may interfere with the effectiveness of the chemotherapy drug asparaginase.

How is it promoted for use?

The claims for amino acids in regard to cancer are complex and somewhat confusing. Some alternative medicine practitioners maintain that restricting dietary intake of certain amino acids, such as phenylalanine and tyrosine, may stop tumor growth. At the same time, they claim that while dietary restriction of the amino acids methionine and arginine may inhibit the growth of some cancers, supplements of these amino acids and two others, tryptophan and glutamine, may stimulate the growth of other cancers.

Some claim the amino acid cysteine may protect people with cancer from the toxic effects of certain chemotherapy drugs, including cyclophosphamide and doxorubicin. Others say the amino acid glutathione may inhibit the development and progression of cancer and protect patients from damaging side effects of radiation therapy and certain chemotherapy drugs, such as fluorouracil and cisplatin. There is no clinical evidence to support these claims.

What does it involve?

Foods high in protein, especially meat and seafood, are excellent sources of amino acids. Once protein is ingested, the human digestive system breaks it down to amino acids, absorbs the amino acids, and then uses the acids to build new proteins.

Amino acid supplements are also available. Some proponents suggest they be taken on an empty stomach with fruit juice to help the body absorb the amino acids.

What is the history behind it?

The use of amino acid supplements is part of a form of therapy known as orthomolecular medicine, a term coined in 1968 by Nobel Prize winner Linus Pauling. He and others have recommended high doses of vitamins, minerals, and amino acids to treat a variety of illnesses, including cancer. More conventional medical practitioners have cautioned that high doses of vitamin, mineral, and amino acid supplements may be harmful, not beneficial, to human health.

What is the evidence?

The scientific evidence for the various effects of amino acids on cancer is based mostly on limited animal and laboratory studies that have not been confirmed in human trials. The conflicting evidence from these studies makes it difficult to draw definitive conclusions about the effects of amino acids on cancer.

One randomized clinical trial in Japan published in 1998 found that glutamine supplements given to 7 patients with advanced esophageal cancer helped them maintain their levels of glutamine and preserved their lymphocyte count for a short period of time. Lymphocytes are a type of white blood cells that help the body fight infection. The number of patients involved in this study was small, and the conclusions need to be confirmed by other studies.

Some laboratory studies have found differences in metabolism of some amino acids between normal cells and cancer cells. With one notable exception, these observations have not lead to useful anticancer treatments. The exception is the use of asparaginase in treating a type of childhood leukemia. Asparaginase breaks down the amino acid asparagine in the blood stream. The normal cells are better able to produce their own asparagine than the leukemia cells.

Are there any possible problems or complications?

Amino acids ingested in foods are safe and necessary for human growth and development. Conflicting evidence suggests both possible beneficial and harmful effects from amino acid supplements on the development, progression, and treatment of cancer. There have been reports that amino acid supplements may interfere with the effectiveness of the chemotherapy drug asparaginase. Supplements are not recommended unless advised by a physician.

References

Sugiyama K, Yu L, Nagasue N. Direct effect of branched-chain amino acids on the growth and metabolism of cultured human hepatocellular carcinoma cells. *Nutr Cancer.* 1998; 31:62-68.

Wu D, Keller WL, Park CS. Lipotrope deficiency inhibits cell growth and induces programmed cell death in human breast cancer cell line MCF-7. *Nutr Cancer.* 1998; 32:13-19.

Yoshida S, Matsui M, Shirouzu Y, Fujita H, Yamana H, Shirouzu K. Effects of glutamine supplements and radiochemotherapy on systemic immune and gut barrier function in patients with advanced esophageal cancer. *Ann Surg.* 1998;227:485-491.

Broccoli

Other common name(s)	Scientific/medical name(s)
None	*Brassica oleracea italica*

DESCRIPTION

Broccoli is a cruciferous vegetable that belongs to the cabbage and mustard families, which also includes arugula, cauliflower, collards, bok choy, kale, mustard greens, radishes, turnips, watercress, rutabaga, and brussel sprouts. It is identified primarily by its dense clusters of green flower buds.

OVERVIEW

Broccoli contains certain chemicals that may reduce the risk of colorectal cancer, although it is not clear which individual compounds are responsible for the protective effects. The best evidence suggests that eating a wide variety of vegetables reduces cancer risk.

How is it promoted for use?

Broccoli is considered one of the best sources of nutrients because it is rich in vitamin C, beta carotene, fiber, calcium, and folate (see Beta Carotene, Folic Acid, and Vitamin C). It is the source of many phytochemicals, which are thought to stimulate the production of anti-cancer enzymes and chemicals (see Phytochemicals). Strong evidence suggests that people who eat five or more servings of fruits and vegetables a day can cut their risk of cancer from 20% to 50% when compared to those who consume one serving or less. The chemical composition of cruciferous vegetables is complex, which makes it difficult to determine which compound or combination of compounds may provide protection against cancer. Eating a wide variety of plant-based foods is the best way to get the necessary components.

Some researchers suggest that small amounts of broccoli sprouts may protect against the risk of cancer as effectively as much larger amounts of the mature vegetable. There have been no studies conducted in humans to verify this claim.

What does it involve?

Broccoli can be eaten raw, boiled, or steamed. It can be purchased fresh or frozen in most grocery and organic food stores. Broccoli retains the most nutrients when eaten raw. Cooking reduces some of the benefits of broccoli because the heating process seems to destroy some beneficial anticarcinogenic compounds.

What is the history behind it?

Broccoli has been around for over 2,000 years but has only been commercially grown in the United States since the 1920s. Today, over 90% of the broccoli harvested in the United States comes from California although it is also grown in other parts of the country.

Almost two decades ago, researchers first suggested that cruciferous vegetables (a group of plants that have four flowers resembling a cross) might be associated with a decreased risk for cancer. However, it was not until the completion, review, and publication of scientific studies in the 1990s that certain chemicals found in broccoli were identified as possible cancer-prevention compounds. Raw broccoli may have a slightly bitter taste. Ironically, the bitter taste can be traced to the same chemicals thought to provide cancer protection. As a result, scientists have developed different types of broccoli, such as broccolini, a cross between broccoli and Chinese kale, which looks like asparagus and tastes sweeter than broccoli.

What is the evidence?

Recent investigations have shown that the frequent consumption of cruciferous vegetables is associated with a decreased risk for cancer. A recent population-based study found that high levels of the carotenoid lutein (obtained from vegetables such as broccoli, spinach, and lettuce) were associated with fewer cancers of the colon. An epidemiologic study published in 1999 in the *Journal of the National Cancer Institute* revealed that eating cruciferous vegetables seemed to reduce bladder cancer risk, while other vegetables and fruits did not appear to have the same benefit. Randomized clinical trials are needed to determine the exact nature of the association.

Researchers at Johns Hopkins University have suggested that sulforaphane, which is present in the broccoli sprouts before the vegetable matures, may be the primary cancer-prevention agent. A study showed that cancer development was reduced by 60% to 80% in laboratory animals that were fed sulforaphane. The compound is thought to prompt the body into manufacturing an enzyme that prevents tumor formation.

The effects of broccoli on the growth of specific cancers have also been studied. For example, scientists at the University of California at Berkeley found that a chemical component of broccoli, indole-3-carbinol, inhibited the growth of cultured breast cancer cells in a laboratory study. Animal and laboratory studies may show a certain compound holds promise as a beneficial treatment, but further studies are necessary to determine if the results apply to humans.

Scientists caution that as promising as broccoli may be as an excellent food for preventing cancer, the results of studies cannot be considered in isolation. The anticancer effects of any single food cannot be completely under-stood without evaluating it as part of a bigger dietary picture. The glucosinolates (a type of phytonutrient) in broccoli, for example, appear to have no benefit of their own. It is still unclear whether it is the vitamin C, beta carotene, folate, or other compounds that, working together and in the right quantities, protect individuals against cancer development. A balanced diet that includes five or more servings a day of fruits and vegetables along with foods from a variety of other plant sources such as breads, cereals, grain products, rice, pasta, and beans is more effective than eating one particular food in large amounts.

Are there any possible problems or complications?

Broccoli is safe to eat. Since it is a food high in fiber, eating large amounts of it may cause gas. High fiber foods should be reduced or avoided in people with diarrhea and some other colon problems.

References

Cao G, Booth SL, Sadowski JA, Prior RL. Increases in human plasma antioxidant capacity after consumption of controlled diets high in fruit and vegetables. *Am J Clin Nutr.* 1998; 68:1081-1087.

Cover CM, Hsieh SJ, Tran SH, et al. Indole-3-carbinol inhibits the expression of cyclin-dependent kinase-6 and induces a G1 cell cycle arrest of human breast cancer cells independent of estrogen receptor signaling. *J Biol Chem.* 1998;273:3838-3847.

Fahey JW, Zhang Y, Talalay P. Broccoli sprouts: an exceptionally rich source of inducers of enzymes that protect against chemical carcinogens. *Proc Natl Acad Sci U S A.* 1997;94:10367-10372.

Gamet-Payrastre L, Li P, Lumeau S, et al. Sulforaphane, a naturally occurring isothiocyanate, induces cell cycle arrest and apoptosis in HT29 human colon cancer cells. *Cancer Res.* 2000;60:1426-1433.

Hasler CM. Functional foods: their role in disease prevention and health promotion. Quackwatch Web site. Available at: http://www.quackwatch.com. Accessed May 8, 2000.

Michaud DS, Spiegelman D, Clinton SK, Rimm EB, Willett WC, Giovannucci EL. Fruit and vegetable intake and incidence of bladder cancer in a male prospective cohort. *J Natl Cancer Inst.* 1999;91:605-613.

Nestle M. Broccoli sprouts in cancer prevention. *Nutr Rev.* 1998;56:127-130.

Shapiro TA, Fahey JW, Wade KL, Stephenson KK, Talalay P. Human metabolism and excretion of cancer chemoprotective glucosinolates and isothiocyanates of cruciferous vegetables. *Cancer Epidemiol Biomarkers Prev.* 1998;7:1091-1100.

Slattery ML, Benson J, Curtin K, Ma KN, Schaeffer D, Potter JD. Carotenoids and colon cancer. *Am J Clin Nutr.* 2000;71:575-582.

Zhang Y, Kensler TW, Cho CG, Posner GH, Talalay P. Anticarcinogenic activities of sulforaphane and structurally related synthetic norbornyl isothiocyanates. *Proc Natl Acad Sci U S A.* 1994;91:3147-3150.

Cassava

Other common name(s)	Scientific/medical name(s)
Cassava Plant, Tapioca, Tapioca Plant, Manioc	*Manihot esculenta*, Crantz

DESCRIPTION

The cassava plant is a staple crop in Africa, Asia, and South America. Tapioca is a starch found in the roots of the plant. Different parts of the plant such as the root, leaves, and sometimes the whole plant, are used in herbal remedies.

OVERVIEW

There is no scientific evidence that cassava or tapioca is effective in preventing or treating cancer. However, a theory to explain how an enzyme in the cassava plant may possibly treat cancer has been proposed. This approach has not been scientifically tested.

How is it promoted for use?

Some researchers have found that through the breakdown of a chemical called linamarin, cassava plants produce hydrogen cyanide. They believe if linamarase (the enzyme that breaks down linamarin to release hydrogen cyanide) could be selectively introduced into cancer cells, it could kill cancer cells by producing cyanide as it does in the cassava plant. Since normal cells cannot convert linamarin into cyanide, only the cancer cells would be killed by this gene therapy, according to this theory.

In folk medicine, the cassava plant is promoted for the treatment of abscesses, snakebites, boils, diarrhea, dysentery, flu, hernia, inflammation, conjunctivitis, sores, and several other problems including cancer and tumors. There is no evidence to support these claims.

What does it involve?

In herbal remedies, the roots of the cassava are made into a poultice and applied directly to the skin to alleviate sores. The leaf, root, and flour obtained from the plant can also be used in a wash that is applied to the skin.

Tapioca starch made from the cassava plant is used as an oral hydration agent (to help restore body fluids) in developing countries. Tapioca starch or the chemical linamarin are not currently used in the prevention or treatment of cancer.

The parts of cassava used for food are the tubers, which are usually eaten raw, boiled, or fried. A form of flour is also made from the cassava plant. In Western countries, tapioca is usually found in baby foods and eaten as a dessert.

What is the history behind it?

Cassava has been used as a food source by many countries for centuries. Today, it is consumed by millions of people in developing countries and sometimes used as an herbal medicine.

Professor Monica Hughes of the University of Newcastle upon Tyne, England identified the cassava genes involved in the production of hydrogen cyanide seven years ago. In collaboration with cancer specialists at the University of Autonoma in Madrid, Spain, she has conducted studies of the linamarase gene from the cassava plant. They added this genetic to a virus, which was then injected into rat brain tumors. These tumors were killed when the rats were infused with linamarin. They claim that if studies go well, this treatment strategy may be available in 5 to 10 years. However, this form of gene therapy is quite different from the use of the cassava plant as an herbal remedy.

What is the evidence?

There is no scientific evidence to support the claims made for the cassava plant. Many scientists around the world are currently developing gene therapy methods for introducing DNA selectively into the tumor cells of cancer patients. More research is needed to determine if the approach using linamarin and linamarase to kill cancer cells is feasible or beneficial for people with cancer.

Are there any possible problems or complications?

The cassava plant produces cyanide when it is damaged or improperly harvested for food. It is a serious potential health hazard if not handled correctly. The breakdown of linamarin by linamarase releases hydrogen cyanide, which can be deadly to humans. Some of the signs of cyanide poisoning are headache, vertigo, agitation, confusion, coma, and convulsions. Some people in developing countries have been poisoned by eating parts of the cassava plant that were not harvested or prepared properly. Cyanide poisoning can lead to death.

References

Borron SW, Baud FJ. Acute cyanide poisoning: clinical spectrum, diagnosis, and treatment. *Arh Hig Rada Toksikol.* 1996;47:307-322.

Hughes J, Keresztessy Z, Brown K, Suhandono S, Hughes MA. Genomic organization and structure of alpha-hydroxynitrile lyase in cassava (Manihot esculenta Crantz). *Arch Biochem Biophys.* 1998;356:107-116.

Hughes M. Cyanogenesis in Manihot esculenta Crantz. University of Newcastle Web site. Available at: http://www.ncl.ac.uk/sbg/monica/mahform.html. Accessed December 20, 1999.

Manihot esculenta Crantz. Purdue University Center for New Crops & Plants Products Web site. Available at: http://www.hort.purdue.edu/newcrop/duke_energy/Manihot_esculenta.html. Accessed March 3, 2000.

Wapnir RA, Wingertzahn MA, Moyse J, Teichberg S. Proabsorptive effects of modified tapioca starch as an additive of oral rehydration solutions. *J Pediatr Gastroenterol Nutr.* 1998;27:17-22.

White WLB, Arias-Garzon DI, McMahon JM, Sayre RT. Cyanogenesis in cassava. The role of hydroxynitrile lyase in root cyanide production. *Plant Physiol.* 1998;116:1219-1225.

Wingertzahn MA, Teichberg S, Wapnir RA. Modified starch enhances absorption and accelerates recovery in experimental diarrhea in rats. *Pediatr Res.* 1999;45:397-402.

Coriolus Versicolor

Other common name(s)	Scientific/medical name(s)
Turkey Tail, PSK	*Coriolus versicolor, Trametes versicolor*

DESCRIPTION

Coriolus versicolor is a mushroom used in traditional Asian herbal remedies (see Chinese Herbal Medicine). A protein-bound polysaccharide K (PSK) from the mushroom, is being studied as a possible cancer treatment. A polysaccharide is a starch-like carbohydrate formed by a large number of sugar molecules.

OVERVIEW

There is some scientific evidence from clinical trials which suggests that PSK may provide benefit to people with cancer, including increased survival rates and longer disease-free periods, without causing significant side effects.

How is it promoted for use?

Proponents claim that PSK, the primary active ingredient in *Coriolus versicolor,* has strong anti-cancer properties–perhaps equal to the effects of some conventional chemotherapy drugs. Supporters also say that PSK has antimicrobial and antiviral properties and that it stimulates cells in the blood that destroy invading microorganisms. PSK is also believed to be a strong antioxidant, a compound that blocks the action of activated oxygen molecules, known as free radicals, that can damage cells. There is some clinical evidence that PSK may be helpful when used in addition to conventional treatments.

Herbalists claim *Coriolus versicolor* and its extracts can be used to stimulate the immune system. The mushroom is also promoted in traditional Asian medicine to treat cancer. There is no evidence the mushroom itself is effective.

What does it involve?

Coriolus versicolor can be taken in capsules, as an extract, or as a tea. The dose ranges from 1,000 to 9,000 mg/day, depending on the patient's condition. *Coriolus versicolor* can be obtained in herbal medicine shops and through the Internet.

What is the history behind it?

Coriolus versicolor has been a component of traditional Asian medicine for centuries. In the 1980s, the Japanese government approved the use of PSK for treating several types of cancers. In Japan, PSK is a best-selling anticancer drug. It is currently used as a cancer treatment in Japan in conjunction with surgery, chemotherapy, and radiation therapy.

What is the evidence?

No clinical trials with the *Coriolus versicolor* have been reported in peer-reviewed journals. However, there have been many studies assessing the usefulness of PSK. These studies have been done with PSK and not the mushroom. More than two dozen human studies have been reviewed by experts at the University of Texas Center for Alternative Medicine Research in Cancer. A number of the studies found that people with cancer benefited from PSK. A review of 8 randomized clinical trials, found that people who received PSK, along with chemotherapy or radiation therapy, generally experienced longer disease-free periods and increased survival rates compared with patients who underwent only chemotherapy or radiation therapy. The researchers also noted that 2 of the 3 studies found that PSK contributed to significantly better survival times for people with cancer of the esophagus.

Another study reviewed by University of Texas experts, the only study that compared PSK to a placebo, found that patients who underwent surgery for colorectal cancer and who received PSK had longer disease-free periods and higher survival rates than patients who did not receive PSK. In a study involving more than 260 patients who underwent surgery for stomach cancer at 46 hospitals in Japan, those who received PSK along with chemotherapy, experienced a higher 5-year disease-free rate and 5-year survival rate than subjects who underwent chemotherapy alone. Another Japanese study involving 227 patients with operable breast cancer found that the combination of PSK and chemotherapy resulted in a 10-year survival rate of 81%, compared with 64.5% for patients who received chemotherapy alone.

Are there any possible problems or complications?

No serious risks are associated with the use of PSK. Side effects that occur infrequently include nausea, vomiting, and diarrhea. Even less common are skin pigmentation, anorexia, anemia, liver dysfunction, leukopenia (abnormally low white blood cell count), and thrombocytopenia (abnormally low level of platelets in the blood).

References

Nakazato H, Koike A, Saji S, Ogawa N, Sakamoto J. Efficacy of immunochemotherapy as adjuvant treatment after curative resection of gastric cancer. Study group of immunochemotherapy with PSK for gastric cancer. *Lancet*. 1994;343:1122-1126.

PSK: A non-toxic natural cancer treatment. WellnessWeb Homepage. Available at: http://www.wellweb.com/altern/cancer/psk/contents.htm. Accessed May 8, 2000.

Torisu M, Hayashi Y, Ishimitsu T, et al. Significant prolongation of disease-free period gained by oral polysaccharide K (PSK) administration after curative surgical operation of colorectal cancer. *Cancer*. 1990;31:261-268.

University of Texas Center for Alternative Medicine Research in Cancer. Coriolus versicolor summary. University of Texas-Houston Health Science Center Web site. Available at http://www.sph.uth.tmc.edu/utcam/therapies/cor_ver.htm. Accessed May 8, 2000.

Ellagic Acid

Other common name(s)	Scientific/medical name(s)
None	None

DESCRIPTION

Ellagic acid is a compound found in raspberries, strawberries, cranberries, walnuts, pecans, pomegranates, and other plant foods.

OVERVIEW

Research in animal and laboratory models has found that ellagic acid inhibits the growth of tumors caused by certain carcinogens. Studies in humans are underway to determine the effect of long-term daily consumption of raspberries on cell activity in the human colon.

How is it promoted for use?

Ellagic acid has been found to cause apoptosis (cell death) in cancer cells in the laboratory. How it works is not yet well understood. Some also claim it prevents the binding of carcinogens to DNA, and strengthens connective tissue, which may keep cancer cells from spreading. Ellagic acid has also been said to reduce heart disease, birth defects, liver fibrosis, and to promote wound healing. Many of these claims are currently under investigation.

What does it involve?

The highest levels of ellagic acid are found in raspberries, strawberries, and pomegranates, especially when they are freeze-dried. Red raspberry leaves, which also contain ellagic acid, are available in capsule, powder, or liquid form. The correct dosage of these preparations are not known.

What is the history behind it?

Early studies of nutrition and cancer focused on macronutrients (eg, protein, carbohydrates, and fat) and micronutrients (eg, vitamins and minerals). More recently, studies have begun focusing on phytochemicals, which are compounds produced by plants (see Phytochemicals). There is an enormous amount of folklore that surrounds phytochemicals, and scientific investigation is currently in the early stages. Early published research on ellagic acid appeared in the 1970s and 1980s, and the first studies began in 1993.

What is the evidence?

Ellagic acid has been demonstrated in animal models to inhibit tumor growth caused by carcinogens. A human study is being completed at the Medical University of South Carolina Hollings Cancer Center. Twelve participants, some of whom had undergone surgery to have cancerous polyps removed, ate one cup of red raspberries daily for a year with some continuing for longer. The study was to determine if eating red raspberries could prevent colon cancer by both inhibiting the abnormal division of cells and promoting the normal death of healthy cells. The results of the study have not yet been published.

Other studies have also found positive effects. A recent animal study found that ellagic acid protected mice against chromosome damage from radiation therapy. A separate study of ellagic acid indicated that it was effective at inhibiting tumor growth from esophageal cancer cells in mice. Animal studies may show a certain substance holds promise as a beneficial treatment, but further studies are necessary to determine if the results apply to humans.

A balanced diet that includes five or more servings a day of fruits and vegetables along with foods from a variety of other plant sources such as breads, cereals, grain products, rice, pasta, and beans is more effective than eating one particular food, such as raspberries, in large amounts.

Are there any possible problems or complications?

Ellagic acid is not available in supplement form; however, eating berries is considered safe. The raspberry leaf, or preparations made from it, should be used with caution during pregnancy because they may initiate labor.

References

Agricultural Research Services. Boosting ellagic acid in strawberries. United States Department of Agriculture Web site. Available at: http://www.ars.usda.gov. Accessed October 8, 1999.

Ahn D, Putt D, Kresty L, Stoner GD, Fromm D, Hollenberg PF. The effects of dietary ellagic acid on rat hepatic and esophageal mucosal cytochromes P450 and phase II enzymes. *Carcinogenesis*. 1996;17:821-828.

Fetrow CW, Avila JR. *Professional's Handbook of Complimentary and Alternative Medicines*. Springhouse, PA: Springhouse Corp; 1999.

Harttig U, Hendricks JD, Stoner GD, Bailey GS. Organ specific, protocol dependent modulation of 7,12-dimethylbenz-[a]anthracene carcinogenesis in rainbow trout (Oncorhyncus mykiss) by dietary ellagic acid. *Carcinogenesis*. 1996;17:2403-2409.

Medical Economics. *PDR for Herbal Medicines*. Montvale, NJ: Medical Economics Company; 1998.

Narayanan BA, Geoffroy O, Willingham MC, Re GG, Nixon DW. P53/p21 (WAF1/CIP1) expression and its possible role in G1 arrest and apoptosis in ellagic acid treated cancer cells. *Cancer Lett*. 1999;136:215-221.

Stoner GD, Morse MA. Isothiocyanates and plant polyphenols as inhibitors of lung and esophageal cancer. *Cancer Lett*. 1997;114:113-119.

Thresiamma KC, George J, Kuttan R. Protective effect of curcumin, ellagic acid and bixin on radiation induced genotoxicity. *J Exp Clin Cancer Res*. 1998;17:431-434.

Fasting

Other common name(s)	**Scientific/medical name(s)**
None	None

DESCRIPTION
Fasting involves not consuming any foods and drinking only water or juice for 2 to 5 days (or longer). Sometimes, tea or broth may be part of the fasting process.

OVERVIEW
Instead of being beneficial to health, even a short-term fast can produce negative effects. Fasting over a longer period of time could cause serious health problems.

How is it promoted for use?
Metabolic practitioners believe the body contains many toxins and harmful substances that can be removed by fasting or detoxifying the body (see Metabolic Therapy). They claim that fasting allows the body to focus energy on cleansing and healing itself. According to these practitioners, fasting allows the immune system to work more efficiently, more oxygen and white blood cells to flow through the body, more fat to be burned, energy to increase, and other healing functions to improve. They also believe that total body toxicity is reduced because the body decreases the intake of new toxins and eliminates stored toxins in the body.

Illnesses and conditions that have been treated by fasting include acne, allergies, arthritis, asthma, cancer, digestive disorders, fever, headaches, glaucoma, heart disease, hypertension, inflammatory diseases, non-cancerous tumors, pain, polyps, and ulcers. Fasting is also promoted to rejuvenate the body, help maintain normal body weight, increase longevity and sex drive, and to improve mental clarity, self-awareness, and self-esteem. It is also said to be helpful in quitting or cutting back on use of tobacco, alcohol, caffeine, or non-prescription drugs. Some practitioners claim it can heighten spiritual awareness and compassion for the poor.

There is no scientific evidence to support any of these claims.

What does it involve?
Short fasts, lasting from 2 to 5 days, are done at home. Other than drinking only water or juice, fasting involves a lot of rest periods. Sometimes, an enema is recommended as part of the regimen, as is sun exposure (see Colon Therapy). Longer fasts require professional supervision and take place at a spa, resort, or similar facility.

What is the history behind it?
Ancient cultures believed fasting could purify the soul. The belief that fasting can also purify or cleanse the body is a modern idea, gaining popularity in the second half of the 20th century.

What is the evidence?
There is no medical basis for using fasting as a treatment for any disease or condition. In fact, researchers find that the body cannot distinguish between fasting and starvation. Studies related to cancer suggest that fasting could actually lead to the promotion of tumors.

A brief fast (eg, 8-12 hours) is often advised by medical professionals in preparation for certain diagnostic tests. In this case, the fast helps to produce more accurate test results.

Fasting may also be necessary for a period of time following surgery, especially if digestive system organs are involved. As for maintaining proper weight, experts recommend restricting calories instead of fasting.

Are there any possible problems or complications?

Even proponents acknowledge that fasting can produce immediate negative effects, such as headaches, dizziness, fatigue, nausea, body odor, and an unpleasant taste in the mouth. Fasting interferes with the immune system, vital bodily functions, and can damage vital organs, such as the liver, kidneys, and other organs. Women who are pregnant or breast-feeding should not fast.

References

Berg FM. 'Detoxification' with pills and fasting. Quackwatch Web site. Available at http://www.quackwatch.com. Accessed May 8, 2000.

Cassileth B. *The Alternative Medicine Handbook*. New York, NY: W. W. Norton & Co; 1998.

Hikita H, Nuwaysir EF, Vaughan J, et al. The effect of short-term fasting, phenobarbital and refeeding on apoptotic loss, cell replication and gene expression in rat liver during the promotion stage. *Carcinogenesis*. 1998;19:1417-1425.

Hikita H, Vaughan J, Pitot HC. The effect of two periods of short-term fasting during the promotion stage of hepatocarcinogenesis in rats: the role of apoptosis and cell proliferation. *Carcinogenesis*. 1997;18:159-166.

Legro RS, Finegood D, Dunaif A. A fasting glucose to insulin ratio is a useful measure of insulin sensitivity in women with polycystic ovary syndrome. *J Clin Endocrinol Metab*. 1998;83:2694-2698.

Premoselli F, Sesca E, Binasco V, Franchino C, Tessitore L. Cell death and cell proliferation contribute to the enhanced growth of foci by fasting in rat medial colon. *Boll Soc Ital Biol Sper*. 1997;73:71-76.

Sesca E, Premoselli F, Binasco V, Bollito E, Tessitore L. Fasting-refeeding stimulates the development of mammary tumors induced by 7,12-dimethylbenz[a]anthracene. *Nutr Cancer*. 1998;30:L25-30.

Garlic

Other common name(s)	Scientific/medical name(s)
Garlic Clove, Garlic Powder, Garlic Oil, Allium	*Allium sativum*

DESCRIPTION

Garlic is a member of the lily family and is closely related to onions, leeks, and chives. Extracts and oils made from garlic are sometimes used as herbal remedies.

OVERVIEW

The health benefits of the allium compounds contained in garlic and other vegetables in the onion family have been widely publicized. Garlic is currently under study for its ability to reduce cancer risk, but there is insufficient evidence to support a specific role for this vegetable in cancer prevention.

How is it promoted for use?

Garlic is promoted for use as a preventive measure against the formation of cancer. Although several compounds in garlic may have anti-cancer properties, the allyl sulfur compounds are said to play a major role. These compounds are reported to prevent cancer by decreasing the activation of carcinogens within the body, reducing the production of carcinogens, and increasing the body's ability to repair damaged DNA. There have been claims that garlic has certain immune boosting properties that may help the body fight off diseases, such as colds or the flu, as well as reduce cancer cell growth. These claims are currently under investigation.

Proponents claim garlic also has strong antibacterial and antifungal properties, and can be used to treat fungal infections, bacterial infections, hyperglycemia, and roundworms. They also say it has medicinal properties that may help stomach and abdominal problems. The use of garlic has also been claimed to reduce risk of heart disease, lower serum cholesterol, and reduce blood pressure. There is no scientific evidence to support these claims.

What does it involve?

There is considerable debate as to how the form and amount of garlic used might influence health. Proponents disagree as to whether garlic is more beneficial when eaten raw or cooked, or if the garlic extracts, powders, and oils that are available in tablet form are more or less effective.

Garlic is on the Commission E (Germany's regulatory agency for herbs) list of approved herbs, and they suggest a dosage of fresh garlic equal to 4 gm/day, or about one large clove per day. Garlic is sold as a supplement in health food stores, drug stores, and over the Internet.

What is the history behind it?

Garlic has been used in cooking throughout recorded history in many cultures around the world, especially those in the Orient, Middle East, and the Mediterranean. Garlic is believed to be one of the first cultivated plants, with initial cultivation thought to begin about 5,000 years ago in the Middle East. Garlic has also been used medicinally for thousands of years and continues to be popular today.

What is the evidence?

It is very difficult to link the exact role of a particular food in the cancer process. It is even more difficult when the food in question is typically used in small amounts, as is garlic. A balanced diet that includes five or more servings a day of fruits and vegetables along with foods from a variety of other plant sources such as breads, cereals, grain products, rice, pasta, and beans is more effective than eating one particular food in large amounts.

Several studies from around the world have found that people who consumed higher levels of garlic had a lower risk of certain types of cancers. In particular, human studies have suggested that garlic may play a protective role in stomach, prostate, and colorectal cancers, but have failed to demonstrate an effect in breast and lung cancer. Randomized clinical trials are needed to make definitive conclusions about the role of garlic in cancer prevention.

Laboratory studies suggest garlic may be of benefit in reducing tumor growth. An oil-soluble sulfur compound in processed garlic has been shown to kill human colon cancer cells in mice. Another compound found in aged garlic extract has also been shown to kill rapidly growing tumor cells. Significant antitumor activity was also found by injections of garlic into carcinoma of the bladder in mice. More work is needed to determine if this antitumor activity holds true for cancers in humans. Research is also needed to identify the specific compounds in garlic that may be of benefit in cancer prevention.

Although widely prescribed for reducing blood cholesterol, a well-controlled study published in a major medical journal concluded that garlic therapy was not effective for treating high cholesterol.

Are there any possible problems or complications?

Consumption of large amounts of garlic may lead to irritation of the gastrointestinal tract, causing stomach pain, gas, and vomiting. One study suggests that the use of garlic may increase the risk of bleeding due to its anti-blood clotting properties. People on blood thinner medication, such as warfarin, should consult with their physician before taking garlic supplements.

References

Berthold HK, Sudhop T, von Bergmann K. Effect of a garlic oil preparation on serum lipoproteins and cholesterol metabolism: a randomized controlled trial. *JAMA.* 1998;279:1900-1902.

Blumenthal M, ed. *The Complete German Commission E Monographs: Therapeutic Guide to Herbal Medicines.* Austin, Tx: American Botanical Council; 1998.

Hasler CM. Functional foods: their role in disease prevention and health promotion. *Food Technol.* 1998;52:57-62.

Levi F, Pasche C, La Vecchia C, Lucchini F, Franceschi S. Food groups and colorectal cancer risk. *Br J Cancer* 1999;79:1283-1287.

Miller LG. Herbal medicinals: selected clinical considerations focusing on known or potential drug-herb interactions. *Arch Intern Med.* 1998;158:2200-2211.

Milner JA. Garlic: its anticarcinogenic and antitumor properties. *Nutr. Rev.* 1996;54:S82-S86.

Riggs DR, DeHaven JI, Lamm DL. Allium sativum (garlic) treatment for murine transitional cell carcinoma. *Cancer.* 1997;79:1987-1994.

Sundaram SG, Milner JA. Diallyl disulfide induces apoptosis of human colon tumor cells. *Carcinogenesis.* 1996;17:669-673.

Steinmetz KA, Kushi LH, Bostick RM, Folsom AR, Potter JD. Vegetables, fruit, and colon cancer in the Iowa Women's Health Study. *Am J Epidemiol.* 1994;139:1-15.

You WC, Blot WJ, Chang YS, et al. *Allium* vegetables and reduced risk of stomach cancer. *J Natl Cancer Inst.* 1989;81:162-164.

Gerson Therapy

Other common name(s)	Scientific/medical name(s)
Gerson Diet, Gerson Method, Gerson Treatment, Gerson Program	None

DESCRIPTION

Gerson therapy involves coffee enemas and a special diet with supplements claimed to cleanse the body and stimulate metabolism (see Metabolic Therapy).

OVERVIEW

There is no scientific evidence that Gerson therapy is effective in treating cancer. Gerson therapy can be very harmful to the body. Coffee enemas have been associated with serious infections, dehydration, constipation, colitis (inflammation of the colon), electrolyte (salt and mineral) imbalances, and even death (see Colon Therapy).

How is it promoted for use?

Gerson therapy is considered a metabolic therapy, and is based on the theory that disease is caused by the body's accumulation of toxic substances (see Metabolic Therapy). Practitioners believe that chemical fertilizers, insecticides, and herbicides contaminate food by lowering the potassium content and raising the sodium content of fruits and vegetables. Food processing and cooking adds more sodium which changes the metabolism of cells in the body, eventually causing cancer.

According to practitioners, people with cancer have an excess amount of sodium, far outweighing the potassium in their bodies. The fruit and vegetable diet, which is part of Gerson therapy, is used to correct this imbalance and revitalize the liver so it can begin to rid the body of malignant cells. Coffee enemas are claimed to eliminate dead cancer cells (detoxification), and relieve pain.

The goal of metabolic therapy is to eliminate toxins from the body and enhance immune function so that the body can "fight off" cancer. Liver extract injections, pancreatic enzymes, and various supplements are said to stimulate metabolism. Proponents of metabolic therapy claim that it addresses the underlying cause of disease rather than treating the symptoms. There is no scientific evidence to support these claims.

What does it involve?

Gerson therapy requires following a strict diet that involves eating a low salt, low fat, vegetarian diet, and drinking juice from approximately 20 pounds of freshly crushed fruits and vegetables. In addition, patients are given 3 or 4 coffee enemas a day. Various other supplemental substances, such as pepsin, potassium, niacin, pancreatin (a digestive enzyme), and thyroid extracts, are ingested to stimulate various organ functions, particularly the liver and thyroid. Sometimes other treatments such as laetrile, hydrogen peroxide, hyperbaric oxygen therapy, and shark cartilage are also recommended (see Laeterile, Hydrogen Peroxide, Hyperbaric Oxygen Therapy, Shark Cartilage).

The Gerson Institute does not own or operate any medical facilities; however, it refers patients to clinics they license. Individual clinic fees often exceed $4,000 per week, and treatment may last from a few months to 10 years or more. The Gerson Institute also offers a home therapy package.

What is the history behind it?

One of the oldest nutritional approaches to cancer treatment, the Gerson therapy was developed by Max Gerson, MD, a German doctor who emigrated to the United States in the late 1930s. He designed the dietary program in order to treat his own migraine headaches. He later expanded his method to treat other conditions such as arthritis, tuberculosis, and cancer. In 1945, Gerson published a preliminary report of his results in treating cancer in the *Review of Gastroenterology.* The National Cancer Institute and New York County Medical Society examined records of his patients and found no evidence that the method was effective against cancer. Gerson's malpractice insurance was discontinued in 1953. After his death in 1959, his work was carried on by his daughter, Charlotte Gerson Strauss, who established the Gerson Institute in 1977.

What is the evidence?

There have been no well-controlled studies to support the beliefs and practices of the Gerson therapy. The Gerson Research Organization conducted a retrospective review and reported that survival rates were higher for patients with melanoma, colorectal and ovarian cancers who participated in the Gerson program compared to those who did not at another institution.

According to a critique in a major peer-reviewed journal, the explanation for how the method is supposed to work does not follow the established scientific principles of basic nutrition, biology, and cancer immunology.

Are there any possible problems or complications?

There are a number of significant problems that may develop from the use of this therapy. Serious illness and death have occurred from some of the components of the treatment, such as the coffee enemas that remove potassium from the body leading to electrolyte imbalances. Continued home use of enemas may cause the colon's normal function to weaken, worsening constipation problems and colitis. Enemas should be given only under medical guidance. Some metabolic diets, used in combination with enemas, cause dehydration. Serious infections from poorly administered liver extracts may result. Thyroid supplements may cause severe bleeding in patients with liver metastases. This method may be especially hazardous to women who are pregnant or breast-feeding. Relying on this treatment alone, and avoiding conventional medical care, may have serious health consequences.

References

Alternative Medicine: Expanding Medical Horizons. *A Report to the National Institutes of Health on Alternative Medical Systems and Practices in the United States.* Washington, DC: US Government Printing Office; 1994. NIH publication 94-066.

American Cancer Society. Questionable methods of cancer management: 'nutritional' therapies. *CA Cancer J Clin.* 1993;43:309-319.

Green S. A critique of the rationale for cancer treatment with coffee enemas and diet. *JAMA.* 1992;268:3224-3227.

Hildenbrand GL, Hildenbrand LC, Bradford K, Cavin SW. Five-year survival rates of melanoma patients treated by diet therapy after the manner of Gerson: a retrospective review. *Altern Ther Health Med.* 1995;1:29-37.

Murphy GP, Morris LB, Lange D. Informed Decisions: *The Complete Book of Cancer Diagnosis, Treatment, and Recovery.* New York, NY: Viking; 1997.

University of Texas Center for Alternative Medicine Research in Cancer. Gerson summary. University of Texas-Houston Health Science Center Web site. Available at: http://www.sph.uth.tmc.edu/utcam/summary/gerson.htm. Accessed May 8, 2000.

US Congress, Office of Technology Assessment. *Unconventional Cancer Treatments.* Washington, DC: US Government Printing Office; 1990. Publication OTA-H-405.

Grapes

Other common name(s)	Scientific/medical name(s)
The Grape Diet, The Grape Cure, Grape Seed Extract, Grape Skins	*Vitis vinifera, Vitis coignetiae*

DESCRIPTION

Grapes grow wild on vines or are cultivated. They are believed to be native to northwest Asia although they are currently grown throughout Europe and the United States. The seeds, skin, leaves, stems, and grape itself are used in herbal remedies. Some chemicals found in grape extracts or grape skin (resveratrol and proanthocynadins) are currently being studied for possible uses in the prevention and treatment of cancer and other illnesses.

OVERVIEW

There is no scientific evidence that a grape diet is effective for treating cancer or any other disease. Some evidence suggests that a chemical in grape seed extract may help to promote antioxidant activity, but more clinical trials are needed to understand the long-term benefits. Some studies suggest the skins of red grapes may help prevent cardiovascular disease and cancer; however, more research is needed to confirm these results.

How is it promoted for use?

Proponents claim the chemicals found in grape seed extract (proanthocyanidins) contain powerful antioxidants. Antioxidants are compounds that block the action of activated oxygen molecules, known as free radicals, that can damage cells. Some claim that these antioxidants inhibit the development of some types of cancer, protect against heart disease, and are useful for treating a variety of medical conditions such as arthritis, allergies, circulatory problems, diabetes, water retention, and vision problems. The compound found in the skins of red grapes (resveratrol) is being studied to see how it affects the development and progression of heart disease and cancer.

Alternative practitioners recommend the use of grapes and parts of the grape plant internally for high blood pressure, menopause, varicose veins, high cholesterol, skin rashes, and urination problems. They also claim it works for inflammation of the gums, throat, eyes, and mouth. There is no scientific evidence to support these claims.

Although now rarely promoted, the grape diet was used as a treatment to flush toxins from the body and protect the body against cancer and virtually all other diseases. Some supporters believed that the diet cured cancer.

What does it involve?

Fresh, preserved, and dried grapes are used in the form of liquid extracts, tinctures, gargles, enemas, douches, and compresses. Grape skins are used to make wine. Grape seed extract and resveratrol are available in tablets and capsule supplements. The dosages vary depending on the manufacturer.

The complete grape diet begins with a period of fasting and eating only grapes for 1 or 2 weeks. Then, fresh fruits and sour milk can also be consumed. The next stage of the diet includes raw vegetables, salads, nuts, dairy products, honey, and olive oil. During the final stage of the diet, if a person is doing well, they may be given one cooked meal per day but no liquids, salad, or fruit is allowed.

What is the history behind it?

Grapes have been associated with health for many centuries. Evidence of fossilized grape leaves, stems, and seeds that date back 10 to 12 million years ago have been found in the Northern hemisphere. Grapes, from the *Vitis vinifera* species, were cultivated for thousands of years in the Old World before they were brought to the United States.

Johanna Brandt, a South African dietitian, proposed the grape diet in 1925. Brandt claimed to have cured herself of cancer by following the diet. After immigrating to the United States in 1927, she opened the Harmony Healing Centre in New York City and began promoting the treatment. She wrote a book that was first published in 1928. Brandt and some of her followers who prescribed or promoted the grape diet as a cure for cancer became the targets of intense criticism and even legal action, because no scientific evidence supported their claims that the treatment benefited health or cured disease.

After that time period, interest began to grow in understanding the role of antioxidants in health, and proanthocyanidins were extracted from grape seeds in 1970. In the mid 1990s, the compound found mostly in the skins of red grapes (resveratrol) was thought to be responsible for the low occurrence of heart disease among people in France who tend to eat a high-fat diet.

What is the evidence?

While grape extracts may hold some positive benefit for people with cancer, there is no scientific evidence that eating grapes or following the grape diet can cure cancer or any other disease.

A balanced diet that includes five or more servings a day of fruits and vegetables along with foods from a variety of other plant sources such as breads, cereals, grain products, rice, pasta, and beans is more effective than eating one particular food in large amounts.

In one randomized clinical trial, researchers found that capsules containing one of the chemicals in grape seed extract increased antioxidant activity, but they concluded that more randomized clinical trials are needed to understand the long-term effects in humans.

Laboratory and animal studies have shown

that resveratrol may help prevent cardiovascular disease and cancer, but randomized clinical trials are needed to make conclusions about how the findings apply to humans. One review article concluded that while moderate drinking of red wine might protect some older people against coronary heart disease, it is associated with increased risk of stroke, certain cancers, accidents and injuries, and a range of social problems. Resveratrol is currently being studied to determine its potential as an antioxidant and as an inhibitor of several enzymes that promote cell proliferation.

Are there any possible problems or complications?

An exclusive grape diet is unhealthy and does not supply the body with adequate amounts of protein and important nutrients, such as vitamin B_{12}. Grape seed extract is believed to be safe, but additional research is needed for confirmation.

The amount of resveratrol in red wine varies greatly, and increased consumption of wine to increase resveratrol intake poses certain health risks. Alcohol is associated with increased risks of cancers of the mouth, esophagus, pharynx, larynx, and liver in both men and women, and of breast cancer in women. Cancer risk also increases with the amount of alcohol consumed. However, the cardiovascular benefits of moderate drinking may outweigh the risk of cancer in men over age 50 and in women over age 60.

References

American Cancer Society. Unproven methods of cancer management. Grape diet. *CA Cancer J Clin.* 1974;24:144-146.

Ashley MJ, Ferrence R, Room R, Bondy S, Rehm J, Single E. Moderate drinking and health. Implications of recent evidence. *Can Fam Physician.* 1997;43:687-694.

Bown D. *Encyclopedia of Herbs & Their Uses.* New York, NY: DK Publishing Inc; 1995.

Fetrow CW, Avila JR. *Professional's Handbook of Complementary and Alternative Medicines.* Springhouse, Pa: Springhouse Corp; 1999.

McElderry MQB. Grape expectations: the resveratrol story. Quackwatch Web site. Available at: http://www.quackwatch.com. Accessed October 21, 1999.

Mitchell SH, Zhu W, Young CY. Resveratrol inhibits the expression and function of the androgen receptor in LNCaP prostate cancer cells. *Cancer Res.* 1999;59:5892-5895.

Moss RW. *Herbs Against Cancer.* New York, NY: Equinox Press; 1998.

Nuttall SL, Kendall MJ, Bombardelli E, Morazzoni P. An evaluation of the antioxidant activity of a standardized grape seed extract, Leucoselect. *J Clin Pharm Ther.* 1998;23:385-389.

Subbaramaiah K, Michaluart P, Chung WJ, Tanabe T, Telang N, Dannenberg AJ. Resveratrol inhibits cyclooxygenase-2 transcription in human mammary epithelial cells. *Ann NY Acad Sci.* 1999;889:214-223.

Inositol Hexaphosphate

Other common name(s)	Scientific/medical name(s)
Inositol, Phytic Acid, Phytate	IP6

DESCRIPTION

Inositol hexaphosphate (IP6) is a chemical found in beans, brown rice, corn, sesame seeds, wheat bran, and other high fiber foods. It aids in the metabolism of insulin and calcium, hair growth, bone marrow cell metabolism, eye membrane development, and helps the liver transfer fat to other parts of the body.

OVERVIEW

Animal and laboratory research has found that IP6 may be effective in decreasing tumor incidence and growth. However, clinical trials are needed to determine the anticancer effects in humans.

How is it promoted for use?

Proponents call IP6 a "natural cancer fighter" and claim the chemical inhibits or reverses the growth of various forms of cancers, including breast, colon, and prostate cancers. It is thought to be an antioxidant, a compound that blocks the action of activated oxygen molecules, known as free radicals, that can damage cells. Some believe IP6 slows abnormal cell division and can sometimes transform tumor cells into normal cells. Supporters also claim it effectively prevents kidney stones, high cholesterol, heart disease, and liver disease. These theories have not been scientifically tested in humans.

What does it involve?

Many high fiber food sources contain IP6, and it is also available as a supplement. Scientists do not know enough about the chemical to recommend a standardized dose. The supplemental pill form is found in a formula which combines inositol and IP6. It is not known if taking a supplement provides the same effect as when eaten from food sources.

What is the history behind it?

The existence of IP6 has been known for several decades. Interest in its potential anticancer properties emerged in the mid-1980s when AbulKalam Shamsuddin, MD, PhD, at the University of Maryland, began to conduct research studies on inositol. He published a consumer book in 1998, and continues to study the effects of IP6.

What is the evidence?

All of the evidence regarding the anticancer effects of IP6 has come from laboratory and animal studies. A recent study found that dietary myo-inositol (a derivative of IP6) significantly reduced the growth of lung cancer in mice. One recent review of two tumor model studies concluded that IP6 has the potential to play a role in the treatment of cancer and high cholesterol. Animal and laboratory studies may show a certain compound holds promise as a beneficial treatment, but further studies are necessary to determine if the results apply to humans.

A randomized clinical trial involving women with polycystic ovary syndrome, a condition that inhibits insulin action was recently done. D-chiro-inositol (a derivative of IP6) appeared to reverse insulin resistance and improve ovulatory function by causing a decrease in the production of androgens (male hormones), blood pressure, and plasma triglycerides (a type of fat found in blood) concentrations.

Inositol hexaphosphate and its derivatives has also been studied for treatment of panic disorders, autism, obsessive-compulsive disorders, Alzheimer's disease, post-traumatic stress disorders, and depression, but researchers have reached no firm conclusions regarding its impact on any of these conditions.

Are there any possible problems or complications?

When taken in moderate amounts, IP6 appears to be safe. However, no studies have been conducted to determine its safety. Experts advise individuals who wish to increase their intake of IP6 to incorporate inositol-rich foods into their diets before resorting to supplements. Women who are pregnant or breast-feeding should not use IP6.

References

Dong Z, Huang C, Ma WY. PI-3 kinase in signal transduction, cell transformation, and as a target for chemoprevention of cancer. *Anticancer Res.* 1999;19:3743-3747.

Hecht SS, Kenney PM, Wang M, et al. Evaluation of butylated hydroxyanisole, myo-inositol, curcumin, esculetin, resveratrol and lycopene as inhibitors of benzo[a]pyrene plus 4-(methylnitrosamino)-1-(3-pyridyl)-1-butanone-induced lung tumorigenesis in A/J mice. *Cancer Lett.* 1999;137:123-130.

Jariwalla RJ. Inositol hexaphosphate (IP6) as an anti-neoplastic and lipid-lowering agent. *Anticancer Res.* 1999;19:3699-3702.

Nestler JE, Jakubowicz DJ, Reamer P, Gunn RD, Allan G. Ovulatory and metabolic effects of D-chiro-inositol in the polycystic ovary syndrome. *N Engl J Med.* 1999;340:1214-1320.

Samsuddin AM. Nonisoflavone soybean anticarcinogens: Inositol phosphates have novel anticancer function. *J Nutr.* 1995;125:725S-732S.

Juicing

Other common name(s)	Scientific/medical name(s)
Juice therapy	None

DESCRIPTION / OVERVIEW

Juicing involves extracting juices from fresh fruit and uncooked vegetables as a primary part of the diet. Juice extractors are used to grind food into small pieces that are spun to extract juice from the pulp. It is promoted as a way to prevent and treat a wide variety of conditions by enhancing the immune system. According to practitioners, "unnatural" dietary habits cause imbalances in the body's cell composition, which are corrected and re-balanced with the nutrients that the juice delivers. This treatment method is frequently used to sustain the body during long fasts, or as part of the Gerson regimen (see Gerson Therapy).

Juicing first became popular in the early 1990s when proponents claimed that it could reverse everything from the natural aging process to chronic diseases such as cancer. It can cause severe diarrhea, which is actually thought to be "cleansing" because "toxins" are supposedly removed from the body during this process. There is no scientific evidence that extracted juices are healthier than whole foods. Juice extractors remove the fiber-containing pulp from the fruits and vegetables, so it is important to maintain a diet that includes an adequate amount of fiber.

Kombucha Tea

Other common name(s)	Scientific/medical name(s)
Manchurian Tea, Kargasok Tea	None

DESCRIPTION

Kombucha tea is made from the flat, pancake-like culture known as the Kombucha mushroom. It is actually not a mushroom but is called one because of its appearance. The culture or mushroom sac used in Kombucha tea consists of several species of yeast and bacteria including Saccharomycodes ludwigii, Schizosaccharomyces pombe, Bacterium xylinum, Bacterium gluconicum, Bacterium xylinoides, Bacterium katogenum, Pichia fermentans, and Torula sp. After the tea is made, it becomes highly acidic and contains alcohol, ethyl acetate, acetic acid, and lactate.

OVERVIEW

There is no scientific evidence that Kombucha tea is effective in treating cancer or any other disease. No data exist showing that it helps promote good health or prevents any ailments. There have been some serious side effects reported with the consumption of Kombucha tea.

How is it promoted for use?

Kombucha tea is promoted as a cure-all for a wide variety of conditions including baldness, insomnia, intestinal disorders, arthritis, chronic fatigue syndrome, multiple sclerosis, AIDS, and cancer. Supporters assert that Kombucha tea can boost the immune system and reverse the aging process. Kombucha tea is said to contain antioxidants, compounds that block the action of activated oxygen molecules, known as free radicals, that can damage cells. For people with cancer, proponents claim the tea can detoxify (cleanse) the body and enhance the immune system thereby improving the body's defenses, especially in the early stages of cancer. After the body is cleansed, the tea is said to help repair and balance the body, and fight off disease. There is no scientific evidence to support these claims.

What does it involve?

Kombucha tea is made by steeping the mushroom culture in tea and sugar for about a week. During this process, the original mushroom floats in the tea and produces a "baby" mushroom on its surface. These new mushrooms can be passed along to other people for starting their own cultures or be kept to make new batches of the tea when the original mushroom goes bad (turns dark brown).

In order to increase the detoxifying abilities of the tea, people are told to remove chemicals from their diets and eat only fresh fruits and vegetables. They are also told to avoid caffeine, soft drinks, alcohol, hormone-fed meat, fertilized or sprayed foods, preservatives, artificial coloring and flavoring, and to quit smoking.

Kombucha mushroom cultures can be obtained from commercial manufacturers in the United States; however, many people have obtained Kombucha mushrooms from friends because they are easily passed along.

What is the history behind it?

Kombucha tea originated in East Asia and was introduced into Germany at the turn of the century. Since the early 19th century, Kombucha tea has been promoted as an immunity-boosting tea, which could strengthen the body against many ailments. It has become prevalent in the United States because it can be grown and harvested at home. It is especially popular among people with HIV and the elderly due to its immunity-boosting and anti-aging claims.

What is the evidence?

There is no scientific evidence to support any of the claims made for Kombucha tea. There have been reports of some serious complications associated with the tea. In April 1995, two women who had been consuming the tea daily for two months, were hospitalized with severe acidosis—an abnormal increase in the acidity in the body fluids. Both had high levels of lactic acid upon hospitalization. One woman died of cardiac arrest two days after admission. The second woman also suffered a heart attack but was stabilized and eventually released. The mushrooms used by both women came from the same "parent" mushroom. While no direct link to Kombucha tea was proven in this case, the FDA has warned consumers to use caution when making and drinking the tea.

Are there any possible problems or complications?

Kombucha tea is highly acidic. Deaths have been reported from acidosis linked with the tea. Drinking excessive amounts of the tea is not recommended. Several experts warn that since home-brewing facilities vary significantly, the tea could become contaminated with harmful bacteria which could be especially detrimental to people with HIV or other immune disorders. Because the acid in the tea could absorb harmful toxins, it should not be brewed in ceramic, lead crystal, or painted containers. Since the potential health risks of Kombucha tea are unknown, anyone with a preexisting medical condition should consult a physician before consuming the tea. Women who are pregnant or breast-feeding should not use this tea.

References

Boik J. *Cancer & Natural Medicine: A Textbook of Basic Science and Clinical Research*. Princeton, Minn: Oregon Medical Press; 1996.

Cassileth B. *The Alternative Medicine Handbook*. New York, NY: W. W. Norton & Co;1998.

Centers for Disease Control and Prevention. *Unexplained severe illness possibly associated with consumption of Kombucha tea-Iowa, 1995. JAMA* 1996;275:96-98.

Spaulding-Albright N. *A review of some herbal and related products commonly used in cancer patients. J Am Diet Assoc.* 1997;97:S208-215.

US Food and Drug Administration. *FDA Talk Paper: FDA cautions consumers on "Kombucha mushroom tea."* Rockville, Md: National Press Office; March 23, 1995. Talk Paper T95-15.

Lycopene

Other common name(s)	Scientific/medical name(s)
None	None

DESCRIPTION

Lycopene is the compound that gives tomatoes and certain other fruits and vegetables their color. It is one of the major carotenoids in the diet of North Americans and Europeans.

OVERVIEW

People who have diets rich in tomatoes, which contain lycopene, appear to have a lower risk of certain types of cancer, especially cancers of the prostate, lung, and stomach. Further research is needed to determine what role, if any, lycopene has in the prevention or treatment of cancer. It is currently thought that the preventive effect of diets high in fruits and vegetables cannot be explained by just one single component in the diet.

How is it promoted for use?

Proponents claim that lycopene may lower the risk of heart disease (atherosclerosis and coronary heart disease), macular degenerative disease (an age-related illness which can lead to blindness), and serum lipid oxidation. It is also said to lower low-density lipoprotein (LDL) cholesterol, enhance the body's defenses, and protect enzymes, DNA, and cellular lipids. A major claim for lycopene's benefits is in the treatment of cancers of the lung, prostate, stomach, bladder, cervix, and skin. These claims are currently under investigation.

Some researchers believe lycopene may be valuable in the prevention and growth of cancers of the prostate, lung, and stomach. These scientists believe lycopene to be a powerful antioxidant, a compound that blocks the action of activated oxygen molecules, known as free radicals, that can damage cells. The antioxidant activity of lycopene is at least twice as great as beta carotene, another carotenoid that is also thought to be an effective cancer-preventing nutrient (see Beta Carotene). Lycopene is considered one of the more effective antioxidants because it is not converted to vitamin A when ingested (see Vitamin A). Conversion to vitamin A weakens the antioxidant properties of carotenoids like beta carotene.

What does it involve?

Dietary lycopene comes primarily from tomatoes, although apricots, guava, watermelon, papaya, and pink grapefruit are also significant sources. Tomatoes are the best source of lycopene. Initial studies have suggested that cooked tomatoes (ie, tomato sauce or paste) are a better source of available lycopene than raw tomato juice because the heating action allows the body to quickly absorb the lycopene. Lycopene can also be taken in the form of soft-gel capsule supplements. Dosages vary according to manufacturer.

What is the history behind it?

In recent years, the role of the diet in preventing the occurrence of cancer has been a popular and important area of research. The examination of the role of other carotenoids, specifically beta carotene, in preventing cancer began in the 1920s. However, interest in lycopene did not really begin until the late 1980s when it was found that the antioxidant activity of lycopene was twice that of beta carotene. By the late 1990s, over 70 studies have looked for a link between diets high in tomatoes (as a source of lycopene) and a lower risk of cancer.

What is the evidence?

Studies suggest that diets rich in tomato intake may account for a reduction in the risk of several different types of cancer. The strongest evidence is for a protective effect against cancers of the lung, stomach, and prostate gland. There may also be a protective benefit against cancers of the cervix, breast, oral cavity, pancreas, colorectum, and esophagus. However, eating a balanced diet that includes five or more servings a day of fruits and vegetables along with foods from a variety of other plant sources such as breads, cereals, grain products, rice, pasta, and beans is more effective than eating one particular food in large amounts.

Population studies from many countries have shown that the risk of developing some cancers are lower in people who either have diets high in tomato products or have higher levels of lycopene in their blood. A population-based case-control study recently found that lycopene from tomato-based foods was associated with a small reduction in risk for prostate cancer. However, a direct relationship has not yet been proven. Other compounds in tomatoes or those diets high in tomato products, either acting alone or with lycopene, may be responsible for the protective effects currently associated with lycopene.

Since interest in lycopene is relatively recent, there have only been a few experimental studies on the role of lycopene in preventing or treating cancer. One animal study found that lycopene treatment reduced the growth of brain tumors. Another animal study showed that chronic intake of lycopene considerably suppressed breast tumor growth. The application of this study to human disease is cautioned since 95% of human breast cancers do not have the same characteristics that mice have. Lycopene has also been shown to interfere with the growth of many different human cancer cell lines in the laboratory, especially those that grow in

response to insulin-like growth factor I. Animal and laboratory studies may show a certain substance holds promise as a beneficial treatment, but further studies are necessary to determine if the results apply to humans.

Results of a small clinical study presented at the 1999 annual meeting of the American Association for Cancer Research suggested that lycopene supplements may benefit those with prostate cancer. Among 15 men who had taken two capsules of lycopene every day for about three weeks before surgery, five had smaller, less advanced lesions and the cancer was less likely to have spread beyond the prostate than the men who received a placebo (inactive substance). Although these results are encouraging, this was a very small study. Also, the daily dose of the lycopene supplements equaled the amount of lycopene in about four pounds of tomatoes. More research is needed to find out whether lycopene treatment before surgery has any impact on long-term survival, whether continuing treatment after surgery is helpful, and what doses are most effective.

Are there any possible problems or complications?

Lycopene obtained from eating fruits and vegetables has no known side effects and is thought to be safe for humans. The potential side effects of lycopene supplements are not known.

References

American Cancer Society. Chemical in tomatoes may slow prostate cancer growth. News Today. American Cancer Society Web site. Available at: http://www.cancer.org. Accessed December 10, 1999.

Clinton SK. Lycopene: chemistry, biology, and implications for human health and disease. *Nutr Rev.* 1998;56:35-51.

Gerster H. The potential role of lycopene for human health. *J Am Coll Nutr.* 1997;16:109-126.

Giovannucci E. Tomatoes, tomato-based products, lycopene, and cancer: review of the epidemiologic literature. *J Natl Cancer Inst.* 1999;91:317-331.

Nagasawa H, Mitamura T, Sakamoto S, Yamamoto K. Effects of lycopene on spontaneous mammary tumour development in SHN virgin mice. *Anticancer Res.* 1995;15:1173-1178.

Norrish AE, Jackson RT, Sharpe SJ, Skeaff CM. Prostate cancer and dietary carotenoids. *Am J Epidemiol.* 2000;151:119-123.

Paiva SA, Russell RM. Beta-carotene and other carotenoids as antioxidants. *J Am Coll Nutr.* 1999;18:426-433.

Porrini M, Riso P. Lymphocyte lycopene concentration and DNA protection from oxidative damage is increased in women after a short period of tomato consumption. *J Nutr.* 2000;130:189-192.

Rao AV, Agarwal S. Bioavailability and in vivo antioxidant properties of lycopene from tomato products and their possible role in the prevention of cancer. *Nutr Cancer.* 1998;31:199-203.

Macrobiotic Diet

Other common name(s)	Scientific/medical name(s)
Macrobiotics	None

DESCRIPTION

A macrobiotic diet is generally vegetarian and consists largely of whole grains, cereals, and cooked vegetables.

OVERVIEW

There is no scientific evidence that a macrobiotic diet is effective in treating cancer. It can lower fat intake and increase fiber, so it can provide general health benefits associated with low-fat/high fiber diets. However, macrobiotic diets can lead to poor nutrition if not properly planned. Some earlier versions of the diet may actually pose a danger to health. Research is underway to determine whether a macrobiotic diet may play a role in preventing cancer.

How is it promoted for use?

Proponents of the macrobiotic diet claim that it can prevent and cure disease, including cancer, and enhance spiritual and physical well being. An important goal of a macrobiatic diet is to balance the yin and yang. These are the two elementary and complementary forms of energy that, according to ancient Asian spiritual traditions, are present within all people. These two forces must be in equilibrium to achieve health and vitality. A macrobiotic diet is considered a more comprehensive way of life rather than just a diet.

What does it involve?

A macrobiatic diet combines elements of Buddhism with dietary principles that are based on simplicity and avoidance of "toxins" that come from eating dairy products, meats, and oily foods. Older versions of the macrobiotic diet were quite restrictive. One variation allowed only the consumption of whole grains.

The standard macrobiotic diet of today consists of 50% to 60% organically grown whole grains, 20% to 25% locally and organically grown fruits and vegetables, 5% to 10% soups made with vegetables, seaweed, grains, beans, and miso (a fermented soy product). Other elements may include occasional helpings of fresh whitemeat fish, nuts, seeds, pickles, Asian condiments, and nonstimulating and nonaromatic teas. Early versions of the diet included no animal products at all. Some vegetables are excluded, such as potatoes, tomatoes, eggplant, peppers, asparagus, spinach, beets, zucchini, and avocados. The diet also advises against eating fruits that do not grow locally, such as bananas, pineapples and other tropical fruits. The eating of dairy products, eggs, coffee, sugar, stimulant and aromatic herbs, red meat, poultry, and processed foods is discouraged.

Macrobiotic principles also prescribe specific ways of cooking food using pots, pans, and utensils made only from certain materials such as wood, glass, ceramic stainless steel, and enameled pieces. People who practice the diet do not usually cook with microwaves or electricity, nor do they consume vitamin or mineral supplements, or heavily processed foods. The food is chewed until it is fluid in order to help with digestion. Since food is thought to be sacred, it is prepared in a peaceful setting.

A specific macrobiotic diet prescription is determined by a person's age, sex, level of physical activity, and native climate. Although macrobiotic dietary guidelines are only one aspect of a larger philosophical and spiritual system, it is the diet that has drawn the most attention in the West.

What is the history behind it

The word "macrobiotic" comes from Greek roots and means "long life," reflecting the view toward long-term health and spirituality embodied by the macrobiotic philosophy. The macrobiotic philosophy and diet were developed by George Ohsawa, a Japanese philosopher who sought to integrate Zen Buddhism, Asian medicine, Christian teachings, and some aspects of Western medicine. Ohsawa believed simplicity in diet was the key to good health. He also believed macrobiotic diets could cure cancer and other serious illnesses. In the 1930s, he began advocating his philosophy of health and healing through proper diet and natural medicine. Ohsawa brought his teachings to the United States in the 1960s. His diet involved 10 stages that were progressively more restrictive.

The last stage consisted only of brown rice and water. This restrictive diet was found to be unhealthy, and is no longer promoted by macrobiotic counselors.

An early disciple, Michio Kushi, adopted and expanded Ohsawa's ideas and became a leader of the macrobiotic lifestyle. Kushi opened the Kushi Institute in Boston in 1978 to promote the philosophy and its practices. According to Kushi, a macrobiatic diet is a common-sense approach to daily living, not just a type of therapy. Although macrobiotic diets were not developed primarily as cancer treatments, they have been widely promoted for that purpose. During the 1980s, interest in the diet grew through a book written by a physician and president of Philadelphia Hospital named Anthony Sattilaro who felt that his prostate cancer remitted due to the diet.

Recently, an item in the *Associated Press* reported that a macrobiatic diet counselor at the Amsterdam-based headquarters of the Kushi Institute is being prosecuted in the alleged deaths of three of his clients. As their macrobiatic diet counselor, he allegedly told these clients that a macrobiotic diet could cure their illnesses instead of relying on conventional medical treatment.

What is the evidence?

There have been no randomized clinical studies to show the macrobiotic diet can be used to prevent or cure cancer. One of the earlier macrobiotic diets that involves eating only brown rice and water has been associated with severe nutritional deficiencies and even death. However, diets that consist primarily of plant products that are low in fat and high in fiber are believed to reduce the risk of cardiovascular disease and some forms of cancer. One review concluded that dietary macro and micronutrients play an important role in estrogen metabolism. This may have an impact on hormone related cancers. The National Institutes of Health Office of Alternative Medicine has funded a pilot study to determine if a macrobiotic diet may prevent cancer.

Are there any possible problems or complications?

Strict macrobiotic diets that include no animal products may result in nutritional deficiencies, such as inadequate intake of protein, vitamin D, zinc, calcium, iron, and vitamin B_{12} (see Calcium, Vitamin B, Vitamin D, and Zinc). The danger may be magnified for people with cancer, who often have increased nutritional and caloric requirements. Relying on this type of treatment alone, and avoiding conventional medical care, may have serious health consequences.

One of the earlier macrobiotic diets, which calls for eating 100% grains, has been associated with severe nutritional deficiencies and even death. Children may be particularly vulnerable to nutritional deficiencies resulting from a macrobiotic diet. Women who are pregnant or breastfeeding should not use this diet.

References

Alternative Medicine: Expanding Medical Horizons. *A Report to the National Institutes of Health on Alternative Medical Systems and Practices in the United States.* Washington, DC: US Government Printing Office; 1994. NIH publication 94-066.

Cassileth B. *The Alternative Medicine Handbook.* New York, NY: W. W. Norton & Co; 1998.

Dutch authorities prosecuting a macrobiatic diet practitioner. *Associated Press.* March 1, 2000. AP World Stream. Cancer Research News.

Murphy GP, Morris LB, Lange D. *Informed Decisions: The Complete Book of Cancer Diagnosis, Treatment, and Recovery.* New York, NY: Viking; 1997.

University of Texas Center for Alternative Medicine Research in Cancer. Macrobiotic summary. University of Texas-Houston Health Science Center Web site. Available at: http://www.sph.uth.tmc.edu/utcam/therapies/macrobiotic.htm. Accessed October 25, 1999.

US Congress, Office of Technology Assessment. *Unconventional Cancer Treatments.* Washington, DC: US Government Printing Office; 1990. Publication OTA-H-405.

Maitake Mushroom

Other common name(s)	Scientific/medical name(s)
Maitake, Maitake Extract, Maitake D-Fraction	*Grifola frondosa*

DESCRIPTION

Maitake is an edible mushroom from the species Grifola frondosa. Maitake D-fraction® is an extract of the mushroom marketed as a food supplement in the United States and Japan.

OVERVIEW

Research has shown that a maitake extract (maitake D-fraction) has some immune system effects in animal and laboratory studies. There is no scientific evidence that the maitake mushroom is effective in treating or preventing cancer in humans.

How is it promoted for use?

Promoters claim that maitake mushroom extract boosts the human immune system and limits or reverses tumor growth. It is also thought to enhance the benefits of chemotherapy and lessen some side effects of anti-cancer drugs, such as hair loss, pain, and nausea. There is no scientific evidence to support these claims.

What does it involve?

D-fraction is a polysaccharide called beta-glucan that is found in several mushrooms used in Asian medicine. A polysaccharide is a large and complex molecule made up of smaller sugar molecules. The beta-glucan polysaccharide is believed to stimulate the immune system and activate certain cells and proteins that attack cancer, including natural killer cells (a type of white blood cell) and interleukin-1 and -2. Maitake D-fraction is one of the only medicinal mushroom extracts said to be effective when taken orally. It is available in liquid, tablet, and capsule form in health food stores. Maitake mushrooms are available in grocery stores.

What is the history behind it?

For thousands of years, Asian healers have used certain edible mushrooms to promote health and long life in tonics, soups, teas, prepared dishes, and herbal formulas. Until recently, the healing properties of mushrooms have been the subject of folklore only. In the past couple of decades, however, researchers in Japan have been studying the medicinal effects of mushrooms on the immune system, cancer, blood pressure, and cholesterol levels.

The Japanese word "maitake" means dancing mushroom because people in ancient times were said to dance for joy when they found these mushrooms–the mushrooms were literally worth their weight in silver. Modern research on the maitake mushroom and its D-fraction extract began in Japan in the mid-1980s and has only recently spread to the United States.

What is the evidence?

There is little research on maitake mushrooms or the extract (maitake D-fraction). Most of the research on maitake D-fraction has been done in Japan in mice and laboratory studies using an injectable form of the extract. A 1997 study published in the *Annals of the New York Academy of Science* found that maitake D-fraction extract was able to enhance the immune system and inhibit the spread of tumors in mice that had been implanted with breast cancer. In a 1995 report published in the same journal, researchers concluded that maitake D-fraction extract was able to activate the immune response in mice injected with liver cancer cells to prevent the spread of tumors to the liver, and prevent the development of cancer in normal cells.

Animal and laboratory studies may show a certain compound holds promise as a beneficial treatment, but further studies are necessary to determine if the results apply to humans. Human studies are under way in Japan and the United States to determine the extract's effects on breast and prostate cancer. More studies are needed to determine maitake's potential usefulness in preventing or treating cancer.

Are there any possible problems or complications?

The mushroom itself has been used in cooking and herbal medicine without harm for centuries. So far, studies have not shown any adverse effects from maitake D-fraction, but human studies have not yet been completed.

References

Nanba H. Activity of maitake D-fraction to inhibit carcinogenesis and metastasis. *Ann NY Acad Sci.* 1995;768:243-245.

Nanba H, Kubo K. Effect of maitake D-fraction on cancer prevention. *Ann NY Acad Sci.* 1997;833:204-207.

Metabolic Therapy

Other common name(s)	**Scientific/medical name(s)**
Kelley's Treatment, Gonzalez Treatment, Issel's Whole Body Therapy	None

DESCRIPTION

Metabolic therapy uses a combination of special diets and nutritional supplements in an attempt to remove "toxins" from the body and strengthen the body's defenses against disease.

OVERVIEW

There is no scientific evidence that metabolic therapy is effective in treating cancer or any other disease. Some aspects of metabolic therapy may be harmful.

How is it promoted for use?

Metabolic therapists believe toxic substances in food and the environment create chemical imbalances that lead to diseases such as cancer, arthritis, and multiple sclerosis. They say that metabolic therapy eliminates these toxins and strengthens the body's resistance to invading microorganisms. Some practitioners claim that a special diet can cure serious illnesses, including cancer. Others claim that by evaluating a patient's metabolism they can diagnose cancer before symptoms appear, locate tumors, and assess a tumor's size and growth rate. There is no scientific evidence to support these claims.

What does it involve?

Metabolic therapy varies a great deal depending on the practitioner, but all are based on special diets that usually emphasize fruits, vegetables, vitamins, and mineral supplements. Other components may include coffee enemas, enzyme supplements, visualization, and stress-reduction exercises. At least one metabolic therapy system also includes the drug laetrile (see Colon Therapy, Enzyme Therapy, Imagery, and Laetrile).

Among the better known types of metabolic therapy are Gerson therapy, Kelley's treatment, and the Gonzalez treatment. Gerson therapy involves a strict dietary program, coffee enemas, and various mineral or chemical supplements. Additional alternative therapies may also be involved (see Gerson therapy).

Kelley's treatment includes dietary supplements (eg, enzymes and large doses of vitamins, minerals, and amino acids), detoxification (eg, fasting, exercising, and using laxatives or coffee enemas), a restricted diet, chiropractic adjustments, and prayer. Practitioners classify people into different metabolic types, which form the basis for specific dietary and supplement recommendations.

The Gonzalez treatment is similar to Kelley's treatment, except that it adds the consumption of organ concentrates such as thymus and liver (taken from beef or lamb) and digestive enzyme supplements to the plan. It also does not use neurological stimulation or prayers. However, the focus remains on detoxifying the body and bringing it into balance.

Another form of metabolic therapy is Issels' whole body therapy, which focuses on strengthening the body's natural defenses. Patients are asked to remove teeth that contain mercury dental fillings, follow a strict diet, and eliminate the use of tobacco, coffee, tea, and other substances that are considered harmful (see Biological Dentistry). Some patients are encouraged to undergo psychotherapy to relieve stress and deal with anger and emotional distress (see Psychotherapy).

What is the history behind it?

Metabolic therapy techniques first appeared during the 20th century. Gerson therapy was introduced by Max Gerson, MD, a German-born physician who immigrated to the United States in 1936. The Kelley treatment was developed in the 1960s by William Donald Kelley, an orthodontist from Washington State. In 1970, Dr. Kelley was convicted of practicing medicine without a license, and in 1976 a court suspended his dental license for five years.

In the 1970s and 1980s Harold Manner, PhD, a biology professor, was also a major proponent of metabolic therapy. He claimed to have cured cancer in mice with injections of laetrile, enzymes, and vitamin A. Dimethyl sulfoxide, which is an unproven alternative method, was often given along with his metabolic cancer therapy (see DMSO). He moved to Tijuana, Mexico in the early 1980s to treat patients in a clinic that is still open despite his death in 1988.

Nicholas Gonzalez, MD, became interested in metabolic therapy when asked to review Dr. Kelley's work when he was a medical student in 1981. He came to adopt Kelley's plan and added raw beef organs and digestive enzyme supplements to the diet. In 1994, US Government officials investigated Dr. Gonzalez and concluded that he had treated patients incompetently, failed to interpret signs of disease progression, and kept inadequate records. He was placed on probation for three years. In a 1997 lawsuit, a patient suffered spinal damage and went blind while under Dr. Gonzalez' care. She brought a lawsuit and was awarded more than $2.5 million dollars in damages.

What is the evidence?

There is general agreement that there are differences in the metabolism of cells in people with cancer compared to people without cancer. However, there is no evidence published in peer-reviewed medical journals that supports the claims made for metabolic therapy or any of its components. The treatment has not been shown to have any positive effects for patients with serious illnesses. Some aspects of metabolic therapy may, in fact, be harmful.

One uncontrolled study was recently reported by Dr. Gonzalez. It was reported that large doses of pancreatic enzymes increased survival times among patients with inoperable pancreatic cancer. This was a small pilot study conducted on 10 patients. A randomized clinical trial sponsored by the National Cancer Institute is reported to be underway to evaluate the use of pancreatic enzymes with nutritional support for treating pancreatic cancer.

Are there any possible problems or complications?

Some aspects of metabolic therapy are considered dangerous. There are reports of complications related to liver cell injections and diets that contained too little salt. Several deaths have been directly linked to injecting live cells from animals (cell therapy). Also, a number of deaths have been linked to coffee enemas. The drug laetrile may cause nausea, vomiting, headache, dizziness, and even cyanide poisoning, which can be fatal. Care should be taken to make sure that any diet containing raw meat or raw meat juice is free from bacterial contamination. Women who are pregnant or breast-feeding should not use this method. Relying on this type of treatment alone, and avoiding conventional medical care, may have serious health consequences.

References

American Cancer Society. Unproven methods of cancer management. The metabolic therapy of Harold W. Manner, Ph.D. *CA Cancer J Clin* 1986;36:185-189.

Barrett S, Herbert V. Questionable cancer therapies. Quackwatch Web site. Available at: http://www.quackwatch.com. Accessed May 8, 2000.

Gonzalez NJ, Isaacs LL. Evaluation of pancreatic proteolytic enzyme treatment of adenocarcinoma of the pancreas, with nutrition and detoxification support. *Nutr Cancer.* 1999;33:117-124.

Green S. Nicolas Gonzalez treatment for cancer: gland extracts, coffee enemas, vitamin megadoses, and diets. Quackwatch Web site. Available at: http://www.quackwatch.com. Accessed May 8, 2000.

Murphy GP, Morris LB, Lange D, eds. *Informed Decisions: The Complete Book of Cancer Diagnosis, Treatment, and Recovery.* New York, NY: Viking; 1997.

University of Texas Center for Alternative Medicine Research in Cancer. Therapies not reviewed. University of Texas-Houston Health Science Center Web site. Available at: http://www.sph.uth.tmc.edu/utcam/summary/greentea.htm. Accessed May 8, 2000.

US Congress, Office of Technology Assessment. *Unconventional Cancer Treatments.* Washington, DC: US Government Printing Office; 1990. Publication OTA-H-405.

Modified Citrus Pectin

Other common name(s)	Scientific/medical name(s)
Citrus Pectin, Pecta-Sol®, MCP	None

DESCRIPTION

Modified citrus pectin (MCP) is a form of pectin that has been altered so that it can be more easily absorbed by the digestive tract. Pectin is a carbohydrate found in most plants, and is particularly plentiful in fruits such as apples, grapefruits, and plums.

OVERVIEW

Animal studies have found that MCP inhibits the spread of prostate cancer and melanoma to other organs, however, there have been no clinical studies done to determine whether MCP has the same effect in humans.

How is it promoted for use?

Proponents claim that MCP slows or stops the growth of metastatic prostate cancer (prostate cancer that has spread) and melanoma, a dangerous form of skin cancer. Some also claim that a compound found in MCP strengthens the cancer cell-killing ability of T-cells (cells that also protect against viruses).

What does it involve?

Modified citrus pectin is available in capsules or a powder. The dose suggested by manufacturers for the powder is 5 g mixed with water or juice taken 3 times/day with meals. For capsules, the suggested dose is 800 mg for 3 times/day with meals.

What is the history behind it?

Pectin is commonly used as a gelling agent for canning foods. It is also used widely in the production of food and cosmetics and as an ingredient in some antidiarrhea medicines. During the last decade, the modified form of pectin has been investigated for anticancer properties.

What is the evidence?

One animal study found that MCP inhibits the

spread of prostate cancer in rats. The rats with prostate cancer received MCP orally and were found to have a much lower risk of the tumor spreading to the lungs.

A second study examined the effects of MCP on lung metastases from melanoma cells. Researchers injected mice with melanoma cells that were given MCP and found that they developed significantly fewer metastatic lung tumors than mice who didn't receive the drug. When lung tumors did develop in MCP-treated mice, they tended to be smaller than those which formed in untreated animals.

The results from these two studies appear to show that MCP makes it difficult for cancer cells that break off from the main tumor to join together and form colonies in other organs. However, the study results also showed that MCP had no effect on the main tumor and that it may only be useful for preventing or slowing the growth of metastatic tumors that are in the very early stages of development. Animal and laboratory studies may show a certain substance holds promise as a beneficial treatment, but further studies are necessary to determine if the results apply to humans.

Are there any possible problems or complications?

Modified citrus pectin is generally considered safe by the FDA. Side effects rarely occur. However, people who are allergic or sensitive to MCP may experience stomach discomfort after taking it.

References
Pienta KJ, Naik H, Akhtar A, et al. Inhibition of spontaneous metastasis in a rat prostate cancer model by oral administration of modified citrus pectin. *J Natl Cancer Inst.* 1995;87:348-353.

Platt D, Raz A. Modulation of the lung colonization of b16-f1 melanoma cells by citrus pectin. *J Natl Cancer Inst.* 1992;84:438-442.

University of Texas Center for Alternative Medicine Research in Cancer. Modified citrus pectin. University of Texas-Houston Health Science Center Web site. Available at: http://www.sph.uth.tmc.edu/utcam/therapies/citrus.htm. Accessed May 10, 2000.

Noni Plant

Other common name(s)	Scientific/medical name(s)
Noni Fruit, Noni Juice, Indian Mulberry, Morinda, Hog Apple, Meng Koedoe, Mora De La India, Ruibarbo Caribe, Wild Pine	*Morinda citrifolia*

DESCRIPTION

The noni or morinda plant is an evergreen tree that grows 10 to 20 feet tall in open coastal regions, and in forests with altitudes up to 1,300 feet. It is commonly found in Tahiti and other Pacific Islands, as well as in parts of Asia and Australia. The juice and whole fruit are used in herbal remedies.

OVERVIEW

There is no scientific evidence that noni juice is effective in preventing or treating cancer or any other disease. Although animal and laboratory studies have shown some positive effects, there have been no studies done in humans. Research is underway to study various compounds found in the noni plant to determine if they produce useful effects on body tissues.

How is it promoted for use?

Proponents claim that the noni fruit and its juice can be used to treat cancer, diabetes, heart disease, cholesterol, high blood pressure, HIV, rheumatism, psoriasis, allergies, infection, and inflammation. Some proponents believe that the fruit can relieve a wide range of conditions, including sinus infections, menstrual cramps, arthritis, ulcers, sprains, injuries, depression, senility, poor digestion, atherosclerosis, addiction, colds, flu, and headaches. It is further claimed that the juice can heal scratches on the cornea of the eye. There is no scientific evidence to support these claims.

In India, proponents use noni as a remedy for asthma and dysentery. Some noni juice distributors also promote it as a general tonic, stress reliever, facial and body cleanser, and a dietary and nutritional aid.

What does it involve?

Parts of the noni plant are used as a juice, a tonic, a poultice, and in tea. Tea made from leaves of the plant is used as a remedy for tuberculosis, arthritis, rheumatism, and anti-aging. The leaves and bark are sometimes made into a liquid tonic for urinary complaints and muscle or joint pain. The juice, which has an unpleasant taste and odor, is used on the scalp as a treatment for head lice. The unripe noni fruit is mashed together with salt and applied on cuts and broken bones. Ripe fruit is used as a poultice for facial blemishes or as a remedy for skin sores, boils, or infections.

Noni products are sold in various forms including juice, extract, powder, capsules (nutritional supplements and diet aids), facial cleansers, bath gels, and soaps.

What is the history behind it?

The noni fruit has been popular among Polynesians for centuries. They originally introduced the noni plant to Hawaii, where it can be found growing near lava flows. During World War II, soldiers stationed in the South Pacific ate the fruit for added sustenance. Over the past few years, juice from the noni plant has become available in health food stores in the United States.

In 1998, the company that manufactures noni juice and other noni products for distribution was charged by the Attorneys General of Arizona, California, New Jersey, and Texas with making unfounded claims. The company claimed that the juice could treat, cure, or prevent many diseases including cancer, HIV, diabetes, rheumatism, blood pressure, cholesterol, psoriasis, allergies, heart rhythm abnormality, chronic inflammation, and joint pain. They were ordered to discontinue advertising these health claims until they received approval from the FDA and could provide scientific evidence of their claims. In the same year, juice marketed under the name of "Noni" was banned in Finland until brochures advertising the juice could be revised to eliminate claims for preventing, treating, or curing illness.

What is the evidence?

A researcher in Hawaii claims to have identified the main active ingredients in noni fruit called xeronine and proxeronine. Only a small amount of xeronine is found in the fruit. Researchers do not know whether xeronine has any direct effects on cells or their function.

Several animal and laboratory experiments have been done on different compounds taken from the noni plant. A group of Hawaiian researchers caused tumors to grow in experimental mice and then investigated the results of treatment using specially prepared injections of noni juice. Mice who received the treatment survived 123% longer than the untreated mice.

Another team of investigators reported that damnacanthal, a compound removed from the root of the noni plant, may inhibit a chemical process which turns normal cells into cancer cells. They stated that damnacanthal caused cells to return to their normal shape and structure. Other scientists studying lyophilised aqueous extract from the roots of the plant found that the substance appeared to prevent pain and induce sleep in mice.

Animal and laboratory studies may show a certain substance holds promise as a beneficial treatment, but further studies are necessary to determine if the results apply to humans. More research is needed before it can be determined what role, if any, noni plant compounds may play in the treatment of cancer or any other health condition. A balanced diet that includes five or more servings a day of fruits and vegetables along with foods from a variety of other plant sources such as breads, cereals, grain products, rice, pasta, and beans is more effective than consuming one particular food or juice in large amounts.

Are there any possible problems or complications?

The safety and long-term effects of noni juice and other noni products are not known. However, relying on this type of treatment alone, and avoiding conventional medical care, may have serious health consequences.

References

Attorneys General put curb claims for "Tahitian Noni." Quackwatch Web site. Available at: http://www.quackwatch.com. Accessed October 21, 1999.

Hiramatsu T, Imoto M, Koyano T, Umezawa K. Induction of normal phenotypes in ras-transformed cells by damnacanthal from Morinda citrifolia. *Cancer Lett.* 1993;73:161-166.

Hirazumi A, Furusawa E. An immunomodulatory polysaccharide-rich substance from the fruit juice of Morinda citrifolia (noni) with antitumor activity. *Phytother Res.* 1999;13:380-387.

Hirazumi A, Furusawa E, Chou SC, Hokama Y. Anticancer activity of Morinda citrifolia (noni) on intraperitoneally implanted Lewis lung carcinoma in syngeneic mice. *Proc West Pharmacol Soc.* 1994;37:145-146.

Younos C, Rolland A, Fleurentin J, Lanhers MC, Misslin R, Mortier F. Analgesic and behavioral effects of Morinda citrifolia. *Planta Med.* 1990;56:430-434.

Omega-3 Fatty Acids

Other common name(s)	Scientific/medical name(s)
None	Alpha-linolenic acid, eicosapentaenoic acid, docosahexaenoic acid

DESCRIPTION

Omega-3 fatty acids are important nutrients that are involved in many human biological processes. The body cannot make these chemicals and must obtain them from dietary sources or from supplements. Three fatty acids compose the Omega-3 family: alpha-linolenic acid, eicosapentaenoic acid, and docosahexaenoic acid.

OVERVIEW

Studies in animals have found that fish fats rich in omega-3 fatty acids suppress cancer formation. However, there is no direct evidence that they have similar protective effects in humans. Omega-3 fatty acids may increase cholesterol and reduce blood clotting.

How is it promoted for use?

Some clinicians believe that omega-3 fatty acids protect against the spread of solid-tumor cancers that are related to hormone production, particularly breast cancer, and that they inhibit the growth of colon, pancreatic, and prostate cancers. Omega-3s may reduce cachexia, the physical wasting and malnourishment that can occur during later stages of some cancers.

Some people assert that omega-3 fatty acids protect against cardiovascular disease and heart attacks, arthritis, and kidney failure. Low levels of omega-3s are also linked to depression, according to some practitioners.

What does it involve?

Diet is the best source of omega-3 fatty acids. Oils from some cold-water fish, such as sardines, salmon, herring, mackerel, halibut, stripped bass, tuna, shark and cod, have high concentrations of omega-3s. Oil from flaxseed contains more alpha-linolenic acid (one of the three omega-3 fatty acids) than any other known plant source (see Flaxseed Oil). Other plant sources of omega-3 fatty acids include great northern beans, kidney beans, navy beans, and soybeans.

Omega-3 supplements, such as salmon oil, are available at pharmacies and natural food stores. Some nutritionists recommend eating a diet rich in fish containing omega-3 fatty acids, eating 1-2 teaspoons of flaxseed or flaxseed oil daily, or taking daily supplements containing 1-2 g of omega-3s. Omega-3 fatty acids are very unstable and spoil easily, so food manufacturers often remove them from foods to increase shelf life.

What is the history behind it?

A German scientist, Johanna Budwig, PhD, discovered essential fatty acids in the 1950s and developed a diet that she said would fight cancer. Dr. Budwig claimed that many of her patients experienced tumor reduction within 3 months, and some experienced even more dramatic results. Dr. Budwig has reportedly used omega-3 fatty acids in combination with other nutrients to treat thousands of people with cancer and other diseases.

What is the evidence?

Although some research supports the anticancer claims made for omega-3 fatty acids, far more investigation is needed before researchers reach any conclusions. The relationship between omega-

3 fatty acids, cancer, and other diseases is not known. Eating a balanced diet that includes five or more servings a day of fruits and vegetables along with foods from a variety of other plant sources such as breads, cereals, grain products, rice, pasta, and beans is more effective than consuming one particular type of food in large amounts.

The evidence from the few clinical studies published in peer-reviewed medical journals is mixed. A limited study conducted at Harvard Medical Center suggested that one of the omega-3 fatty acids limited the recurrence of colon cancer. A preliminary study of omega-3s published in the *Journal of the National Cancer Institute* said that even though there appears to be a biological reason for omega-3s to fight cancer, clinical findings didn't prove that fish oil containing omega-3 fatty acids prevented cancer or its recurrence. A clinical study published recently in the journal *Cancer* concluded that omega-3 fatty acids seemed to prolong the survival of people with cancer who were also severely malnourished.

In societies that consume a lot of fish, researchers have noticed links between high intake of omega-3s and lower rates of breast cancer. For example, a study of people who live on the typical Mediterranean diet, which tends to contain high amounts of omega-3 fatty acids, concluded that the food they eat may offer some protection against heart disease and cancer. But the evidence is not conclusive and the subject needs further study. One researcher found evidence that major depression and cardiovascular disease were associated with low levels of omega-3 fatty acids which implied that omega-3s may possess the ability to maintain steady heart rates, therefore reducing the risk of sudden cardiac death.

Research is also focusing on the role of omega-3 fatty acids in relation to omega-6 fatty acids. Omega-6 is another essential fatty acid, and it can be found in many vegetable oils (corn, safflower, and sunflower), cereals, snack foods, and baked goods. Some researchers believe one of the reasons why Americans suffer high rates of cardiovascular disease and certain cancers, may be due to an imbalance in the ratio of omega-3 to omega-6 fatty acids. Ideally, the ratio of omega-3 to omega-6 fatty acids in the human body is 1-to-1.

However, because the typical American diet is low in omega-3s and high in omega-6s, many people have 10 to 20 times more omega-6 fatty acids than omega-3 fatty acids in their systems. Studies show that women with breast cancer have 2 to 5 times more omega-6 fatty acids than omega-3 fatty acids in their systems.

Laboratory experiments suggest that omega-3 fatty acids may delay or reduce tumor development in animals. Other laboratory evidence shows that the balance between omega-3 and omega-6 fatty acid levels plays a role in the formation of breast cancer. One laboratory experiment, however, showed that both omega-3 and omega-6 fatty acids may promote the spread of colon cancer. Animal and laboratory studies may show that a substance has certain effects, but further studies are necessary to determine if the results apply to humans.

Are there any possible problems or complications?

Not enough is known about omega-3 fatty acids to determine if they are safe in large quantities or in the presence of other drugs. Omega-3s may increase total blood cholesterol and inhibit blood clotting. People who take anticoagulant drugs or aspirin should not consume additional amounts of omega-3 due to the risk of excessive bleeding.

The source of omega-3 fatty acids may be a health concern. Because of pollution, many fish caught in the wild contain toxins absorbed from pollution. Experts recommend varying the type of fish eaten to reduce the chances of ingesting poisonous substances. Swordfish and shark, for instance, both of which are high in omega-3 fatty acids, may also contain high levels of mercury. Farm-raised fish tend to carry fewer toxins than fish in the wild.

Supplements may cause fishy breath odor, belching, or abdominal bloating. They may also increase a tendency toward anemia in menstruating women. Women who are pregnant or breast-feeding should consult their physician before adding extra omega-3 to their diets.

References

Bagga D, Capone S, Wang HJ, et al. Dietary modulation of omega-3/omega-6 polyunsaturated fatty acid ratios in patients with breast cancer. *J Natl Cancer Inst.* 1997;89:1123-31.

de Lorgeril M, Salen P, Martin JL, Monjaud I, Boucher P, Mamelle N. Mediterranean dietary pattern in a randomized trial: Prolonged survival and possible reduced cancer rate. *Arch Intern Med.* 1998;158:1181-1187.

Godley PA, Campbell MK, Gallagher P, Martinson FE, Mohler JL, Sandler RS. Biomarkers of essential fatty acid consumption and risk of prostatic carcinoma. *Cancer Epidemiol Biomarkers Prev.* 1996;5:889-895.

Gogos CA, Ginopoulos P, Salsa B, Apostolidou E, Zoumbos NC, Kalfarentzos F. Dietary omega-3 polyunsaturated fatty acids plus vitamin E restore immunodeficiency and prolong survival for severely ill patients with generalized malignancy. *Cancer.* 1998;82:395-402.

Huang YC, Jessup JM, Forse RA, et al. n-3 fatty acids decrease colonic epithelial cell proliferation in high-risk bowel mucosa. *Lipids.* 1996; 31:S313-5317.

Selected Vegetable Soup

Other common name(s)	Scientific/medical name(s)
SV, Sun Soup	None

DESCRIPTION / OVERVIEW

Selected vegetable soup (SV), is promoted as a treatment for cancer. It is a freeze-dried brown powder that contains a specific selection of vegetables and herbs, including soybean, mushroom (shiitake), red date, scallion, garlic, lentil bean, leek, mung bean, hawthorn fruit, onion, American ginseng, angelica root, licorice, dandelion root, senegal root, ginger, olive, sesame seed, and parsley (see Garlic, Ginger, Ginseng, Licorice, Shiitake Mushroom, and Soybean). One study has been published, and was conducted by the developer of the soup, Alexander Sun, PhD. This recent randomized clinical trial found daily consumption of SV, along with conventional cancer treatment, to be nontoxic and associated with improvement in weight maintenance and survival of patients with advanced non-small cell lung cancer. The study involved a very small sample size (eg, 12 patients). More research is needed to determine the effectiveness of SV.

Shiitake Mushroom

Other common name(s)	Scientific/medical name(s)
Japanese Mushroom	*Lentinus edodes*

DESCRIPTION

A shiitake mushroom is an edible fungus native to Asia and grown in forests. Shiitake mushrooms are the second most commonly cultivated edible mushrooms in the world. Extracts from the mushroom, and sometimes the whole mushroom itself, are used in herbal remedies.

OVERVIEW

Animal studies have found antitumor, cholesterol-lowering, and virus-inhibiting effects of the active compounds in shiitake mushrooms. However, clinical studies are needed to determine if these effects can be beneficial for people with cancer and other diseases.

How is it promoted for use?

Shiitake mushrooms are promoted to fight the development and progression of cancer and AIDS by boosting the body's immune system. These mushrooms are also said to help prevent heart disease by lowering cholesterol levels in the blood and treating infections by producing interferon (a group of natural proteins that inhibits viruses from multiplying). Promoters claim that eating the whole mushroom (cap and stem), may have therapeutic value, but they do not say how much must be eaten to have an effect. They say the content and activity of the compounds depend on how the mushroom is prepared and consumed. Research shows, however, that eating a balanced diet that includes five or more servings a day of fruits and vegetables along with foods from a variety of other plant sources such as breads, cereals, grain products, rice, pasta, and beans is more effective than consuming one particular food in large amounts.

A compound contained in shiitake mushrooms, lentinan, is believed to stop or slow tumor growth. Another component, activated hexose-containing compound, is also said to reduce tumor activity and lessen the side effects of cancer treatment. The mushrooms also contain the compound eritadenine, which is thought to lower cholesterol by blocking the way cholesterol is absorbed into the bloodstream. These claims are currently under investigation.

What does it involve?

The natural mushroom is widely available in grocery stores, while extracts of the mushroom are sold in capsule form in health food stores and on the Internet.

The extracts of the active compounds in shiitake mushrooms are usually used for medicinal purposes, rather than the natural mushroom itself. For example, some Japanese researchers give lentinan along with chemotherapy to treat patients with lung, nose, throat, and stomach cancers. Extracts of the active compounds, such as lentinan and eritadenine, are mainly sold in Japan. Activated hexose-containing compound is sold in the United States, Europe, and Japan as a nutritional supplement.

What is the history behind it?

The use of shiitake mushrooms as medicine dates at least to 100 AD in China (see Chinese Herbal Medicine). The mushrooms have been widely consumed as a food for thousands of years in the East and more recently in the West.

Today, shiitake mushrooms are a major source of protein in Japan and are very popular in the United States as well. Research into the anti-cancer properties of shiitake mushrooms has been going on since at least the 1960s.

What is the evidence?

Animal studies have found some positive results regarding the antitumor, cholesterol-lowering, and virus-inhibiting effects of the active compounds in shiitake mushrooms. At least one randomized clinical trial of lentinan has shown it to be effective against advanced and recurrent stomach and colorectal cancer. Research has been done on the specific compounds that have been cultivated in laboratories. It is not known whether these results apply to the mushrooms bought in supermarkets.

More human trials are necessary to confirm the health claims made for shiitake mushrooms, and to understand which compounds have antitumor effects for which type of cancers and at what dosages. Researchers at the University of California at Davis are studying one of the compounds extracted from the mushroom (hexose-containing compound) to see if it can reduce tumor activity in men with prostate cancer. Animal studies found that the compound may reduce tumor growth and side effects of cancer treatment. Animal studies may show a certain therapy holds promise as a beneficial treatment, but further studies are necessary to determine if the results apply to humans.

Are there any possible problems or complications?

Shiitake mushrooms and their extracts are generally considered safe, but some people have been known to develop allergic reactions affecting the skin, nose, throat, and lungs.

References

Borchers AT, Stern JS, Hackman RM, Keen CL, Gershwin ME. Mushrooms, tumors, and immunity. *Proc Soc Exp Biol Med.* 1999;221:281-293.

Chihara G, Hamuro J, Maeda Y, et al. Antitumor and metastasis-inhibitory activities of lentinan as an immunomodulator: an overview. *Cancer Detect Prev.* 1987;1:423-443.

Chung R. Functional properties of edible mushrooms. *Nutr Rev.* 1996;54:S91-S93.

Ikekawa T, Uehara N, Maeda Y, Nakanishi M, Fukuoka F. Antitumor activity of aqueous extracts of edible mushrooms. *Cancer Res.* 1969;29:734-735.

Matsushita K, Kuramitsu Y, Ohiro Y, et al. Combination therapy of active hexose correlated compound plus UFT significantly reduces the metastasis of rat mammary adenocarcinoma. *Anticancer Drugs.* 1998;9:343-350.

Taguchi T. Clinical efficacy of lentinan on patients with stomach cancer: end-point results of a four-year follow-up survey. *Cancer Detect Prev Suppl.* 1987;1:333-349.

Soybean

Other common name(s)	Scientific/medical name(s)
Soy, Soy Protein, Soy Powder	*Glycine soja*

DESCRIPTION

The soybean plant is an annual plant that is indigenous to east Asia. It has oblong pods that contain 2 to 4 seeds. Soy lecithin is the part that is extracted from the soya bean, soya oil, and soya seed.

OVERVIEW

Isoflavones in soy have been found to have protective effects against breast and prostate cancer in laboratory, animal, population, and case control studies. Randomized clinical trials are needed to understand how these findings apply to cancer prevention in humans. Results of research on the effects of consuming isoflavones on colon cancer risk have been mixed. Human studies on individual soy components are currently underway.

How is it promoted for use?

Soybean products are promoted for their protective properties against breast, prostate, colon, and lung cancer. The effects of soy are considered to be due to the isoflavones that many soy products contain. Isoflavones are sometimes called phytoestrogens or plant estrogens that act like weak forms of estrogens naturally produced in the body. Genistein and daidzein, both soy isoflavones, are thought to be responsible for the protective effects of soy.

As a protein source, soybean products are promoted as a healthier protein alternative to eating meat and as an aid to weight loss. Soy products are also used to lower cholesterol and blood pressure, and relieve symptoms of menopause and osteoporosis. Research suggests that including soy protein in a diet low in saturated fat and cholesterol may help reduce the risk of heart disease. Eating a balanced diet that includes five or more servings a day of fruits and vegetables along with foods from a variety of other plant sources such as breads, cereals, grain products, rice, pasta, and beans is more effective than consuming one particular food in large amounts.

What does it involve?

Soybean can be consumed in many forms with tofu, soy milk, and soy powder being three of the most popular. The amount of isoflavones varies between different types of tofu and soy milk products. Soy is also available in the form of dietary supplements. Soy protein powders and bars are available in nutrition stores and health food markets. The powders can be added to liquids and are also used in cooking.

Soy lecithin, an extract from the seeds of the soya bean has been approved by Commission E (Germany's regulatory agency for herbs) for use in lowering cholesterol.

What is the history behind it?

The soybean has been used as a food source for over 5,000 years. Today, there are over 2,500 varieties of soybeans cultivated throughout the world. It was not until relatively recently that studies began on the potential medicinal properties of the soybean.

Plant estrogens were first identified in the early 1930s, when it was discovered that soybeans, willows, dates, and pomegranates contained compounds similar in structure to estrogens. Scientists began studying the role isoflavones play in reducing the risk of breast cancer in the 1960s. In a 1981 prospective study in Japan, researchers found that daily intake of miso (soybean paste) was associated with significantly reduced death rates from stomach cancer in more than 260,000 men and women. Other studies related to soy also began to be published in the United States at that time. In October 1999, the FDA agreed to allow health claims to be made about the role of soy in reducing heart disease on food products containing soy protein.

What is the evidence?

Researchers believe that the isoflavones in soy (such as genistein and daidzein) possibly play a role in reducing the risk of cancer. A number of laboratory and animal experiments and population studies have found that soy isoflavones have the potential to reduce the risk of developing several types of cancer including breast, prostate, and colon cancer. However, these results have not yet been reflected in human clinical trials, so no definite conclusions can be made.

There is enough evidence, scientists believe, for phytoestrogens to be used in clinical trials as potential chemopreventive agents (to prevent the development of cancer) or as an addition to breast or prostate cancer treatment. Human studies sponsored by the National Cancer Institute (NCI) are currently underway.

Are there any possible problems or complications?

The consumption of soybeans is generally considered safe. Side effects are rare, but may include occasional gastrointestinal problems such as stomach pain, loose stool, and diarrhea.

The isoflavones in soy have weak estrogen-like activity, and it remains uncertain how this affects the growth of estrogen receptor-positive breast cancers. Some researchers suggest they may act as anti-estrogens and reduce cancer growth, while others suggest their estrogenic activity could cause cancers to grow faster. Until this issue is resolved, many oncologists recommend that people who take tamoxifen or people with estrogen-sensitive breast tumors should avoid the addition of large amounts of soy to their diets.

References

Fournier DB, Erdman JW Jr, Gordon GB. Soy, its components, and cancer prevention: a review of the in vitro, animal, and human data. *Cancer Epidemiol Biomarkers Prev.* 1998;7:1055-1065.

Jacobsen BK, Knutsen SF, Fraser GE. Does high soy milk intake reduce prostate cancer incidence? The Adventist Health Study. *Cancer Causes Control.* 1998;9:553-557.

Medical Economics. *PDR for Herbal Medicines.* Montvale, NJ: Medical Economics Company; 1998.

Messina M. Soy, soy phytoestrogens (isoflavones), and breast cancer. *Am J Clin Nutr.* 1999;70:574-575.

Messina M, Bennink M. Soyfoods, isoflavones and risk of colonic cancer: a review of the in vitro and in vivo data. *Baillieres Clin Endocrinol Metab.* 1998;12:707-728.

Moyad MA. Soy, disease prevention, and prostate cancer. *Semin Urol Oncol.* 1999;17:97-102.

Stoll BA. Eating to beat breast cancer: potential role for soy supplements. *Ann Oncol.* 1997;8:223-225.

US Food and Drug Administration. *FDA Talk Paper: FDA approves new health claim for soy protein and coronary heart disease.* Rockville, Md: National Press Office; October 20,1999. Talk Paper T99-48.

Vegetarianism

Other common name(s)	Scientific/medical name(s)
Lactovegetarian, Lacto-Ovo-Vegetarian, Semivegetarian, Vegan	None

DESCRIPTION

Vegetarianism is the practice of eating a diet consisting mainly or entirely of food that comes from plant sources such as fruits and vegetables. Vegetarian diets vary widely. Some include no animal products, while others include dairy products, eggs, and fish.

OVERVIEW

Some studies have linked vegetarian diets to lower risk for heart disease, diabetes, high blood pressure, obesity, and certain types of cancer (ie, colon cancer). However, physicians point out that a totally vegetarian diet may not provide all the necessary nutrients if it is not well planned.

How is it promoted for use?

Many vegetarianism proponents believe a vegetarian diet promotes health because it contains less fat, protein, and cholesterol and more fiber, vitamins, minerals, antioxidants, and phytochemicals (plant chemicals) than a diet containing meat (see Phytochemicals, and Herbs, Vitamins, and Minerals chapter). Some vegetarians believe it is more natural for humans to consume plant-based foods. Still others choose to eliminate or reduce their consumption of animal products because of religious, cultural, moral, or philosophical reasons.

What does it involve?

All vegetarian diets include plant-based foods, but vary according to the kinds of animal products consumed. A vegan does not eat any meat. A lacto-ovo-vegetarian will eat dairy products and eggs, and a lacto-vegetarian will eat dairy products. One small group of vegetarians, fruitarians, eat only raw fruits and fruit vegetables, like tomatoes, because they believe that cooking fruit damages its nutritional properties.

What is the history behind it?

Vegetarianism has long been a part of many cultures. In the United States, the vegetarian movement began in the middle of the 1900s. The American Vegetarian Society was founded in 1850. Today, vegetarianism is very popular in the United States and abroad because it is thought to be a more healthy approach to diet and nutrition.

Currently, the American Cancer Society's (ACS) nutrition guidelines recommend a mostly vegetarian diet including five or more servings a day of fruits and vegetables along with regular consumption of breads, cereals, grain products, rice, pasta, and beans. The ACS recommends limiting intake of high-fat foods, particularly from animal sources. The National Cancer Institute (NCI) also recommends a diet low in fat and high in plant foods such as fruits and vegetables in order to decrease cancer risk.

What is the evidence?

Population studies have linked vegetarian diets with a decreased risk of heart disease, diabetes, high blood pressure, obesity, and colon cancer.

A review of research on the effects of vegetarian diets among Seventh-Day Adventists, whose religious doctrine advises against eating animal flesh, was presented to the National Institutes of Health (NIH). The report stated that Seventh-Day Adventists experienced less heart disease and fewer cases of some cancers than the general population. On average, Seventh-Day Adventist males had lower-than-average serum cholesterol levels and blood pressure and their overall cancer death rate was about half that of the general population. The overall cancer death rate of females was also lower. A couple of studies indicated an increased risk of colon and prostate cancer with increased animal fat intake. An increase in the consumption of beans and lentils appeared to decrease the risk of colon cancer and prostate cancer. The report cautioned that abstinence from tobacco and alcohol may have contributed to some of the health effects associated with vegetarian diets in the Seventh-Day Adventist community.

A population study in Germany found the death rate for colon cancer was lower among moderate and strict vegetarians compared with that of the general population. The authors of the study noted vegetarians tend to be more health conscious than average. In Great Britain, a 17-year population study that followed 11,000 vegetarians and health-conscious people, concluded that the daily consumption of fresh fruit was associated with a significant reduction in mortality from ischemic heart disease, cerebrovascular disease (stroke), and all causes of death combined. Another population study found a diet rich in grains, cereals, and nuts protected against prostate cancer.

In 1991, two nutritionists studying the benefits and risks of vegetarian diets reported that vegetarians are not necessarily healthier than non-vegetarians and that well-planned omnivorous diets (animal and vegetable products) can provide health benefits as well. They also pointed out that since many vegetarians adopt a healthier lifestyle–more physical exercise and no smoking–this factor may help improve their overall health.

Are there any possible problems or complications?

Strict vegetarians (those who eat no animal products at all) must be careful to consume adequate amounts of protein. Other nutrients which may be missing from a vegetarian diet include vitamin B_{12}, vitamin D, calcium, zinc, and iron (see Calcium, Vitamin B, Vitamin D, and Zinc). Vegan diets must be carefully planned to ensure adequate amounts of required nutrients are consumed. Many health care professionals consider vegan diets risky, especially for infants and toddlers.

Switching to a vegetarian diet may increase the amount of dietary fiber consumed, which could cause intestinal problems. Dietitians suggest a gradual rather than quick change in diet.

References

Alternative Medicine: Expanding Medical Horizons. *A Report to the National Institutes of Health on Alternative Medical Systems and Practices in the United States.* Washington, DC: US Government Printing Office; 1994. NIH publication 94-066.

Dingott S, Dwyer J. Vegetarianism: healthful but unnecessary. Quackwatch Web site. Available at: http://www.quackwatch.com. Accessed May 10, 2000.

Frentzl-Beyme R, Chang-Claude J. Vegetarian diets and colon cancer: The German experience. *Am J Clin Nutr.* 1994;59:1143S-1152S.

Healthscout Library. Vegetarianism. Healthscout Web site. Available at: http://www.healthscout.com. Accessed May 10, 2000.

Hebert JR, Hurley TG, Olendzki BC, Teas J, Ma Y, Hampl JS. Nutritional and socioeconomic factors in relation to prostate cancer mortality: a cross-national study. *J Natl Cancer Inst.* 1998;90:1637-1647.

Key TJ, Thorogood M, Appleby PN, Burr ML. Dietary habits and mortality in 11,000 vegetarians and health conscious people: results of a 17 year follow up. *BMJ.* 1996;313:775-779.

Singh PN, Fraser GE. Dietary risk factor for colon cancer in a low-risk population. *Am J Epidemiol.* 1998;148:761-764.

Wheatgrass

Other common name(s)	Scientific/medical name(s)
Wheatgrass Diet	*Agropyron*

DESCRIPTION

Wheatgrass is a member of the genus Agropyron, which includes a wide variety of wheat-like grasses. Wheatgrass is tall grass (12-40 inches) commonly found in temperate regions of Europe and the United States. It is a perennial, which can be grown outdoors or indoors. The roots and rhizomes (underground stems) are used in herbal remedies.

OVERVIEW

There have been no scientific studies in humans to support any of the claims made for wheatgrass or wheatgrass diet programs.

How is it promoted for use?

Wheatgrass is promoted for oral use to treat a number of conditions, including the common cold, coughs, bronchitis, fevers, infections, and inflammation of the mouth and pharynx. Proponents also use wheatgrass liquid preparations to irrigate inflammatory disease of the urinary tract and to prevent kidney stones. In folk medicine, practitioners used wheatgrass to treat cystitis, gout, rheumatic pain, chronic skin disorders, and constipation.

Proponents further claim that a dietary program based on wheatgrass commonly called "the wheatgrass diet" can cause cancer to go into regression and extend the life of people with cancer. They believe that the wheatgrass diet strengthens the immune system, kills harmful bacteria in the digestive system, and rids the body of toxins and waste matter. There is no scientific evidence to support these claims.

What does it involve?

Wheatgrass is available in its natural state and in tablets, capsules, liquid extracts, tinctures and juices. It can also be used to make tea. The wheatgrass diet excludes all meat, dairy products, and cooked foods, and emphasizes "live foods," such as uncooked sprouts, raw vegetables and fruits, nuts, and seeds.

What is the history behind it?

The wheatgrass diet was developed by Boston resident Ann Wigmore, who emigrated to the United States from Lithuania. Wigmore believed strongly in the healing power of nature. Wigmore's notion that wheatgrass had therapeutic value came from her interpretation of the bible and observations that dogs and cats eat grass when they feel ill. Wigmore claimed that the wheatgrass diet could cure disease.

In 1982, the Massachusetts Attorney General sued Wigmore for claiming that her program could reduce or eliminate the need for insulin in diabetics. Afterward, she retracted her claims. In 1988, the Massachusetts Attorney General sued Wigmore again, this time for claiming that an "energy enzyme soup" she invented could cure AIDS. Wigmore was ordered to stop representing herself as a physician or person licensed to treat disease.

What is the evidence?

There is no scientific evidence to suggest that wheatgrass or the wheatgrass diet can cure or prevent disease. There are only anecdotal reports that describe tumor regression and extended survival among people with cancer who followed the wheatgrass diet. However, eating a balanced diet that includes five or more servings a day of fruits and vegetables along with foods from a variety of other plant sources such as breads, cereals, grain products, rice, pasta, and beans is more effective than consuming one particular food in large amounts.

Are there any possible problems or complications?

Wheatgrass is generally considered safe. Wheatgrass should not be used to flush out the urinary tract if the patient has swelling caused by heart or kidney insufficiency. Women who are pregnant or breast-feeding should not use wheatgrass.

References

Blumenthal M, ed. *The Complete German Commission E Monographs: Therapeutic Guide to Herbal Medicines.* Austin, Tx: American Botanical Council; 1998.

Fetrow CW, Avila JR. *Professional's Handbook of Complementary and Alternative Medicines.* Springhouse, Pa: Springhouse Corp; 1999.

Medical Economics. *PDR for Herbal Medicines.* Montvale, NJ: Medical Economics Company; 1998.

NCAHF Newsletter. Volume 17, Number 5, September-October 1994. National Council Against Health Fraud Web site. Available at: http://www.ncahf.org/newslett/n117-5.html. Accessed May 10, 2000.

US Congress, Office of Technology Assessment. *Unconventional Cancer Treatments.* Washington, DC: US Government Printing Office; 1990. Publication OTA-H-405.

Willard Water

Other common name(s)	Scientific/medical name(s)
None	None

DESCRIPTION / OVERVIEW

Manufacturers describe Willard Water as "catalyst altered water," meaning that it is a diluted water solution. Proponents claim that Willard Water eases the burning caused by radiation therapy, relieves sores in the mouth and on the lips, eliminates bad breath, removes plaque from teeth, heals minor skin irritations (eg, scrapes, bruises, cuts, insect bites, burns), prevents hangovers, and eases pain from arthritis and muscle sprains. They also claim it flushes toxins from the body and eliminates harmful free radical molecules. Willard Water was reportedly created around 1970 by Dr. John Willard, a professor at the South Dakota School of Mining and Technology. The liquid can be swallowed, sprayed directly on the skin or in the mouth, added to herbal remedies or bath water, or used as an ointment. Since no scientific studies have been conducted on Willard Water, there is no evidence to support these claims. It has not been proven useful for any medical condition and the exact contents are not known. Not enough is known about Willard Water to know whether it is safe.

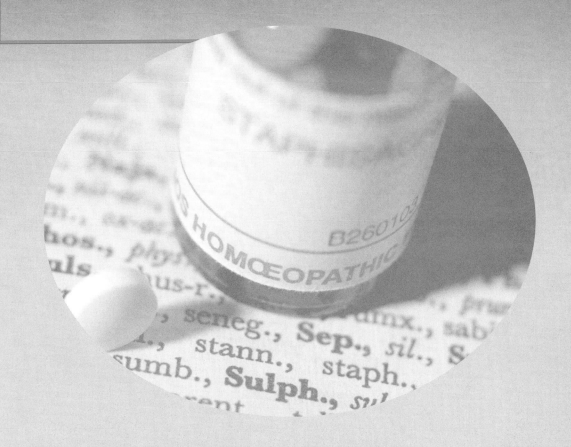

Chapter 9

Pharmacological and Biological Treatment Methods

This category provides information about substances

that are synthesized and produced from chemicals or

concentrated from plants and other living things.

Extracted chemicals are not the same as the

raw plant or a plant in its natural state.

Antineoplaston Therapy

Other common name(s)	Scientific/medical name(s)
Antineoplastons	None

DESCRIPTION

Antineoplaston therapy is an alternative form of cancer treatment that involves using a group of synthetic chemicals called antineoplastons to protect the body from disease. Antineoplastons are made up mostly of peptides and amino acids originally taken from human blood and urine.

OVERVIEW

There is no scientific evidence that antineoplaston therapy is effective in treating cancer or any other disease.

How is it promoted for use?

Supporters claim antineoplastons are a part of something called the body's natural biochemical defense system. This system is said to operate independently from the body's immune system and protect against diseases like cancer, which involve a breakdown in the chemistry of the body's cells.

Proponents claim antineoplaston therapy has been successful in treating many forms of cancer. They claim people with cancer have a deficiency of naturally occurring antineoplastons, and that this therapy replenishes the body's supply allowing the biochemical defense system of the body to convert cancer cells into normal cells. There is no scientific evidence to support these claims.

What does it involve?

Antineoplastons are given orally or by injection into a vein. The duration of treatment ranges from 4 to 12 months. A year of treatment can cost from $36,000 to $60,000, depending on the type of treatment, number of consultations, and the need for surgery to implant a catheter for drug delivery.

What is the history behind it?

Antineoplaston therapy was developed in 1967 by Stanislaw Burzynski, MD, PhD, a Polish physician and researcher. In 1970, while working at Baylor College of Medicine, Burzynski isolated chemicals in the blood and urine of healthy people, which he believed were a natural form of anticancer protection he called antineoplastons. He later manufactured these naturally occurring substances in his laboratory. Shortly afterwards, Dr. Burzynski opened his own clinic and has used antineoplaston therapy to treat patients for a variety of cancers. He claims that the therapy has cured many patients of their illnesses.

In 1995, Burzynski was indicted by a federal grand jury for mail fraud, marketing his unapproved drug, and with the false billing of insurance companies for his treatment. His clinical trials have been criticized for not following approved scientific standards.

In the United States today, antineoplaston therapy can only be given to patients who go to Dr. Burzynski's clinic and enroll in his clinical trials approved by the FDA

What is the evidence?

There is no scientific evidence showing that antineoplaston therapy cures cancer. A recent review of 17 small clinical series (less than 25 patients in some cases) found some promising results for the use of antineoplaston therapy. However, most of the studies were directed by Dr. Burzynski himself.

During the 1980s, the NCI reviewed cases of cancer patients that Dr. Burzynski had treated with antineoplaston therapy. The NCI found no evidence that these patients benefited in any way from the therapy. Burzynski's research process was criticized and it was reported that his definitions of complete and partial remission were not used in accordance with generally accepted definitions.

In 1985, the Canadian Bureau of Prescription Drugs examined the records of Canadian doctors who had treated patients at Dr. Burzynski's clinic in Houston. Out of 36 patients, 32 had died without showing signs of improvement. Of the remaining four, one patient died after slight improvement while one patient died after stabilizing for a year. The two remaining patients had widespread cancer.

In 1991, the NCI again reviewed several of Burzynski's cases and concluded that the results warranted further investigation through clinical trials. Because of the inability to gather enough patients, and lack of agreement on proposed changes to increase patient participation, the clinical trials were canceled in 1995. Due to the lack of scientific evidence and the popularity of this therapy among some people with cancer, the FDA has recently granted Burzynski permission to conduct clinical trials of antineoplaston therapy at his clinic. The NCI is also conducting laboratory experiments on the peptides involved in antineoplaston therapy.

Are there any possible problems or complications?

Proponents claim that antineoplaston therapy is non-toxic. Side effects may include stomach gas, slight rashes, chills, fever, change in blood pressure, and unpleasant body odor during treatment. High levels of blood sodium can also be a significant problem with this therapy. Relying on this type of treatment alone, and avoiding conventional medical care, may have serious health consequences.

References

Alternative Medicine: Expanding Medical Horizons. *A Report to the National Institutes of Health on Alternative Medical Systems and Practices in the United States.* Washington, DC: US Government Printing Office; 1994. NIH publication 94-066.

Barrett S, Herbert V. Questionable cancer therapies. Quackwatch Web site. Available at http://www.quackwatch.com. Accessed October 19, 1999.

Cassileth B. *The Alternative Medicine Handbook.* New York, NY: W. W. Norton & Co; 1998.

Green S. 'Antineoplastons'. An unproved cancer therapy. *JAMA.* 1992;267:2924-2928.

University of Texas Center for Alternative Medicine Research in Cancer. Antineoplastons summary. University of Texas-Houston Health Science Center Web site. Available at: http://www.sph.uth.tmc.edu/utcam/summary/anti.htm. Accessed October 19, 1999.

US Congress, Office of Technology Assessment. *Unconventional Cancer Treatments.* Washington, DC: US Government Printing Office; 1990. Publication OTA-H-405.

Pharmacological / Biological

Apitherapy

Other common name(s)	Scientifi/medical name(s)
Bee Venom Therapy, Bee Venom, Venom Immunotherapy	None

DESCRIPTION

Apitherapy refers to the use of various products of the common honeybee in alternative remedies. These include venom, propolis (waxy substance produced by honeybees that is used to solidify hives), raw honey, royal jelly, and pollen.

OVERVIEW

While research is being performed on the anti-tumor properties of some of the active ingredients in bee products, there have been no studies in humans showing that bee venom or other honeybee components are effective in preventing or treating cancer.

How is it promoted for use?

Some researchers believe some of the active ingredients in bee products may have possible anticancer effects, however, there is no clinical evidence to support these claims.

Practitioners claim bee venom relieves chronic pain, and can be used to treat various rheumatic diseases, including several types of arthritis, neurological diseases (multiple sclerosis, low back pain, and migraine), and skin conditions (eczema, psoriasis, and herpes).

Other proponents claim raw honey has antifungal, antibacterial, anti-inflammatory, and antitumor properties. They say it is an energy building source, with minerals and seven vitamins from the B complex group, however, this has not been scientifically proven (see Vitamin B Complex).

Pieces of honeycomb containing pollen are said to be successful for treating allergies. Ingesting bee pollen is also claimed to increase endurance, energy, and overall performance. Proponents claim bee pollen contains 22 nutrients required by the human body, and that it has 5 to 7 times more protein than beef. There is no scientific evidence to support these claims.

What does it involve?

The usual application of bee venom involves using a live bee to sting the patient at a specific site, and repeating this procedure over a period of time. Injections can also be used. For example, it is suggested that the venom be injected into arthritic patients at trigger points on a daily course of treatment that lasts 4 to 6 weeks.

The two most popular forms of delivery for other apitherapy applications (ie, honey and pollen) are pills and injections. In China, raw honey is applied directly to burns as an antiseptic and painkiller.

Bee products are widely available in pharmacies, health food stores, and shops that specialize in bee products.

What is the history behind it?

Various forms of apitherapy have been used since ancient times. There is even a reference in the Koran about its medicinal properties. The cultivation of the hive has been written about as early as 800 BC. Charlemagne (742-814 AD) is said to have had himself treated with bee stings. In 1888, Austrian physician Phillip Terc advocated the deliberate use of bee stings as a treatment for rheumatism.

What is the evidence?

Most research in this area has focused on immunotherapy (preventing allergic reactions to bee venom). However, several animal and laboratory studies have examined the anticancer effects of some active ingredients contained in bee products (mellitin and propolis). Propolis, a natural resin produced by honeybees, has been found to contain ingredients (caffeic esters), which may inhibit the development of colon cancer in rats.

In the laboratory, mellitin has been combined with certain antibodies to target cancer cells. According to researchers in Germany, mellitin has been shown to exhibit anti-tumor activity in tumor-derived cell lines. Scientists at the Oncology Research Centre at Prince of Wales Hospital in Australia claim to have killed cancer cells in a test-tube using synthesized mellitin, which destroys cells by creating a hole in their outer membranes. They further claim they have modified the structure of the mellitin molecule by removing the part that causes allergic reactions in some patients, while maintaining its cell-killing ability. This research has not yet been published. Animal and laboratory studies may show a certain substance holds promise as a beneficial treatment, but further studies are necessary to determine if the results apply to humans.

Are there any possible problems or complications?

Some people have extreme allergic reactions to bee stings, the most severe of which can prove fatal. Asthmatic attacks and the death of one young girl have been attributed to the use of royal jelly.

References

Alternative Medicine: Expanding Medical Horizons. *A Report to the National Institutes of Health on Alternative Medical Systems and Practices in the United States.* Washington, DC: US Government Printing Office; 1994. NIH publication 94-066.

Cassileth B. *The Alternative Medicine Handbook.* New York, NY: W. W. Norton & Co; 1998.

CSIRO Media Release. Bees: latest weapon in cancer fight. CSIRO Web site. Available at: http://www.csiro.au. Accessed March 31, 2000.

Rao CV, Desai D, Simi B, Kulkarni N, Amin S, Reddy BS. Inhibitory effect of caffeic acid esters on azoxymethane-induced biochemical changes and aberrant crypt foci formation in rat colon. *Cancer Res.* 1993;53:4182-4188.

Winder D, Gunzburg WH, Erfle V, Salmons B. Expression of antimicrobial peptides has an antitumour effect in human cells. *Biochem Biophys Res Commun.* 1998;242:608-612.

Pharmacological / Biological

Bovine Cartilage

Other common name(s)	Scientific/medical name(s)
None	None

DESCRIPTION / OVERVIEW

Bovine cartilage is cartilage that has been extracted from various parts of a cow, such as the trachea. It is promoted as a treatment for cancer, osteoporosis, and other conditions. The therapeutic potential of various types of cartilage have been studied for more than 40 years (see Shark Cartilage). The first reported use of bovine cartilage to treat a person with cancer was in 1972. It has been proposed that bovine cartilage boosts the immune system and inhibits tumor cell growth. Some claim it contains a protein that inhibits angiogenesis, which in theory involves stopping the blood supply to cancer cells. There is no scientific evidence to support these claims of immunotherapeutic or antiangiogenic activity, however. Clinical trials are currently underway to evaluate the effectiveness of bovine cartilage in many types of solid tumors.

Cancell

Other common name(s)	Scientific/medical name(s)
Entelev, Cantron, Sheridan's Formula, Jim's Juice, Crocinic Acid, Radic	None

DESCRIPTION

Cancell is a dark liquid made up of common chemicals, including nitric acid, sodium sulfite, potassium hydroxide, sulfuric acid, inositol, and catechol (see Inositol Hexaphosphate).

OVERVIEW

There is no scientific evidence that cancell has any effect on cancer or any other disease. The FDA received a permanent injunction against its manufacturers making it illegal to sell cancell across state lines.

How is it promoted for use?

Cancell is promoted as a cure for all forms of cancer and a wide variety of other diseases. According to its manufacturers, it is supposed to cause cancer cells to self-destruct by depriving them of the ability to receive energy. Two theories have been proposed for this activity. The original theory was that the proteins in cancer cells are different than normal cells and that cancell causes cells with these different proteins to revert to the "primitive state" where they self-destruct. A later theory held that all cancers are due to an altered anaerobic cell (a cell that does not require oxygen for respiration). This theory claimed that cancell changes the "vibrational frequency" and energy of the cancer cell, which then causes the cancer cell to self-digest.

Cancell has also been promoted to be effective against AIDS, herpes, chronic fatigue syndrome, lupus, endometriosis, Crohn's disease, fibromyalgia, diabetes, emphysema, scleroderma, Lou Gehrig's disease, multiple sclerosis, cystic fibrosis, muscular dystrophy, Parkinson's disease, Alzheimer's disease, hemophilia, high and low blood pressure, mental illness, and some forms of epilepsy. There is no scientific evidence to support these claims.

What does it involve?
Cancell is promoted for both internal and external use. Manufacturers typically recommend administration by both routes at the same time for 45 days or until all signs of the disease disappear. Cancell or a very similar product is available for purchase in some health food stores or on the Internet.

For internal use, cancell is administered either orally or rectally. Orally, $1/4$ teaspoon is held under the tongue for 5 minutes before swallowing. Rectally, $1/4$ teaspoon is injected into the rectum with a medicine dropper. Both of these procedures must be repeated every 6 hours. For external use, a solvent is first swabbed on the inside of a clean area on the wrist or the ball of the foot and the dose of cancell is applied to a cotton pad. The cotton pad is then secured to the area with tape.

The promoters of cancell also recommend lifestyle and dietary changes including quitting smoking and avoiding high concentrations of certain vitamins. They also strongly discourage patients from using cancell with any other conventional cancer treatment.

What is the history behind it?
The idea for cancell was first developed in 1936 by James Sheridan, a chemist working for Dow Chemical. Sheridan reported that the formula was a cure for all forms of cancer and a wide variety of diseases and came to him in a dream inspired by God. Sheridan called his product "Entelev." In 1984, Sheridan gave the formula to Edward Sopcak for manufacturing and distribution. In 1989, the FDA received a permanent injunction against Sheridan and Sopcak prohibiting them or their agents from distributing entelev or cancell across state lines on the basis that they were adulterated, misbranded, and unapproved new drugs. Supporters today claim that the formula for Sheridan's original product was changed by Sopcak. They claim that cancell is not the equivalent of entelev. Cancell continues to be popular in the United States, especially in Florida and the Midwest.

What is the evidence?
There is no evidence that cancell is effective in treating cancer. Animal studies by the National Cancer Institute (NCI) in 1978 and 1980 found no anticancer activity. The NCI performed another series of tests in 1990 and 1991 using human cancer cells and again found no response. The claims that cancell is effective against other diseases have not been scientifically proven.

Are there any possible problems or complications?

People may experience temporary, moderate fatigue and flu like symptoms after taking the product. Ingredients and strength of the mixtures may vary. Cancell is not produced in conformity with good manufacturing practices. Relying on this type of treatment alone, and avoiding conventional medical care, may have serious health consequences.

References
American Cancer Society. Questionable methods of cancer management: Cancell/Entelev. *CA Cancer J Clin.* 1993;43:57-62.

Cassileth B. *The Alternative Medicine Handbook.* New York, NY: W. W. Norton & Co; 1998.

Spencer JW, Jacobs JJ. *Complementary/Alternative Medicine: An Evidence-Based Approach.* St. Louis, MO: Mosby Inc; 1999.

Pharmacological / Biological

Cell Therapy

Other common name(s)	Scientific/medical name(s)
Cellular Therapy, Fresh Cell Therapy, Live Cell Therapy	None

DESCRIPTION

Cell therapy involves the injection of living tissue from animal organs, embryos or fetuses into patients.

OVERVIEW

There is no scientific evidence that cell therapy is effective in treating cancer or any other disease. Serious side effects can result from cell therapy. In fact, it may be lethal and several deaths have been reported.

How is it promoted for use?

In cell therapy, live or freeze-dried cellular material from the healthy organs, fetuses, or embryos of animals (such as sheep or cows) are injected into patients to supposedly repair cellular damage and heal sick or failing organs. Cell therapy is promoted as an alternative therapy for cancer, arthritis, atherosclerosis, and Parkinson's disease. Cell therapy is also used to counter the effects of aging, to reverse degenerative disease processes, and to improve general health, increase vitality and stamina, and enhance sexual function. Some practitioners have proposed using cell therapy to treat AIDS patients. There is no scientific evidence to support these claims.

The reasoning behind cell therapy is that the healthy cells injected into the body find their way to weak or damaged organs of the same kind and stimulate the body's own healing process. The choice of what type of cells to use depends on which organ is having the problem. For instance, a patient with a diseased liver may receive injections of animal liver cells. Most cell therapists today use cells derived from embryonic animal tissue.

Proponents assert that after the cells are injected, the body transports them directly to where they are most needed and that embryonic and fetal animal tissue contains therapeutic agents that are immunologically active, and therefore assist cell healing within the body.

What does it involve?

First, healthy live cells are harvested from the organs of juvenile or adult live animals, animal embryos, or animal fetuses. These cells may be harvested from the brain, pituitary gland, thyroid gland, thymus gland, liver, kidney, pancreas, spleen, heart, ovary, and testis. Patients might receive one or several types of the animal cells.

Some cell therapists inject fresh cells into their patients. Others freeze them first. Frozen cells have a longer "shelf life" and can be screened for disease. Fresh cells cannot be screened.

A course of cell therapy to address a specific disease might require several injections over a short period of time, whereas cell therapy designed to treat the effects of aging and increase vitality may involve injections received over many months.

Animal organ cells are also sold in pill form

as dietary supplements, usually called glandular supplements. These too are alleged to go to the aid of organs of the same kind in the body to promote healing.

What is the history behind it?

The Swiss physician Paul Niehans, MD invented cell therapy in 1931. During a medical emergency, Dr. Niehans injected a solution containing ground up parathyroid cells from a calf into a patient who had damaged parathyroid glands. The patient recovered, and Dr. Niehans attributed the improvement to the injection. He went on to apply the idea of animal-human cellular transfer to other diseases.

Dr. Niehans claimed that he treated more than 30,000 patients with cell therapy. He also claimed that the death rate from cancer among his patients who received cell therapy was five times less than that of the average population. He believed that injections of cells from animals that were resistant to cancer would increase cancer resistance in humans. A second physician announced similar findings 30 years later. Neither claim has ever been proven. In fact, cell therapy may be harmful, and is not legally available in the United States. The treatment is provided in clinics and spas in Europe, Mexico, and the Bahamas.

What is the evidence?

None of the therapeutic successes claimed by cell therapists have ever been proven through rigorous scientific testing. They are all based on anecdotal reports, testimonials, and publicity issued by practitioners of the therapy. Even proponents of cell therapy admit they don't know how cell therapy works within the body. There are no scientific peer-reviewed publications in medical journals to support the claims of cell therapy.

Are there any possible problems or complications?

Cell therapy may be dangerous and several cases have been reported in the medical literature of patient deaths directly linked to the therapy. Patients may contract bacterial and viral infections carried by the animal cells, and have experienced life-threatening and even fatal allergic reactions. Animal cells may seriously compromise the immune system. Other reports list complications such as immune vasculitis, encephalitis, and polyradiculitis (nerve inflammation) following cellular treatment. Serious immunological reactions resulting in death have also been reported.

This treatment should be avoided, especially by women who are pregnant or breast-feeding. Relying on this type of treatment alone, and avoiding conventional medical care, may have serious health consequences.

References

American Cancer Society. Unproven methods of cancer management. Fresh cell therapy. *CA Cancer J Clin.* 1991;41:126-128.

Barrett S, Herbert V. Questionable cancer therapies. Quackwatch Web site. Available at: http://www.quackwatch.com. Accessed May 8, 2000.

Cassileth B. *The Alternative Medicine Handbook.* New York, NY: W. W. Norton & Co; 1998.

Gage FH. Cell therapy. *Nature.* 1998;392:18-24.

US Congress, Office of Technology Assessment. *Unconventional Cancer Treatments.* Washington, DC: US Government Printing Office; 1990. Publication OTA-H-405.

Pharmacological / Biological

Chelation Therapy

Other common name(s)	Scientific/medical name(s)
None	None

DESCRIPTION

Chelation therapy involves the injection of ethylene diamine tetraacetic acid (EDTA), a chemical that chelates (binds) heavy metals which include iron, lead, mercury, cadmium, and zinc. The term "chelation" comes from the Greek word "chele," which means claw, referring to the way the chemical grabs onto these metals.

OVERVIEW

Chelation therapy is one of several effective treatments for lead poisoning. However, there is no scientific evidence that it is effective for treating other conditions such as cancer. Chelation therapy can be toxic and has the potential to cause kidney damage, irregular heartbeat, and even death.

How is it promoted for use?

Chelation therapy has been approved by the FDA as a treatment for lead poisoning for more than forty years. The human body can't break down heavy metals, which can accumulate to toxic levels in the body and interfere with normal functioning. Chelating drugs remove poisonous buildups of metals such as lead, mercury, cadmium, and zinc by circulating in the bloodstream and attaching to the heavy metal molecules, helping to remove them from the body in the urine.

Chelation therapy is promoted as an alternative treatment for many unrelated conditions, such as angina, gangrene, thyroid disorders, multiple sclerosis, muscular dystrophy, high cholesterol, psoriasis, hypercalcemia, arthritis, Alzheimer's disease, and the improvement of memory, sight, hearing, and smell. Because chelation drugs can reduce the amount of calcium in the bloodstream, some practitioners consider chelation therapy an effective and inexpensive alternative to coronary bypass surgery and angioplasty for reopening coronary arteries blocked by mineral deposits (hardening of the arteries, or atherosclerosis). Alternative practitioners further claim chelation therapy can be used as a cancer treatment to block the production of a group of harmful molecules called free radicals (unstable oxygen molecules, which can cause cell damage). There is no scientific evidence to support these claims.

What does it involve?

Chelation therapy is given intravenously. Sometimes it is administered as an infusion that drips into the vein over a period of 3 or 4 hours. A typical treatment cycle may include 20 injections or infusions spread over 10 to 12 weeks. Chelation therapy can also be given orally. Because the therapy removes some important minerals from the body, patients often receive vitamin and mineral supplements during treatment. Practitioners recommend a minimum of 20 to 40 treatments initially; however, some may recommend continued therapy for up to 100 treatments over a period of several years.

What is the history behind it?

The chemical solution used in chelation therapy,

EDTA, was first manufactured in Germany in the 1930s. It is now widely accepted as an effective treatment for heavy metal poisoning. In the 1950s, some scientists hypothesized that EDTA could remove calcium from the body (which can build up on artery walls and cause heart disease) and thereby help to unclog blocked arteries. In some early studies, researchers reported positive results among patients with heart disease who received EDTA. Some said that chelation therapy relieved angina (chest pain) caused by blocked arteries. These initial observations lead practitioners to begin using chelation therapy for heart and circulatory problems and later, for several other illnesses. It is estimated that tens of thousands of Americans currently undergo chelation therapy for heart disease.

In 1998, the Federal Trade Commission charged the American College of Advancement in Medicine (ACAM), the principal group promoting chelation therapy, with presenting false advertising and unsubstantiated statements about the benefits of chelation therapy. The ACAM agreed to stop publishing any claims not based on reliable scientific evidence.

What is the evidence?

Chelation therapy is a proven treatment for lead poisoning and poisoning from other heavy metals. However, there is no evidence that the treatment benefits patients with cancer, heart disease, or any medical problems other than heavy-metal poisoning.

In 1998, researchers studied chelation therapy to see if it would reduce the growth of neuroblastoma (a type of cancer in infants and young children) in mice. The study concluded that after chelation therapy, there was no reduction in tumor size. Two randomized clinical trials found that chelation therapy drugs did not benefit patients with impaired circulation in their legs. In 1993, a review of all chelation therapy studies reported during the previous 37 years concluded that scientific data did not support claims that the treatment was useful for treating heart problems.

Several well respected organizations have found no scientific evidence that chelation ther-

apy is an effective treatment for any medical condition except heavy metal poisoning including: the American Heart Association, American Medical Association, Centers for Disease Control and Prevention, American Osteopathic Association, the American Academy of Family Physicians, and the FDA.

Are there any possible problems or complications?

There is no evidence the chelation therapy is a safe treatment for any type of cancer. Chelation therapy may produce toxic effects, including kidney damage, irregular heart beat, and inflammation of the veins. Since the therapy involves the removal of minerals from the body, there is also a risk of hypocalcemia (low calcium) and bone damage. It may also compromise the immune system and decrease the body's ability to produce insulin. People may also experience pain at the site of EDTA injection.

Chelation therapy is often accompanied by the infusion of large doses of vitamins and other minerals, which may actually contribute to the processes that produce dangerous free radicals in the body. Loss of zinc can also lead to mutations in cells. For this reason, chelation therapy may actually increase the risk of cancer. Women who are pregnant or breast-feeding should not use this method. Relying on this type of treatment alone, and avoiding conventional medical care, may have serious health consequences.

References

Cassileth B. *The Alternative Medicine Handbook.* New York, NY: W. W. Norton & Co; 1998.

Green S. Chelation therapy: unproven claims and unsound theories. Quackwatch Web site. Available at: http://www. quackwatch.com. Accessed May 9, 2000.

Grier MT, Meyers DG. So much writing, so little science: a review of 37 years of literature on edetate sodium chelation therapy. *Ann Pharmacother.* 1993;27:1504-1509.

Guldager B, Jelnes R, Jorgensen SJ, et al. EDTA treatment of intermittent claudication: a double-blind placebo-controlled study. *J Intern Med.* 1992;231:261-267.

Selig RA, White L, Gramacho C, Sterling-Levis K, Fraser IW, Naidoo D. Failure of iron chelators to reduce tumor growth in human neuroblastoma xenografts. *Cancer Res* 1998;58:473-478.

Spencer JW, Jacobs JJ. *Complementary/Alternative Medicine: An Evidence-Based Approach.* St. Louis, MO: Mosby Inc; 1999.

van Rij AM, Solomon C, Packer SG, Hopkins WG. Chelation therapy for intermittent claudication. A double-blind, randomized, controlled trial. *Circulation.* 1994;90:1194-1199.

Coenzyme Q10

Other common name(s)	Scientific/medical name(s)
CoQ10	Ubiquinone

DESCRIPTION

Coenzyme Q10 (CoQ10) is an enzyme that regulates numerous chemical reactions in the body. It occurs naturally in the body and can also be obtained from a number of foods, such as mackerel, salmon, sardines, beef, soybeans, peanuts, and spinach (see Enzyme Therapy and Soybean).

OVERVIEW

Dietary or supplemental CoQ10 may promote health and fight some diseases, but more research is needed to determine the role of supplements in health and disease. Results from small studies need to be verified by larger randomized clinical trials to determine CoQ10's role in reducing chemotherapy-induced cardiac toxicity (heart problems resulting from chemotherapy drugs) and in treating cancer.

How is it promoted for use?

Scientists believe CoQ10 is an antioxidant. An antioxidant is a compound that blocks the action of activated oxygen molecules, known as free radicals, that can damage cells. Deficiencies of CoQ10 are thought to contribute to illness. Some studies have found CoQ10 deficiency in people with cancer.

Coenzyme Q10 is promoted as a treatment for cancer, heart disease, stroke, gum disease, and immune deficiencies. Some claim that CoQ10 can reduce pain and weight loss among people with cancer. Supporters also claim CoQ10 supplements protect against the toxic side effects of chemotherapy drugs, such as adriamycin, which can harm the heart. These claims are currently under investigation.

What does it involve?

Coenzyme Q10 occurs naturally in the body. It can also be obtained from a number of foods or as a supplement. The usual supplement dose found in the literature is 90-400 mg/day. Supplements are available in tablets, capsules, and gel caps.

What is the history behind it?

Coenzyme Q10 was first isolated and identified in 1957. Particularly high amounts were found in heart tissue, which is why researchers became interested in the connection between CoQ10 and heart disease. In the 1970s, researchers began experimenting with CoQ10 supplements for treating heart disease, cancer, and other conditions.

What is the evidence?

Although preliminary studies involving small numbers of patients suggest certain anticancer benefits of CoQ10 supplements, the amount of evidence is minimal. More studies are needed with larger groups of patients to compare to conventional cancer treatments.

A review of 25 small human studies by the University of Texas reported mixed results for the use of CoQ10 as a cancer treatment. In one study involving 43 breast and prostate cancer patients, deaths were significantly lower among those who received a CoQ10 supplement with vitamins and minerals compared with those that received no CoQ10. In another study of 32 women with breast cancer that had spread to the lymph nodes and who were treated with a nutritional supplement program of vitamins, minerals, essential fatty acids, and CoQ10, all survived at least 24 months and had stable disease.

Low levels of CoQ10 have been associated with heart damage and chemotherapy treatment for cancer. One randomized clinical trial and four controlled studies found that for people who received CoQ10, there were some protective effects against heart damage related to chemotherapy. No scientific clinical research was found related to pain, weight loss, or increased appetite.

Are there any possible problems or complications?

Few serious reactions to CoQ10 have been reported. Side effects may include headache, heartburn, and fatigue. Very high doses may cause involuntary muscle movements. Some users report mild diarrhea and skin reactions. Little is known about dosage or consequences of long-term use of CoQ10 supplements. There have been reports that CoQ10 may interact with anticoagulant (blood thinning) medications and pose a risk for prolonged bleeding.

References

Alternative Medicine: Expanding Medical Horizons. *A Report to the National Institutes of Health on Alternative Medical Systems and Practices in the United States.* Washington, DC: US Government Printing Office; 1994. NIH publication 94-066.

Fetrow CW, Avila JR. *Professional's Handbook of Complementary and Alternative Medicines.* Springhouse, Pa: Springhouse Corp; 1999.

Folkers K, Brown R, Judy WV, Morita M. Survival of cancer patients on therapy with coenzyme Q10. *Biochem Biophys Res Commun.* 1993;192:241-245.

Hodges S, Hertz N, Lockwood K, Lister R. CoQ10: could it have a role in cancer management? *Biofactors.* 1999;9:365-370.

Lockwood K, Moesgaard S, Hanioka T, Folkers K. Apparent partial remission of breast cancer in 'high risk' patients supplemented with nutritional antioxidants, essential fatty acids and coenzyme Q10. *Mol Aspects Med.* 1994;15:S231-240.

Spigset O. Reduced effect of warfarin caused by ubidecarenone. *Lancet.* 1994;344:1372-1373.

University of Texas Center for Alternative Medicine Research in Cancer. Coenzyme Q10 summary. University of Texas-Houston Health Science Center Web site. Available at: http://www.sph.uth.tmc.edu/utcam/summary/CoQ10.htm. Accessed May 9, 2000.

Pharmacological / Biological

Coley Toxins

Other common name(s)	Scientific/medical name(s)
Coley's Toxins, Mixed Bacterial Vaccines, Issel's Fever Therapy	None

DESCRIPTION

Coley toxins is an alternative form of cancer immunotherapy that involves injections of inactive bacterial cultures (Streptococcus pyogenes and Serratia marcescens). *Immunotherapy is a method of treatment in which a person receives various biologic substances designed to stimulate the immune system and help the body fight off diseases such as cancer.*

OVERVIEW

There is no scientific evidence that Coley toxins alone are effective in treating cancer. Some research has examined combining this immunotherapy with conventional cancer treatments. Some of these studies found this combined treatment approach to be more effective than conventional treatment alone, while other studies did not find any significant benefit to the combined approach. Modern immunotherapy is likely to be more effective.

How is it promoted for use?

Proponents claim Coley toxins stimulate the immune system in people with cancer, which helps to fight off disease. Proponents believe the high fever caused by Coley toxins helps to rid the body of cancer because tumor cells are more sensitive to heat than normal cells.

What does it involve?

Coley toxins are injected into the bloodstream in increasing doses and continue for at least 3 to 4 months. Patients are monitored closely for side effects and to control fevers if they develop.

The original formula for Coley toxins is no longer used in the United States. Coley toxins are used in Central America, Germany, and China; however it is not clear if they are using the original Coley toxins or a combination of Coley toxins and other bacteria.

What is the history behind it?

Coley toxins were developed in the 1890s by William B. Coley, MD, a bone surgeon at Memorial Hospital in New York City (now Memorial Sloan-Kettering Cancer Center). After his attempt to save a young woman from bone cancer failed, Dr. Coley began reviewing bone cancer cases and noted that cancer patients who developed bacterial infections after surgery seemed to have better outcomes than those who did not. He believed the bacterial infection helped to stimulate the immune system, causing it to fight off cancer cells. At first, Coley injected live bacterial cultures into patients with cancer but due to the danger involved, he began using bacterial cultures that had been killed. His treatment was controversial, despite the anecdotal reports of cancer regression associated with its use.

Coley toxins were used to treat patients with a variety of cancers until the 1950s when production of the drug was discontinued in the United States. Dr. Coley's daughter, Helen Coley Nauts, published several papers documenting the results of the treatment between 1976 and 1989. She founded the Cancer Research

Institute in New York in 1953, which is devoted to immunological approaches to the diagnosis and treatment of cancer.

A vaccine of Coley toxins combined with ten other strains of bacteria is being used at the Waisbren Clinic in Milwaukee. One pharmaceutical company and a cancer center are said to be investigating a variation of Coley toxins.

Dr. Coley is credited with pioneering the field of immunotherapy. Some oncologists regard immunotherapy as the "fourth modality" or type of cancer treatment. The other three conventional treatments are surgery, radiation, and chemotherapy. Immunotherapy is usually combined with or after conventional cancer treatments but is sometimes used alone. Immunotherapy has a relatively small role in treating people with the most common types of cancer. However, researchers are optimistic that more effective immunotherapies can be developed that will have a greater impact on the outlook for people with cancer.

What is the evidence?

Scientific evidence suggests Coley toxins or the mixed bacterial vaccine (MBV) may have a therapeutic role in the treatment of cancer in a combined treatment approach. According to a review by researchers at the University of Texas Center for Alternative Medicine, three randomized clinical trials found that people who received Coley toxins or a MBV, in combination with conventional treatment, tended to have higher survival rates than patients who received conventional treatment alone.

However, a recent review comparing 128 patients treated with surgery and Coley toxins between 1890 and 1960 to 1,675 patients treated with conventional methods, suggested that survival rates for Coley patients did not vary significantly from those treated with conventional methods. The researchers point out that the study was limited by small sample size, short duration, and selection bias. More research is needed to determine what benefit, if any, this therapy might have for people with cancer.

Although Coley toxins are often regarded historically as a key step that has led to modern immunotherapy, much has been learned about the science of immunology and practice of immunotherapy since that time. Modern immunotherapy is likely to be of greater value, especially in treating certain cancers, such as renal cell (kidney) cancer, melanoma, and lymphoma.

Are there any possible problems or complications?

The inactive bacteria in Coley toxins can produce fever and nausea. Less common side effects include headache, back pain, chills, chest pain, and shock-like reactions. There may be a danger that the administration of Coley toxins could produce serious infections among patients with weakened immune systems. Women who are pregnant or breast-feeding should not use these toxins.

References

Alternative Medicine: Expanding Medical Horizons. *A Report to the National Institutes of Health on Alternative Medical Systems and Practices in the United States.* Washington, DC: US Government Printing Office; 1994. NIH publication 94-066.

Richardson MA, Ramirez T, Russell NC, Moye LA. Coley toxins immunotherapy: a retrospective review. *Altern Ther Health Med.* 1999;5:42-47.

University of Texas Center for Alternative Medicine Research in Cancer. Immune augmentation therapy summary. Available at: http://www.sph.uth.tmc.edu/utcam/therapies/coley.htm. Accessed May 9, 2000.

DHEA

Other common name(s)	Scientific/medical name(s)
None	Dehydroepiandrosterone

DESCRIPTION

Dehydroepiandrosterone (DHEA) is a steroid hormone produced by the adrenal gland, which is broken down into other important hormones, such as estrogen and testosterone. It is found in humans, plants, and animals.

OVERVIEW

There is no scientific evidence that DHEA is safe or effective. It should not be used for treating cancer, especially in hormone responsive cancers. DHEA may have some usefulness in treating mood and memory problems of older age. People less than 30 years of age run the risk of suppressing the body's production of DHEA if they take supplemental DHEA.

How is it promoted for use?

Advocates claim that DHEA supplements can prevent the growth and recurrence of some cancers, protect against heart disease, improve memory, reduce the risk of osteoporosis in women, and help prevent other diseases such as diabetes, Parkinson's, and Alzheimer's. Since levels of DHEA usually begin to decline after a person reaches 30 years of age, proponents claim that the supplements can help slow the aging process. Proponents also contend that DHEA stimulates the immune system, reduces fat, builds muscle, promotes sleep, increases a person's overall sense of well being and increases sex drive. Some practitioners say that DHEA is an effective treatment for colitis and depression. There is no scientific evidence to support these claims.

What does it involve?

Dehydroepiandrosterone is found in the human body, plants, and animals. The dietary supplements sold in the United States are likely to be made from an extract of the yam plant. DHEA is taken orally and applied topically. It is formulated in tablets, capsules, and creams, and can also be made into a tea. There are no widely accept-

ed dosage guidelines for DHEA.

What is the history behind it?

Dehydroepiandrosterone was banned by the FDA in 1985 due to its unproven safety and effectiveness. The ban was removed by the 1994 Dietary Supplement Health & Education Act. Dehydroepiandrosterone supplements became available to the public in 1995.

What is the evidence?

There is no scientific evidence that DHEA can slow or prevent the growth of cancer, or that the extract from the yam plant will increase DHEA levels in the body. The few clinical research studies that link DHEA with improved health are not considered scientifically valid.

One early human study showed that men who had high levels of DHEA in their blood were less likely to have died of heart disease, but women who had high DHEA levels were at greater risk of dying of heart disease. An analysis of the research published recently found that there was little association with levels of DHEA and heart disease in men or women. An animal study concluded that DHEA had no influence on either cancer or life span.

One clinical study found no relationship between DHEA levels in the blood and the risk of breast cancer in postmenopausal women, while another found that a high level of DHEA in the blood was associated with a higher risk of breast cancer. No clinical research has demonstrated that DHEA supplements increase muscle mass, reduce fat, or prevent disease.

A recent study in humans taking DHEA supplements suggests that it may help treat the autoimmune disease lupus. Clinical trials are underway to study DHEA's ability to stimulate the immune system.

A small pilot study suggested that DHEA may improve mood, energy, libido, and in some cases, memory performance in the elderly. The preliminary results raise the question of DHEA's usefulness in older age individuals with depression. Larger, double-blind clinical trials are currently underway.

Are there any possible problems or complications?

It is not known whether DHEA is safe for long-term use. Some researchers believe DHEA supplements might actually increase the risk of breast cancer, prostate cancer, heart disease, diabetes, and stroke. Dehydroepiandrosterone may stimulate tumor growth in women with cancers related to estrogen, such as breast cancer and uterine cancer and men with prostate cancer. Men with benign prostatic hypertrophy (an enlarged prostate gland) should avoid DHEA because it could increase swelling.

High doses of DHEA may cause aggressiveness, irritability, insomnia, and the growth of body or facial hair on women. It also may stop menstruation and decrease the levels of HDL cholesterol ("good cholesterol"), which increases the risk of heart disease. Other reported side effects include acne, heart rhythm disturbances, hepatitis, scalp hair loss, and oily skin. Women who are pregnant or breast-feeding should not use DHEA.

References

Fetrow CW, Avila JR. *Professional's Handbook of Complementary and Alternative Medicines.* Springhouse, Pa: Springhouse Corp; 1999.

Pugh TD, Oberley TD, Weindruch R. Dietary intervention at middle age: caloric restriction but not dehydroepiandrosterone sulfate increases lifespan and lifetime cancer incidence in mice. *Cancer Res.* 1999;59:1642-1648.

Schardt D. Remembering Gingko & DHEA; claims of dietary supplement have not been proven. *Nutr Action Healthletter.* 1998;25:9.

Skerret PJ. DHEA: ignore the hype. Quackwatch Web site. Available at: http://www.quackwatch.com. Accessed May 8, 2000.

Skolnick AA. Scientific verdict still out on DHEA. *JAMA.* 1996;276:1365-1367.

Pharmacological / Biological

Di Bella Therapy

Other common name(s)	Scientific/medical name(s)
Di Bella Multitherapy	None

DESCRIPTION

Di Bella therapy consists of a mixture of the drugs somatostatin, bromocriptine, as well as vitamins, melatonin, and sometimes other substances combined in varying amounts depending on the patient under treatment (see Melatonin and section on Herbs, Vitamins, and Minerals).

OVERVIEW

There is no scientific evidence that Di Bella therapy is effective in treating cancer. It can cause serious and harmful side effects.

How is it promoted for use?

Proponents of Di Bella therapy claim the drug mixture stimulates the body's self-healing properties and can shrink tumors and even cure cancer. The inventor claims he has treated and cured thousands of people who have had a variety of cancers, and that his formula causes no side effects.

One of the components in Di Bella therapy, bromocriptine (Parlodel®), is a drug approved by the FDA for treating pituitary tumors, Parkinson's Disease, and fertility problems.

What does it involve?

Patients undergoing Di Bella therapy consume the custom-made drug mixture daily. The potency of the mixture and which drugs are involved depends on the type of cancer under treatment.

What is the history behind it?

Di Bella therapy was invented by Professor Luigi Di Bella, a retired physiologist from Modena, Italy. During 1997 and 1998, Di Bella therapy caused an uproar throughout Italy when a judge in the southern city of Maglie ruled that the government must pay for Di Bella therapy to treat a 2-year-old boy with brain cancer. The child's parents had filed a lawsuit against the

Italian Ministry of Health, which had refused to fund the treatment because Di Bella therapy was untested and expensive. The young boy died in July 1998. A number of similar legal actions followed.

Even though there was no scientific evidence to prove Di Bella therapy's benefits, the therapy still had a number of supporters and the Italian media quickly spread news about the professor's claims and about the lawsuits. Di Bella appeared in 50 television interviews and 300 newspaper articles. Demand for Di Bella's formula depleted the supply in many pharmacies, and people with cancer flooded Italian hospitals requesting to participate in clinical trials. Thousands of supporters even held rallies in Rome to support government funding of Di Bella therapy.

Finally, bowing to public pressure, the Ministry of Health ordered a controlled clinical investigation of Di Bella therapy. Some cancer specialists refused to participate for ethical reasons. The results of the clinical trial revealed that Di Bella therapy was ineffective against cancer.

Before the clinical trial began, researchers at the University of Parma surveyed more than 1,100 Italian citizens. Forty-two percent believed that Di Bella therapy worked, 53% said they didn't know, and only 1% said they thought it was a sham. Ninety percent of the respondents said they learned about the treatment from television, and only 5% said they asked a doctor about it. Since then, public interest in the treatment has decreased, but Di Bella therapy still has many supporters despite the lack of evidence that it has any value.

What is the evidence?

Research has shown that Di Bella therapy is not effective in treating cancer. Italy's Health Ministry conducted a multicenter study involving nearly 400 patients with various forms of advanced cancers. Early results showed that none of the first 134 patients treated with Di Bella therapy benefited at all after 2 months of treatment. Half suffered serious side effects and three quarters became sicker or died. The final report that included 397 patients showed that not one tumor went into complete remission and only three went into partial remission. Twenty-five percent of the subjects died and the conditions of more than 50% worsened. The researchers concluded that Di Bella therapy did not deserve further clinical testing in patients with advanced cancer.

A survey was recently published on the survival rates of cancer patients treated with Di Bella therapy during the years 1971 to 1997. A review of 248 records showed that the treatment did not improve their survival.

Bromocriptine, one of the ingredients in the Di Bella formula is approved for use in addition to conventional treatment to reduce the size of some pituitary tumors before surgery and during radiation. It is also used to treat Parkinson's disease and fertility problems.

Are there any possible problems or complications?

Some of the side effects of Di Bella therapy include nausea, vomiting, diarrhea, and neurological symptoms.

Women who are pregnant or breast-feeding should not use this method. Relying on this type of treatment alone, and avoiding conventional medical care, may have serious health consequences.

References

Bertelli G. Di Bella Therapy. Quackwatch Web site. Available at: http://www.quackwatch.com. Accessed May 8, 2000.

Buiatti E, Arniani S, Verdecchia A, Tomatis L. Results from a historical survey of the survival of cancer patients given Di Bella multitherapy. *Cancer*. 1999;86:2143-2149.

Italian Study Group for the Di Bella Multitherapy Trials. Evaluation of an unconventional cancer treatment (the Di Bella multitherapy): results of phase II trials in Italy. *BMJ*. 1999;318:224-228.

Medical Economics. *Physicians' Desk Reference*. Montvale, NJ: Medical Economics Company; 1999.

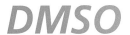
DMSO

Other common name(s)	Scientific/medical name(s)
None	Dimethyl Sulfoxide

DESCRIPTION
Dimethyl sulfoxide (DMSO) is an industrial solvent, produced as a byproduct of paper manufacturing, that has been promoted as an alternative cancer treatment since the 1960s.

OVERVIEW
There is no scientific evidence that DMSO is effective in treating cancer. It is currently under study as a drug carrier used to increase the effectiveness of some chemotherapy agents for the treatment of bladder cancer. If administered in high concentrations, DMSO can cause death.

How is it promoted for use?
Proponents say that DMSO can be used as a cancer treatment to cause malignant cells to become benign and slow or halt the progress of cancers in the bladder, colon, ovary, breast, and skin. Some claim that it is effective in treating leukemia, and it has also been used as a component of some metabolic cancer therapies. This treatment has been used as a cream or ointment applied to the skin to reduce pain, decrease swelling, treat arthritis, and promote healing in normal tissue. Some people have promoted DMSO as a cancer preventative agent. They claim it works by "cleaning" the cell membrane and decreasing the effect of cancer causing substances, however, these claims have not been proven.

Dimethyl sulfoxide is also promoted to reduce the side effects of chemotherapy and radiation treatments in people with cancer. This activity is supposedly due to the ability of DMSO to stimulate the immune system and neutralize free radicals that are produced by these treatments and are a main cause of the side effects. In addition, it has been promoted as a way to control "withdrawal symptoms" experienced by cancer patients when taken off conventional cancer treatment. There is no scientific evidence to support these claims.

What does it involve?
Dimethyl sulfoxide is medically approved only for the treatment of interstitial cystitis (inflammation of the bladder). However, as an alternative therapy for cancer, it is available in many health food stores and mail order outlets. It is typically taken either orally or in an intravenous injection, in many cases with other drugs. For topical applications, DMSO is available in gel, liquid, and roll-on forms. The dosage people use varies widely, from three times a day to once every other day.

What is the history behind it?
Dimethyl sulfoxide was first discovered in the mid- to late 19th century and has been used as an industrial solvent for more than 100 years. In the 1950s, it was discovered that DMSO could protect cells from the damage of freezing. In the 1960s, Dr. Stanley Jacob, one of its main proponents, began to investigate other medicinal properties of DMSO. In 1965, clinical trials of DMSO were ended due to questions about its safety. However, in the 1970s, DMSO was

approved for use as an anti-inflammatory in dogs and horses and as a prescription drug for a type of bladder inflammation in humans.

What is the evidence?

Tests of DMSO for treating human illness began in the mid-1960s, but were discontinued due to questions of safety. Previous research did not find that DMSO was useful in the treatment of cancer. However, more recent research in rats has shown that DMSO deserves further evaluation as a drug carrier used to enhance the effectiveness of some chemotherapy agents for the treatment of bladder cancer.

In a 1988 laboratory study, researchers tested the hypothesis that DMSO might increase the anticancer activity of chemotherapeutic drugs that are instilled in the bladder for the treatment of bladder cancer. The addition of 4% DMSO to the four drugs most frequently used for chemotherapy instilled within the bladder (adriamycin, epodyl, mitomycin C, thiotepa) did not increase the killing of cancer cells in this test tube study.

Three studies in rats, however, found that adding DMSO to some chemotherapeutic agents improved their absorption in the bladder. Animal and laboratory studies may show a certain substances holds promise as a beneficial treatment, but further studies are necessary to determine if the results apply to humans.

Dimethyl sulfoxide is a common chemical used in the laboratory. It is sometimes used to help tumor cells mature and/or differentiate. This use is claimed to be one rationale for DMSO's use as an anticancer agent. However, the concentrations used in the lab would be fatal to a human being. A small amount of DMSO is sometimes also used to dissolve drugs and to deliver them through the skin. However, in these cases, it is the drug, not DMSO, that has biological activity.

Research has shown that DMSO does appear to have some effect in reducing swelling and inflammation. Dimethyl sulfoxide is approved by the FDA to treat a single type of bladder disorder (interstitial cystitis) in humans and as a veterinary therapy to reduce swelling in horses and dogs.

Are there any possible problems or complications?

Clinical trials with DMSO were halted due to questions about its safety, especially with regard to its ability to affect the eye. The most commonly reported side effects include burning and itching upon contact with the skin. It can also cause a powerful garlic-like odor on the breath and skin. In high concentrations, DMSO can be fatal to humans. Women who are pregnant or breast-feeding should not use this treatment.

References

American Cancer Society. Unproven methods of cancer management. Dimethyl sulfoxide (DMSO). *CA Cancer J Clin.* 1983;33:122-125.

Cassileth B. *The Alternative Medicine Handbook.* New York, NY: W. W. Norton & Co; 1998.

Hashimoto H, Tokunaka S, Sasaki M, Nishihara M, Yachiku S. Dimethylsulfoxide enhances the absorption of chemotherapeutic drug instilled into the bladder. *Urol Res.* 1992;20:233-236.

See WA, Xia Q. Regional chemotherapy for bladder neoplasms using continuous intravesical infusion of doxorubicin: impact of concomitant administration of dimethyl sulfoxide on drug absorption and antitumor activity. *J Natl Cancer Inst.* 1992;84:510-515.

US Congress, Office of Technology Assessment. *Unconventional Cancer Treatments.* Washington, DC: US Government Printing Office; 1990. Publication OTA-H-405.

Walker L, Walker MC, Parris CN, Masters JR. Intravesical chemotherapy: combination with dimethyl sulfoxide does not enhance cytotoxicity in vitro. *Urol Res.* 1988;16:329-331.

Yaman O, Ozdiler E, Sozen S, Gogus O. Transmurally absorbed intravesical chemotherapy with dimethylsulfoxide in an animal model. *Int J Urol.* 1999;6:87-92.

Enzyme Therapy

Other common name(s)	Scientific/medical name(s)
Digestive Enzyme Therapy, Pancreatic Enzyme Therapy, Systemic Enzyme Therapy	None

DESCRIPTION

Enzyme therapy involves the consumption of enzyme supplements as an alternative form of treatment. Enzymes are proteins that stimulate and accelerate numerous biological reactions in the body. Digestive enzymes, many of which are produced in the pancreas, break down food and assist with the absorption of nutrients into the bloodstream. Metabolic enzymes build new cells and repair damaged ones in the blood, tissues, and organs.

OVERVIEW

There is no scientific evidence that enzyme supplements are effective in treating cancer or any other disease. There is no information to determine the safety of the supplements. Research funded by the National Cancer Institute (NCI) is currently underway.

How is it promoted for use?

Enzymes are sometimes used in conventional medicine. For example, the approved chemotherapy drug asparaginase is an enzyme. Some enzymes are also important in gene therapy research, which is a new but promising treatment for cancer and other serious illnesses. Pancreatic enzymes may be given to treat digestive problems resulting from surgical removal of the pancreas or certain diseases of the pancreas.

Enzyme therapy, however, involves the use of enzyme supplements by alternative medicine practitioners to fight illness. Digestive enzymes, they claim, not only relieve digestive problems, such as ulcers and food allergies, but also strengthen the immune system, help to destroy viruses, ease the discomfort of sore throats, aid weight loss, and relieve hay fever, ulcers, and rheumatoid arthritis. Proponents also claim certain enzymes remove the protective coating from cancer cells, allowing white blood cells to identify and attack the intruders.

What does it involve?

Human cells naturally produce about 10,000 different enzymes, which are essential in normal metabolism. Enzyme supplements are extracted from animal organs and some plants. Among the most popular enzyme supplements are pancreatic enzymes, which come from animal pancreas.

Enzyme supplements are available in pills, capsules, and powders. Supplements often consist of combinations of several different enzymes. Enzyme therapy is a component of some forms of metabolic therapy, particularly the Kelley and Gonzalez programs (see Metabolic Therapy). There is currently no established safe or effective dosage.

What is the history behind it?

Pancreatic enzymes were reportedly first used to treat cancer in 1902 by John Beard, an English scientist. German researchers later used enzyme therapy to treat patients with multiple sclerosis, cancer, and viral infections. Dr. Edward Howell introduced enzyme therapy to the United States in the 1920s. He believed that by eating raw meat, people created an enzyme surplus, which resulted in better health and increased resistance to disease.

What is the evidence?

There have been no controlled studies showing the effectiveness of enzyme supplements in treating cancer, improving digestion, or curing any other diseases. According to experts, enzymes, regardless of their source, are eventually broken down into amino acids and absorbed in the digestive tract.

One uncontrolled study reported that large doses of pancreatic enzymes increased survival times among patients with inoperable pancreatic cancer. This was a small pilot study conducted on 10 patients. A randomized clinical trial sponsored by the NCI is underway to evaluate the use of pancreatic enzymes with nutritional support for treating pancreatic cancer.

Are there any possible problems or complications?

Some enzymes, like Coenzyme Q10, have been reported to cause side effects (see Coenzyme Q10). There is not a lot of information to determine the safety of enzyme supplements.

References

Cassileth B. *The Alternative Medicine Handbook*. New York, NY: W. W. Norton & Co; 1998.

Gonzalez NJ, Isaacs LL. Evaluation of pancreatic proteolytic enzyme treatment of adenocarcinoma of the pancreas, with nutrition and detoxification support. *Nutr Cancer*. 1999;33:117-124.

Green S. Nicolas Gonzalez treatment for cancer: gland extracts, coffee enemas, vitamin megadoses, and diets. Quackwatch Web site. Available at: http://www.quackwatch.com. Accessed May 8, 2000.

Gamma Linolenic Acid

Other common name(s)	Scientific/medical name(s)
Borage Seed Oil, Black Currant Oil, GLA	γ-Linolenic Acid

DESCRIPTION

Gamma linolenic acid (GLA) is a highly unsaturated fatty acid made in the human body from other essential fatty acids. The main sources of GLA are oils of evening primrose, borage, and black currant plants (see Evening Primrose). Many commercial preparations sell these extracts as GLA. It is also found in human breast milk.

OVERVIEW

Some studies have shown that GLA can inhibit the growth of some cancer cell lines in tissue cultures in the laboratory; however, there is no evidence that it is effective in preventing or treating cancer in humans. Human studies are currently being done to evaluate the role of essential fatty acids on the growth of cancer cells (see Omega-3 Fatty Acids). There is some evidence that GLA may be useful in treating neurological problems related to diabetes. A recent study suggests a promising role for the use of GLA in acute respiratory distress syndrome.

How is it promoted for use?

Gamma linolenic acid is used in the production of prostaglandins (hormone-like substances made in the body). Prostaglandins are believed to be involved in many processes in the body, including regulation of the immune system. It has been proposed that GLA supplements may inhibit the growth of cancer cells. This claim is currently under investigation.

Gamma linolenic acid has been promoted as a fatty acid that also helps people with benign breast disease, skin problems, obesity, rheumatoid arthritis, cardiovascular disease, high blood pressure, premenstrual syndrome, and neurological problems related to diabetes.

What does it involve?

Gamma linolenic acid supplements are available in liquid and capsules. Gamma linolenic acid is usually found in combination with other ingredients (eg, evening primrose supplements contain about 10% GLA). An injectable form of GLA is under study in the United Kingdom. Dosages vary according to manufacturer.

What is the history behind it?

Research in the 1980s began to find that prostaglandins played a role in many biological processes. Since GLA was known to be an intermediate in the production of prostaglandins, it was soon thought that GLA could be beneficial in treating human disease.

What is the evidence?

Most of the research on GLA has been done using evening primrose oil. This makes it difficult to credit the effects to GLA, linolenic acid, Vitamin E, or other components of the oil. A randomized clinical trial found that GLA had a beneficial effect on neurological problems related to diabetes, especially in patients whose condition was well under control. Neither evening primrose oil nor GLA has been shown to be effective in preventing or treating cancer in humans.

Dietary GLA can contribute to prostaglandin synthesis and regulation; however, the types of prostaglandins and their exact role in fighting cancer are still unknown. Gamma linolenic acid can inhibit the growth of certain human tumor cells in the laboratory. Animal and clinical trials have found that dietary GLA has no effect on established tumors. A new injectable form of GLA has been developed and has been used in a single clinical trial with some limited success. However, follow-up studies with animals suggested that this new, injectable form of GLA was only effective when injected directly into the tumor.

A recent randomized clinical trial found that a nutritional formula containing GLA was useful in patients with acute respiratory distress syndrome.

Are there any possible problems or complications?

Gamma linolenic acid does not appear to be toxic. However, it has been reported to aggravate temporal lobe epilepsy and should not be used by people who take anticonvulsant medication. Long-term use of GLA may lead to inflammation, thrombosis (blood clots), or decreased immune system functioning.

References

Fetrow CW, Avila JR. *Professional's Handbook of Complementary and Alternative Medicines.* Springhouse, Pa: Springhouse Corp; 1999.

Gadek JE, DeMichele SJ, Karlstad MD, et al. Effect of enteral feeding with eicosapentaenoic acid, gamma-linolenic acid, and antioxidants in patients with acute respiratory distress syndrome. Enteral Nutrition in ARDS study group. *Crit Care Med.* 1999;27:1409-1420.

Jiang WG, Bryce RP, Horrobin DF, Mansel RE. gamma-Linolenic acid blocks cell cycle progression by regulating phosphorylation of p27kip1 and p57kip2 and their interactions with other cycle regulators in cancer cells. *Int J Oncol.* 1998;13:611-617.

Keen H, Payan J, Allawi J, et al. Treatment of diabetic neuropathy with gamma-linolenic acid. The gamma-Linolenic Acid Multicenter Trial Group. *Diabetes Care.* 1993;16:8-15.

Kleijnen J. Evening primrose oil. *BMJ.* 1994;309:824-825.

Phinney S. Potential risk of prolonged gamma-linolenic acid use. *Ann Intern Med.* 1994;120:692.

Glucarate

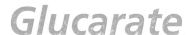

Other common name(s)	**Scientific/medical name(s)**
Calcium Glucarate, D-Glucarate™	D-Glucaric Acid

DESCRIPTION

Glucarate is a phytochemical (plant compound) found primarily in apples, grapefruit, broccoli, brussels sprouts, and bean sprouts (see Broccoli and Phytochemicals). It also occurs naturally in the body in very small amounts.

OVERVIEW

Several laboratory and animal studies found that glucarate has some preventative and anti-cancer effects; however, it has not yet been found to be effective in humans.

How is it promoted for use?

Proponents claim that glucarate supplements reduce the risk of colon, lung, liver, skin, and prostate cancer by increasing the body's ability to eliminate cancer-causing toxins that come from diet and the environment. Supporters also say that glucarate hinders the formation of breast and uterine cancers by removing excess estrogen and other hormones from the body that promote these diseases. These claims are under investigation.

What does it involve?

Glucarate supplements are available in capsules and tablets. There is no standardized dosage.

What is the history behind it?

In 1986, Zbigniew Walaszek, PhD, a cancer researcher, stated that glucarate supplements demonstrated anticancer properties in humans and animals. Dr.. Walaszek and other researchers have since conducted studies to evaluate the effects of glucarate.

What is the evidence?

Glucarate may have potential as an anticancer agent; however, there is no evidence yet to show that the supplement is effective in treating cancer or lowering cancer risk in humans. A number of animal studies published in peer-reviewed medical journals found that dietary glucarate caused rats to develop fewer breast cancer tumors, and shrank some existing tumors. Animal studies also found that dietary glucarate inhibited the development of tumors in the colon, lung, liver, skin, and prostate. These results suggest that dietary glucarate is worthy of further investigation to evaluate its possible role in preventing and treating cancer in humans.

Are there any possible problems or complications?

There are no known side effects associated with the use of glucarate.

References

Abou-Issa H, Moeschberger M, el-Masry W, Tejwani S, Curley RW Jr, Webb TE. Relative efficacy of glucarate on the initiation and promotion phases of rat mammary carcinogenesis. *Anticancer Res.* 1995;15:805-810.

Abou-Issa H, Koolemans-Beynen A, Meredity TA, Webb TE. Antitumour synergism between non-toxic dietary combinations of isotretinoin and glucarate. *Eur J Cancer.* 1992;28A:784-788.

Curley RW Jr, Humphries KA, Koolemans-Beynan A, Abou-Issa H, Webb TE. Activity of D-glucarate analogues: synergistic antiproliferative effects with retinoid in cultured human mammary tumor cells appear to specifically require the D-glucarate structure. *Life Sci.* 1994;54:1299-1303.

Dwivedi C, Oredipe OA, Barth RF, Downie AA, Webb TE. Effects of the experimental chemopreventive agent, glucarate, on intestinal carcinogenesis in rats. *Carcinogenesis.* 1989;10:1539-1541.

Heerdt AS, Young CW, Borgen Pl. Calcium glucarate as a chemopreventive agent in breast cancer. *Isr J Med Sci.* 1995;31:101-105.

Walaszek Z. Potential use of D-glucaric acid derivatives in cancer prevention. *Cancer Lett.* 1990;54:1-8.

Walaszek Z, Szemraj J, Narog M, et al. Metabolism, uptake, and excretion of a D-glucaric acid salt and its potential use in cancer prevention. *Cancer Detect Prev.* 1997;21:178-190.

Greek Cancer Cure

Other common name(s)	Scientific/medical name(s)
METBAL®, Cellbal®	None

DESCRIPTION

This treatment consists of a blood test reportedly used to diagnose cancer, and intravenous therapy designed to cure the disease. The injections are said to contain a combination of organic substances such as sugars, vitamins, amino acids, and other ingredients.

OVERVIEW

There is no scientific evidence that the Greek Cancer Cure is effective in preventing or treating cancer.

How is it promoted for use?

Practitioners of the Greek Cancer Cure claim the regular use of a special intravenous injection (which they refer to as a serum) boosts the patient's immune system, enabling it to fight and destroy tumor cells. The inventor of the Greek Cancer Cure claimed to have cured a high percentage of patients who had cancers of the skin, bone, uterus, stomach, and lymph system.

What does it involve?

The first stage of the Greek Cancer Cure is a blood test that is claimed to determine the nature, location, and seriousness of a patient's tumor. The second stage involves daily intravenous injections of the serum. Treatment lasts from 6 to 30 days. The secret formula is believed to consist of brown sugar, nicotinic acid (also known as niacin or vitamin B3), vitamin C, and alanine, an amino acid (see Amino Acids, Vitamin B Complex, and Vitamin C). An oral supplement is also available.

Patients are also advised to limit their intake of salts and acids, limit physical activities, and avoid drugs such as aspirin and laxatives. They are also asked to stop chemotherapy or radiation therapy before beginning the treatment program.

What is the history behind it?

The Greek Cancer Cure was developed in Athens, Greece during the 1970s by microbiologist Hariton-Tzannis Alivizatos, MD. Dr. Alivizatos was investigated by Greek regulatory officials several times. At one point he lost his license to practice medicine because he failed to submit a sample of his serum to the government for testing. His license was reinstated after he finally agreed, but the Greek government could not establish the serum's effectiveness against cancer and ordered him to stop giving it to patients.

In 1983, Dr. Alivizatos again lost his license, this time for two years, following an investigation by the Hellenic Medical Association. He resumed treating patients after the suspension expired.

On several occasions, the American Cancer Society and the National Cancer Institute asked Dr. Alivizatos to provide scientific documentation or information regarding his treatment, but all requests went unanswered. Throughout his career, Dr. Alivizatos closely guarded the details of his blood test and refused to share information with fellow cancer researchers. In 1979, a surgeon from Seattle traveled to Greece, posed as a cancer patient and underwent treatment by Dr. Alivizatos. He returned with samples of the serum. An analysis conducted at the University of Washington revealed that the formula contained only nicotinic acid and water. Dr. Alivizatos died in 1991. Today, his treatment is reportedly offered in Greece, Poland, and some clinics in North America.

What is the evidence?

There is no scientific evidence that the Greek Cancer Cure has any effect on cancer. No studies have shown that either the blood tests or the injections used in the Greek Cancer Cure result in any measurable benefit in the treatment of people with cancer.

Are there any possible problems or complications?

The safety of this treatment has not been proven. The intravenous serum can contain levels of nicotinic acid high enough to cause burning at the injection site. Relying on this type of treatment alone, and avoiding conventional medical care, may have serious health consequences.

References

American Cancer Society. Unproven Methods of Cancer Management. Greek Cancer Cure. CA Cancer J Clin. 1990;40:368-371.

Barrett S. Alivazatos Greek Cancer Cure. Quackwatch Web site. Available at http://www.quackwatch.com. Accessed May 10, 2000.

British Columbia Cancer Agency. Unconventional therapies: Greek cancer cure. British Columbia Cancer Agency Web site. Available http://www.bccancer.bc.ca/uctm/13.html. Accessed May 10, 2000.

Cancer Facts. Hariton-Tzannis Alivizatos Greek Cancer Cure. National Institutes of Health Web site. Available at: http://rex.nci.nih.gov/INFO_CANCER/Cancer_facts/Section9/FS9_2.html. Accessed May 10, 2000.

Homeopathy

Other common name(s)	Scientific/medical name(s)
Homeopathic Medicine	None

DESCRIPTION

Homeopathy is based on the idea that large doses of a substance cause a symptom, while very small doses of that same substance will cure it. Homeopathic remedies are water (and sometimes alcohol) solutions containing tiny amounts of various naturally occurring plants, minerals, animal products, or chemicals. The term "homeopathy" comes from the Greek words "homoios" (similar) and "pathos" (suffering or sickness).

OVERVIEW

There is no scientific evidence that homeopathic remedies are effective in treating cancer or any other disease.

How is it promoted for use?

Homeopathy is promoted for use to treat problems such as arthritis, asthma, colds, flu, and allergies. However, some advocates believe that homeopathy can be used to treat and cure cancer.

Some practitioners claim homeopathy can help cancer patients by decreasing pain, improving vitality and well being, stopping the spread of cancer, strengthening the immune system, and alleviating certain symptoms and side effects from radiation and chemotherapy such as infections, vomiting, nausea, hair loss, depression, weakness, and ascites (accumulation of serous fluid in peritoneal cavity). There is no scientific evidence to support any of these claims.

Proponents claim that homeopathic solutions, even though they may contain minuscule quantities of the original ingredient, contain a "memory" of the substance that somehow interacts with the body to cure illness. It is also believed that shaking or diluting a homeopathic solution releases the essence, or healing life force, of the material. Some practitioners compare homeopathy to the beliefs of Ayurvedic and traditional Chinese medicine which claim a

need to bring the body into balance in order to restore health and wellness (see Ayurvedia and Chinese Herbal Medicine). Many advocates of homeopathy admit that they do not know how the treatments work, but insist that future research will unlock the mystery.

What does it involve?

Homeopathy is based largely on the "law of similars," or the notion that "like cures like." In other words, a substance that causes symptoms of illness can relieve those same symptoms when administered in very small amounts. A patient complaining of vomiting and diarrhea might receive a solution containing tiny amounts of thorn apple, since larger amounts of that herb cause those symptoms.

When a patient complains of certain symptoms, the homeopath consults a reference guide, which lists thousands of individual symptoms, and searches for an entry that matches the patient's description. The remedy, which is determined by the person's symptoms, is called the "simillium." The practitioner then takes an extract of the plant, mineral, animal product, or chemical remedy that matches the patient's symptoms and repeatedly dilutes it in water. Every time the extract is diluted in water, a part of the diluted water is then added to another sample of water and so on until the final solution contains virtually none of the original extract. Each solution may go through the dilution process as many as 30 to 50 times. After the dilution process is complete, the patient is then given the remedy.

What is the history behind it?

The German physician Samuel Hahnemann developed homeopathy early in the 1800s as a more civilized alternative to some of the harsh medical practices of the time, such as bloodletting and purging. Dr. Hahnemann believed a substance that caused specific symptoms in a healthy person could cure those same symptoms in a sick person, so he gave his patients diluted doses of the offending substances.

To determine the specific effects of each material, Dr. Hahnemann and his assistants conducted "provings," during which they ingested plants, minerals, and other materials, then noted what symptoms resulted. From these experiments, Hahnemann compiled a reference book containing descriptions of the effects of various materials and the recommended homeopathic remedy. Today, homeopathy is popular as an alternative form of therapy in the United States.

What is the evidence?

There is no scientific evidence showing that homeopathic remedies possess any therapeutic value. Some researchers suggest, however, that homeopathy may result in beneficial effects for patients who believe the treatment is working–a phenomenon known as the placebo effect. A placebo is an inactive substance or treatment.

One study on the increased use of complementary therapies by people with cancer showed that while certain complementary therapies had no actual anti-tumor effect, patients reported psychological improvement including increased hope and optimism. The complementary therapies studied included homeopathy.

Are there any possible problems or complications?

Although some homeopathic solutions contain toxic chemicals, they are typically present in amounts too small to present any danger. Relying on this type of treatment alone, and avoiding conventional medical care, may have serious health consequences.

References

Bradley GW, Clover A. Apparent response of small cell lung cancer to an extract of mistletoe and homeopathic treatment. *Thorax.* 1989;44:1047-1048.

Cassileth B. *The Alternative Medicine Handbook.* New York, NY: W. W. Norton & Co; 1998.

Downer SM, Cody MM, McCluskey P, et al. Pursuit and practice of complementary therapies by cancer patients receiving conventional treatment. *BMJ.* 1994;309:86-89.

Holmes OW. Homeopathy and its kindred delusions. Quackwatch Web site. Available at: http://www.quackwatch.com. Accessed May 10, 2000.

Sampson W. Inconsistencies and errors in alternative medicine research. *Skeptical Inquirer.* September/October 1997;21:35-38.

Hydrazine Sulfate

Other common name(s)	Scientific/medical name(s)
None	None

DESCRIPTION

Hydrazine sulfate is a chemical commonly used in industrial processes, such as rare metal refining and the production of rocket fuel, rust-prevention products, and insecticides. It is used as an alternative method to treat some symptoms of advanced cancer. It is usually produced in a laboratory, but does occur naturally in tobacco plants, tobacco smoke, and in some mushrooms.

OVERVIEW

There is some conflicting research on hydrazine sulfate; however, most carefully designed studies have shown it does not help people with cancer live longer or feel better. It may also cause potentially serious side effects.

How is it promoted for use?

Proponents claim hydrazine sulfate may relieve cachexia, one of the most devastating syndromes resulting from cancer and other conditions such as AIDS. Cachexia occurs when cancer disrupts the body's metabolism, leading to progressive loss of appetite, weight loss, weakness, and muscle atrophy (wasting away). Cachexia affects about half of all cancer patients, especially those with advanced cancer of the lung, pancreas, or gastrointestinal system. It is responsible for 10% to 22% of all cancer deaths.

According to some theories, cancer cachexia is due to energy loss resulting from cancerous tumors taking energy from normal body functions, causing a kind of energy "short circuit." For example, energy that should be devoted to maintaining muscle mass is redirected to the tumor. Proponents claim that hydrazine sulfate may block a key enzyme in this process and restore the proper energy circuit, halting the progressive decline of cachexia.

What does it involve?

Hydrazine sulfate is usually given in pills or capsules. It can also be injected. A common dose is 60 mg 4 times/day for several days, then from 2 to 3 times/day for 35 to 40 days. Treatment is then stopped for 2 to 6 weeks and is sometimes repeated for up to 40 times.

Hydrazine sulfate is not approved for use with cancer patients in the United States. It can be obtained by physicians through the investigational new drug (IND) program of the FDA. In Canada, hydrazine sulfate is available by prescription. It is widely used in Europe, and in Russia, where it is known as Sehydrin.

What is the history behind it?

Hydrazine compounds have been studied for more than 90 years as a treatment for cancer and a therapy to reduce the symptoms associated with cancer such as weight loss, fatigue, muscle wasting, and decreased appetite. Hydrazine sulfate was popularized as an unconventional cancer treatment in the mid-1970s by a cancer researcher, Joseph Gold, MD, director of the Syracuse Cancer Research Institute in New York. He based his ideas on the research of Otto Warburg, a Nobel Prize winner in the

1930s. Dr. Gold reported that hydrazine sulfate inhibited the growth of tumors in rodents as well as in people with advanced cancer. He recommended its use for people with several kinds of cancer including breast, colorectal, ovary, lung, thyroid, Hodgkin's disease and other lymphomas, melanomas, and neuroblastomas. He believed it would be most effective if used alongside conventional methods.

Hydrazine sulfate was a popular alternative cancer treatment until the FDA stopped the company from selling it directly to the public in the mid-1970s.

What is the evidence?

Studies show that hydrazine sulfate has many effects in the body. However, research has produced conflicting results. Some studies have found that hydrazine sulfate inhibits the growth of cancerous tumors in laboratory animals, while others report that the chemical can damage DNA and trigger the development of tumors. It also may promote the growth of existing tumors.

Research in humans has not been encouraging. Several randomized clinical trials found that hydrazine sulfate treatment did not reduce the size of tumors, or increase patient survival time. Some patients reported feeling better for brief periods during treatment with hydrazine sulfate including experiencing less pain, lower fever, and increased appetite. Other studies reported that patients treated with the chemical had more normal glucose metabolism, weight gain, and improved appetite. Some patients experienced feelings of euphoria that developed after nearly six months of therapy.

A 1990 study of 65 patients with inoperable lung cancer found that adding hydrazine sulfate to a combination chemotherapy treatment improved patient's nutritional status. Patients were able to consume more calories and showed other positive metabolic changes. Among patients who started the study in better condition, those given hydrazine sulfate lived longer than those taking a placebo. Among those who started in worse condition, hydrazine sulfate did not improve survival. Based on this

study, the National Cancer Institute (NCI) felt that additional studies involving more patients were needed.

Reports published in 1994, based on three studies sponsored by NCI, described treatment involving a total of 636 patients who had advanced lung cancer, colon cancer, or leukemia and who received hydrazine sulfate along with their chemotherapy regimen. None of these well-controlled studies showed that hydrazine sulfate provided any benefit to cancer patients. Nerve damage occurred more often and the quality of life was significantly worse among the group receiving hydrazine sulfate. After the studies were published, proponents of hydrazine sulfate claimed that the studies were flawed. However, a review by the US General Accounting Office, a federal agency, confirmed that the studies were done correctly and that their conclusions were valid.

Are there any possible problems or complications?

Side effects are uncommon, but include mild to moderate levels of nausea, vomiting, itching, dizziness, poor motor coordination, and/or tingling or numbness in the hands and feet. Hydrazine sulfate should not be taken with tranquilizers, barbiturates, alcohol, or foods high in tyramine (eg, aged cheeses and fermented products). Liver damage can be caused by very high doses (ie, over 20 times the regular dose). Women who are pregnant or breast-feeding should not use this therapy.

References

Chlebowski RT, Bulcavage L, Grosvenor M, et al. Hydrazine sulfate influence on nutritional status and survival in non-small-cell lung cancer. *J Clin Oncol.* 1990;8:9-15.

Kaegi E. Unconventional therapies for cancer: 4. Hydrazine sulfate. Task Force on Alternative Therapies of the Canadian Breast Cancer Research Initiative. *CMAJ.* 1998;158:1327-1330.

Kosty MP, Fleishman SB, Herndon JE II, et al. Cisplatin, vinblastine, and hydrazine sulfate in advanced, non-small-cell lung cancer: a randomized placebo-controlled, double-blind phase

III study of the Cancer and Leukemia Group B. *J Clin Oncol.* 1994;12:1113-1120.

Loprinzi CL, Kuross SA, O'Fallon JR, et al. Randomized placebo-controlled evaluation of hydrazine sulfate in patients with advanced colorectal cancer. *J Clin Oncol.* 1994;12:1121-1125.

Loprinzi CL, Goldberg RM, Su JQ, et al. Placebo-controlled trial of hydrazine sulfate in patients with newly diagnosed non-small-cell lung cancer. *J Clin Oncol.*1994;12:1126-1129.

National Cancer Institute PDQ. Complementary/Alternative medicine: hydrazine sulfate. National Cancer Institute Cancernet Web site. Available at: http://cancernet.nci.nih.gov/cam/hydrazine.htm. Accessed May 10, 2000

Tisdale MJ. Biology of cachexia. *J Natl Cancer Inst.* 1997;89:1763-1773.

University of Texas Center for Alternative Medicine Research in Cancer. Hydrazine sulfate summary. University of Texas-Houston Health Science Center Web site. Available at: http://www.sph.uth.tmc.edu/utcam/summary/hydrazine.htm. Accessed May 10, 2000.

US Congress, Office of Technology Assessment. *Unconventional Cancer Treatments.* Washington, DC: US Government Printing Office; 1990. Publication OTA-H-405.

Hydrogen Peroxide Therapy

Other common name(s)	Scientific/medical name(s)
Hydrogen Peroxide	H_2O_2

DESCRIPTION

Hydrogen peroxide is a clear, odorless oxygen solution that is widely available for use in cleaning and disinfecting wounds. In high concentrations (eg, 35%), hydrogen peroxide is used by alternative practitioners as a treatment for cancer and other diseases.

OVERVIEW

Although hydrogen peroxide is well known for its antiseptic properties, there is no evidence that it has value as a treatment for cancer or other diseases. It can be toxic at concentrations above 10%.

How is it promoted for use?

Proponents claim that hydrogen peroxide therapy can be used to oxidize toxins, kill bacteria and viruses, and stimulate the immune system. It is promoted for everything from cleansing the digestive tract to curing cancer and other diseases such as arthritis. Some people advocate cleaning foods with it prior to eating.

Supporters of hydrogen peroxide therapy believe that cancer cells grow rapidly if they are deprived of oxygen. They claim that hydrogen peroxide can cure cancer by bombarding cancer cells with more oxygen than they can handle (see Oxygen Therapy).

What does it involve?

Hydrogen peroxide is used internally or injected. Some practitioners promote it for use rectally, vaginally, as a nasal spray, and as eardrops. It is often used to soak affected parts of the body. The stronger solution recommended by alternative medicine practitioners (about 35%) are sold in some health food stores.

Because of its antiseptic and whitening properties, hydrogen peroxide is found in some toothpastes and mouthwashes, usually at a 3% (or less) solution. In stronger solutions of about 10%, it is used as hair bleach, and in industry to bleach paper and cloth, to manufacture other chemicals, and as an ingredient in some rocket fuels.

What is the history behind it?

One of the earliest accounts of the scientific study of hydrogen peroxide was a short article by I.N. Love, MD, in 1888 in the *Journal of the American Medical Association*. Dr. Love reported that the hydrogen peroxide was useful in treating diseases such as scarlet fever, diphtheria, cancer of the uterus, and pneumonia. In 1920, hydrogen peroxide injections were used to treat patients during an epidemic of viral pneumonia.

Many promoters base their claims on the ideas of Otto Warburg, a Nobel Prize winner in the 1930s. His theory was that cancer cells grow better under conditions where there are lower levels of oxygen. Contemporary use of hydrogen peroxide can be traced to Father Richard Wilhelm, a retired high school teacher and former Army chaplain. He claimed to have discovered the healing potential of hydrogen peroxide through acquaintance with a physician who headed the Mayo Clinic's division of experimental bacteriology, Edward Carl Rosenow, MD.

What is the evidence?

Medical researchers have studied hydrogen peroxide for over a century to determine if it can cure various diseases. In the 1940s, hydrogen peroxide was tested on animals to see if it could treat carbon monoxide poisoning, hemorrhage, and toxic reactions of exposure to certain chemicals. During the next three decades, many researchers studied the effects of hydrogen peroxide on tumors in laboratory animals. When used alone, hydrogen peroxide was not effective.

Some have investigated it as an addition to radiation therapy. Although some patients appeared to benefit, many did not. Attempts to treat patients with hydrogen peroxide injections directly into solid tumors or into the blood system have generally been ineffective. There is currently no scientific evidence that hydrogen peroxide therapy is effective for treating any of the conditions that have been claimed.

Are there any possible problems or complications?

Hydrogen peroxide can be harmful if swallowed. Drinking the concentrated solutions sold in some health food stores (35%) can cause vomiting, severe burns of the throat and stomach, and even death. Direct skin contact or breathing the vapors of hydrogen peroxide can also be harmful.

Hydrogen peroxide injections can have dangerous side effects. High blood levels of hydrogen peroxide create oxygen bubbles that can block blood flow and cause gangrene and death. Acute hemolytic crisis (destruction of blood cells) has also been reported following intravenous injection of hydrogen peroxide. Women who are pregnant or breast-feeding should not use this method.

References

American Cancer Society. Questionable methods of cancer management: hydrogen peroxide and other 'hyperoxygenation' therapies. *CA Cancer J Clin.* 1993;43:47-56.

Cassileth B. *The Alternative Medicine Handbook.* New York, NY: W. W. Norton & Co; 1998.

Cina SJ, Downs JC, Conradi SE. Hydrogen peroxide: a source of lethal oxygen embolism. Case report and review of the literature. *Am J Forensic Med Pathol.* 1994;15:44-50.

Green S. Hyperoxygenation Therapy. Healthcare Reality Check Web site. Available at: http://www.hcrc.org//faqs/hyperox.html. Accessed October 19, 1999.

Hirschtick RE, Dyrda SE, Peterson LC. Death from an unconventional therapy for AIDS. *Ann Intern Med.* 1994;120:694.

Pharmacological / Biological

Murphy GP, Morris LB, Lange D. *Informed Decisions: The Complete Book of Cancer Diagnosis, Treatment, and Recovery.* New York, NY: Viking; 1997.

Sherman SJ, Boyer LV, Sibley WA. Cerebral infarction immediately after ingestion of hydrogen peroxide solution. *Stroke.* 1994;25:1065-1067.

US Congress, Office of Technology Assessment. *Unconventional Cancer Treatments.* Washington, DC: US Government Printing Office, 1990. Publication OTA-H-405.

Immuno-Augmentive Therapy

Other common name(s)	Scientific/medical name(s)
IAT	None

DESCRIPTION
Immuno-augmentative therapy (IAT) is promoted as an alternative form of cancer treatment involving daily injections of a protein mixture made from blood in an attempt to restore normal immune function. Components of the blood products are claimed to contain three tumor antibodies and deblocking proteins, all from healthy donors.

OVERVIEW
There is no scientific evidence that IAT is effective in treating cancer. The IAT serum has not been tested for safety according to widely accepted medical standards.

How is it promoted for use?
Proponents claim IAT causes cancer to stabilize or go into remission. It is not promoted as a cure for cancer, but as a life-long treatment of daily injections. Like diabetics, IAT patients are told that they can live normal lives as long as they continue their daily injections.

Practitioners of IAT believe that cancer cells begin to grow and multiply when a person's immune system is weakened or out of balance. Tumor antibodies attack the cancer and the deblocking proteins remove a "blocking factor" that prevents the patient's immune system from detecting the cancer. Proponents further claim IAT is a safe, non-toxic, and effective treatment for all types of cancer.

What does it involve?
This therapy involves daily self-injections of a protein mixture made from human blood. The initial IAT session requires a trip to an IAT facility. At the facility, a patient is given a physical exam, blood tests, and urinalysis. Once the patient's immune system status is determined, the IAT treatment begins. Patients are given IAT drugs according to their particular situation. Treatment continues until the practitioner determines that the patient's cancer is controlled. The average stay is 10 to 12 weeks. The patient is then shown how to self-inject and is sent home to continue treatment.

Pharmacological / Biological

What is the history behind it?

A zoologist, Lawrence Burton, PhD, developed the theory of IAT in the 1950s, while working at the California Institute of Technology. Based on his research with fruit flies and mice, he developed a mixture of blood proteins that he believed would slow or stop the growth of cancer cells. He claimed that IAT caused cancer in mice to go into remission. The results of these experiments were questioned and the study could not be repeated by other researchers.

Dr. Burton first offered his treatment to cancer patients in 1973, when he established the Immunology Research Foundation in Great Neck, NY. In 1974, Dr. Burton submitted an investigational new drug (IND) application to the Food and Drug Administration (FDA) in order to begin human trials with IAT. He later withdrew his application when the FDA began asking questions about his experimental evidence.

In 1977, Dr. Burton closed his New York Clinic and opened the Immunology Researching Center in the Bahamas. In 1978, representatives of the Bahamian Ministry of Health and the Pan American Health Organization visited his facility and reviewed the charts of several patients. The report filed by these representatives concluded that there was no evidence that IAT was beneficial and recommended that the clinic be closed. They found violations of the conditions for patient admission, treatment, and evaluation. They also could not determine the components of the IAT treatment and found no record of patient survival rates from cancer after treatment with IAT. The clinic remained open despite these findings. In 1985, Bahamian health authorities closed the clinic on charges that the compounds used for IAT injections may have been contaminated with hepatitis virus and HIV. The clinic reopened less than a year later. A decade later Dr. Burton opened additional clinics in West Germany and Mexico.

During the late 70s and early 80s, National Cancer Institute (NCI) officials contacted Dr. Burton asking to evaluate his IAT techniques. No agreement could be reached on research methods and Dr. Burton never disclosed his technique for isolating the blood proteins in IAT, which he had patented. In 1986, the Office of Technology Assessment (OTA), working with Dr. Burton, developed procedures for a clinical trial of IAT on patients with colon cancer. Communication between Dr. Burton and the OTA eventually broke down and the OTA's final report stated that "no reliable data are available on which to base a determination of IAT's efficacy."

The FDA imposed a ban on the import of IAT drugs in 1986 over concerns about the potential contamination of IAT drugs with hepatitis and HIV. Although Dr. Burton died in 1993, his clinics continue to operate.

What is the evidence?

There is no evidence to support claims that IAT has any beneficial effects for people with cancer. Success stories associated with the treatment are based on anecdotal reports provided by Dr. Burton's clinics, and they include little or no supporting evidence.

A contract between Dr. Burton and MetPath, a large biomedical laboratory firm, was terminated because their scientists did not identify and were unable to measure a substance Burton claimed was present. A research team from the University of Pennsylvania Cancer Center collected data on 79 patients who received IAT at Dr. Burton's clinic. Based on the available data, they could make no meaningful comparisons between IAT patients and those treated with conventional cancer treatment. They suggested that a well-controlled prospective study was needed.

The concept that cancer can be treated by enhancing activity of the immune system is reasonable, and is the basis for conventional immunotherapy. Unlike IAT, conventional immunotherapy, founded on scientific principles of immunology and evaluated by randomized clinical trials, has been useful in treating melanoma, lymphoma, kidney cancer, bladder cancer, and others.

Pharmacological / Biological

Are there any possible problems or complications?

The safety of IAT has not been established. Based on anecdotal reports from patients who have received IAT, side effects appear to be minor and include fatigue, pain at the injection site, and flu-like symptoms. Some medical professionals fear infectious agents, such as HIV and hepatitis virus, may contaminate the unregulated compounds used in IAT, which come from human blood. Relying on this type of treatment, and avoiding conventional medical care, may have serious health consequences.

References

Alternative Medicine: Expanding Medical Horizons. *A Report to the National Institutes of Health on Alternative Medical Systems and Practices in the United States.* Washington, DC: US Government Printing Office; 1994. NIH publication 94-066.

American Cancer Society. Questionable methods of cancer management. Immuno-augmentative therapy (IAT). *CA Cancer J Clin.* 1991;41:357-364.

Cassileth B. *The Alternative Medicine Handbook.* New York, NY: W. W. Norton & Co; 1998.

Green S. Immunoaugmentative therapy. An unproven cancer treatment. *JAMA.* 1993;70:1719-1723.

Murphy GP, Morris LB, Lange D. *Informed Decisions: The Complete Book of Cancer Diagnosis, Treatment, and Recovery.* New York, NY: Viking; 1997.

University of Texas Center for Alternative Medicine Research in Cancer. Immune augmentation therapy summary. University of Texas-Houston Health Science Center Web site. Available at: http://www.sph.uth.tmc.edu/utcam/therapies/immune.htm. Accessed May 10, 2000.

US Congress, Office of Technology Assessment. *Unconventional Cancer Treatments.* Washington, DC: US Government Printing Office; 1990. Publication OTA-H-405.

Inosine Pranobex

Other common name(s)	Scientific/medical name(s)
Isoprinosine®, Methisoprinol, Inosiplex, Imunovir®	None

DESCRIPTION

Inosine pranobex is a substance that may mimic the actions of immune stimulating hormones produced in the thymus gland.

OVERVIEW

There is no scientific evidence that inosine pranobex is effective in treating cancer. Experimental data suggests that it may help boost the immune system, however, more studies in humans are needed to determine the benefits. The drug cannot be sold legally in the United States.

How is it promoted for use?

Proponents claim inosine pranobex strengthens the immune system and fights viral infections.

They also say it decreases the risk of infection in people with cancer who undergo chemotherapy, radiation therapy, or surgery, all of which suppress the immune system. Some assert that inosine pranobex intensifies the effects of the anticancer drug interferon and increases the activity of natural killer cells (a type of white blood cell) which can help stop tumors from growing. Some practitioners recommend it as an alternative to conventional cancer therapy. It is also used to treat people with AIDS and other viral diseases, including herpes, shingles, viral hepatitis, influenza, the common cold, and viral encephalitis, although there is not enough clinical evidence to prove its effectiveness.

What does it involve?

Inosine pranobex is administered in 500 mg capsules. Some studies have used a dosage of 3 g/day for 28 days.

What is the history behind it?

Inosine pranobex was introduced about 30 years ago. In 1981, the FDA refused to allow the drug to be marketed in the United States. Today it is sold in Europe and other countries as a treatment for a number of viral diseases including herpes, influenza A, and viral hepatitis.

What is the evidence?

In a large clinical study conducted in Sweden and Denmark researchers concluded that inosine pranobex delays the onset of AIDS in people with HIV infection. However, the FDA pointed out several important flaws in the study and said that more clinical investigation of inosine pranobex is needed before its value for HIV-infected patients can be sufficiently evaluated. The agency added that this and other studies have not demonstrated that the drug slows the progression of HIV.

A French study found no differences in survival or recurrence rates between 60 patients treated with surgery alone and another 60 treated with surgery plus inosine pranobex. In another, much smaller study, researchers concluded that inosine pranobex combined with the chemotherapy drug 5-fluorouracil was not effective in the treatment of metastatic colorectal cancer.

A European study found that inosine pra-

nobex did not protect children against the development of respiratory infections. There is also no clinical evidence showing that inosine pranobex enhances the effects of interferon.

A number of animal and laboratory studies conducted mostly in Europe have found that inosine pranobex increases T helper lymphocytes and natural killer cell activity, which may inhibit the growth of tumors. Animal and laboratory studies may show a certain therapy holds promise as a beneficial treatment, but further studies are necessary to determine if the results apply to humans.

Some studies suggest inosine pranobex may be useful as a treatment for genital warts.

Are there any possible problems or complications?

Not enough is known about inosine pranobex to make conclusions about its safety. Possible side effects include stomach upset and heartburn.

References

Colozza M, Tonato M, Belsanti V, et al. 5-Fluorouracil and isoprinosine in the treatment of advanced colorectal cancer. A limited phase I, II evaluation. *Cancer*. 1988;15:1049-1052.

Isoprinosine update. US Food and Drug Administration Web site. Available at: http://www.fda.gov. Accessed October 8, 1999.

Litzman J, Lokaj J, Krejci M, Pesak S, Morgan G. Isoprinosine does not protect against frequent respiratory tract infections in childhood. *Eur J Pediatr*. 1999;158:32-37.

Pedersen C, Sandstrom E, Petersen CS, et al. The efficacy of inosine pranobex in preventing the acquired immunodeficiency syndrome in patients with human immunodeficiency virus infection. The Scandinavian Isoprinosine Study Group. *N Engl J Med*. 1990;322:1757-1763.

Roeslin N, Dumont P, Morand G, Wihlm JM, Witz JP. Immunotherapy as an adjuvant to surgery in carcinoma of bronchus. Results in three randomised trials. *Eur J Cardiothorac Surg*. 1989;3:430-435.

US National Library of Medicine. Inosine pranobex. AEGIS Web site. Available at http://ww2.aegis.com/pubs/drugs/257.html. Accessed March 23, 2000.

Krebiozen

Other common name(s)	Scientific/medical name(s)
Carcalon, Creatine	None

DESCRIPTION

Krebiozen is the commercial name of an alternative cancer formula originally prepared from the blood of horses that have been injected with bacteria. An analysis by several federal agencies later found Krebiozen to contain mineral oil and a form of creatine. Creatine is a substance that naturally occurs in the human body and is sold as a dietary supplement.

OVERVIEW

There is no scientific evidence that Krebiozen is effective in treating cancer or any other disease. According to the FDA, creatine has been associated with several dangerous side effects.

How is it promoted for use?

Proponents have claimed that Krebiozen cures cancer. They have cited private experiments claiming that Krebiozen stops tumor growth in mice and induces recovery in some people with advanced cancer.

What does it involve?

Krebiozen has been manufactured in powder and liquid forms. The liquid form of Krebiozen is combined with mineral oil and delivered through injection.

What is the history behind it?

Krebiozen was originally developed by Stevan Durovic, a Yugoslavian physician, in Argentina, and brought to the United States in 1949. It drew the attention of Dr. Andrew C. Ivy, at the University of Illinois, who began producing his own version of the drug in mid-1959, calling it Carcalon. Ivy privately published two monographs claiming extensive anti-cancer benefits. Krebiozen therapy grew in popularity during the 1950s and early 1960s.

Durovic claimed his original powder was obtained as an extract from the blood of 2,000 Argentinian horses that had been previously injected with an extract of *Actinomyces bovis*, a microorganism. However, in September 1963, the US Department of Health, Education, and Welfare announced that both government and independent scientists had identified the Krebiozen powder given to the FDA by both Ivy and Durovic as creatine. Later, the FDA found that the Krebiozen solution administered through injection contained no creatine, or any other substance except mineral oil.

Ivy and several colleagues were indicted on a number of criminal charges, including mail fraud, and found guilty, but they were ultimately acquitted on appeal. Although supporters expressed their enthusiasm quite vigorously during this period through protests and sit-ins, the Krebiozen boom ultimately collapsed. It is rarely used today.

What is the evidence?

Federal government agencies that conducted a thorough investigation of Krebiozen concluded that it had no anticancer activity in humans. This conclusion was drawn by a committee of 24 scientists, who studied the completed medical records of 504 cases submitted by the Krebiozen Research Foundation. Following the investigation, the National Cancer Institute agreed, saying that it saw no justification for a clinical trial, and that from a scientific standpoint the case was "closed."

Are there any possible problems or complications?

There is no information on the safety of Krebiozen. However, creatine supplements have been associated with some adverse reactions including vomiting, diarrhea, seizure, anxiety, myopathy (muscle tissue disorder), irregular heartbeat, blood clots, and even death.

References

American Cancer Society. Unproven methods of cancer management. Krebiozen and carcalon. *CA Cancer J Clin.* 1973;23:111-115.

British Columbia Cancer Agency. Unconventional cancer therapies: manual for patients. British Columbia Cancer Agency Web site. Available at: http://www.bccancer.bc.ca/uctm/22.html. Accessed September 8, 1999.

Holland JF. The Krebiozen Story. Quackwatch Web site. Available at: http://www.quackwatch.com. Accessed March 23, 2000.

Jallut O, Guex P, Barrelet L. Unproven methods in oncology. *Sweiz Med Wochenschr.* 1984;114:1214-1220.

Lullinski B. Creatine Supplementation. Quackwatch Web site. Available at: http://www.quackwatch.com. Accessed March 23, 2000.

The SN/AEMS Web Report. Creatine search. US Food and Drug Administration Center for Food Safety and Applied Nutrition Web site. Available at: http://vm.cfsan.fda.gov. Accessed March 23, 2000.

US Congress, Office of Technology Assessment. *Unconventional Cancer Treatments.* Washington, DC: US Government Printing Office; 1990. Publication OTA-H-405.

Laetrile

Other common name(s)	Scientific/medical name(s)
Amygdalin, Vitamin B_{17}	None

DESCRIPTION

Laetrile is a compound produced from amygdalin, a naturally occurring substance found primarily in the kernels of apricots, peaches, and almonds.

OVERVIEW

There is no scientific evidence that Laetrile is effective in treating cancer or any other disease. It contains a small percentage of cyanide and several cases of cyanide poisoning have been linked to its use. The FDA has not issued approval for Laetrile as a medical treatment and its use is illegal in the United States.

How is it promoted for use?

Laetrile was once called "the perfect chemotherapeutic agent" since it was alleged to selectively kill cancer cells while being non-toxic to normal cells. Promoters claim that societies with diets rich in Laetrile, such as the Hunza and the Karakorum, are "cancer-free peoples." Supporters also say that Laetrile can prevent cancer from occurring and can help patients stay in remission. It is also promoted to provide pain relief to people with cancer. Other reported uses for Laetrile have been in the prevention and treatment of high blood pressure and arthritis.

There are two proposed explanations for Laetrile's use. Proponents claim that cancer cells trigger the release of the cyanide found in Laetrile, causing the death of the cancer cells due to cyanide poisoning. The second theory proposed for Laetrile's effectiveness is that cancer is really a "vitamin deficiency" and that Laetrile is the missing "vitamin B-17." There is no scientific evidence to support these claims.

What does it involve?

Laetrile is most commonly extracted from apricot pits. It is usually taken as part of a metabolic therapy involving a specific diet with high doses of other vitamins (see Metabolic Therapy). Although no standard treatment plan for Laetrile therapy exists, a typical treatment consists of daily intravenous administration for 2 to 3 weeks, followed by the use of oral tablets as a maintenance therapy. Laetrile is also used in enemas and in solutions applied directly to skin lesions.

Laetrile treatments may cost thousands of dollars per week and can only be obtained from some hospitals in Mexico because it is illegal in the United States.

What is the history behind it?

"Bitter almonds" have been used for thousands of years by cultures as diverse as the ancient Egyptians, Chinese, and Pueblo Indians as a medical remedy. In 1802, a chemist discovered that the distillation of the water from bitter almonds released hydrocyanic acid. In the 1830s, the source of this hydrocyanic acid was purified and called amygdalin. It was thought to be the active ingredient in bitter almonds.

The current use of Laetrile can be directly attributed to the theories of Ernst T. Krebs, Sr., MD, first made in the 1920s. Around 1952, his son, Ernst T. Krebs, Jr., modified the extraction process of amygdalin from apricot pits and named the product Laetrile. He claimed that the new extract was more potent as an anticancer drug than previously believed. So, what is actually used in Laetrile is amygdalin, and these terms are used interchangeably in many reports.

Beginning in 1957, Laetrile was repeatedly tested against tumor cells implanted in animals. At least a dozen separate sets of experiments were done at seven institutions. Targets included carcinoma, leukemia, sarcoma, lymphoma, and melanoma cells. No anti-tumor activity was found in any of these studies with the use of Laetrile.

In 1971, the FDA placed sanctions against the sale of Laetrile. In 1977, the FDA commissioner stated that there was no evidence for the safety or effectiveness of Laetrile. Due to the risk of cyanide poisoning, the FDA has banned the use of Laetrile.

What is the evidence?

During the 1970s, Laetrile achieved great popularity in the United States as an alternative anticancer therapy. For this reason, despite the lack of scientific evidence for the efficacy of Laetrile, the National Cancer Institute (NCI) evaluated it in 1978 through a retrospective case review. A clinical trial of Laetrile was also performed between 1979 and 1982 at medical centers around the country. Both studies found that Laetrile provided no significant benefit to people with cancer.

In contrast to the findings by the NCI, one of the leading proponents of Laetrile's use claims to have treated nearly 30,000 cancer patients in Phase I, II, and III studies of the drug with promising results. However, these results have not been reviewed nor repeated by the scientific medical community.

There is no scientific evidence that Laetrile is effective as an anti-cancer treatment, either in animal studies or in clinical trials. Cancer cells do not trigger the release of cyanide making them more susceptible to the effects of Laetrile. All of the successes claimed by its supporters are based on anecdotal reports, testimonials, and publicity issued by promoters.

Are there any possible problems or complications?

The use of Laetrile has been directly linked to cyanide toxicity and death in a few cases.

This treatment should be avoided, especially by women who are pregnant or breast-feeding. Relying on this type of treatment alone, and avoiding conventional medical care, may have serious health consequences.

References

American Cancer Society. Unproven methods of cancer management. Laetrile. *CA Cancer J Clin.* 1991;41:187-192.

Ellison NM, Byar DP, Newell GR. Special report on Laetrile: the NCI Laetrile review. Results of the National Cancer Institute's retrospective Laetrile analysis. *N Engl J Med.* 1978;299:549-552.

Fetrow CW, Avila JR. *Professional's Handbook of Complementary and Alternative Medicines.* Springhouse, Pa: Springhouse Corp; 1999.

Moertel CG, Fleming TR, Rubin J, et al. A clinical trial of amygdalin (Laetrile) in the treatment of human cancer. *N Engl J Med.* 1982;306:201-206.

Wilson B. The rise and fall of laetrile. Quackwatch Web site. Available at: http://www.quackwatch.com. Accessed May 8, 2000.

Lipoic Acid

Other common name(s)	Scientific/medical name(s)
Alpha-Lipoic Acid	None

DESCRIPTION

Lipoic acid is an antioxidant found in certain foods, including red meat, spinach, broccoli, potatoes, yams, carrots, beets, and yeast (see Broccoli).

OVERVIEW

Lipoic acid is an antioxidant that plays an important role in metabolism. Recent research has shown that it is beneficial in treating nerve damage in diabetics. There is currently no evidence that lipoic acid prevents the development or spread of cancer.

How is it promoted for use?

Lipoic acid is an antioxidant that is promoted to protect the body against cancer and other diseases. An antioxidant is a compound that blocks the action of activated oxygen molecules, known as free radicals, that can damage cells. Oxidation may also play a role in causing poor health as people age, and some researchers claim that lipoic acid is beneficial to maintaining good health in old age. The nutrient has been used to treat diabetic polyneuropathy, a nerve disease found in many diabetics that causes pain and numbness in the hands and feet. In addition to treating nerve damage in diabetics, researchers claim lipoic acid also lowers blood sugar levels.

Promoted as the most powerful and versatile of all the antioxidants, including vitamin E and vitamin C, lipoic acid is claimed to strengthen the effects of other antioxidants and regenerate antioxidants used up in the fight against free radicals (see Vitamin C and Vitamin E). Some proponents believe that lipoic acid may inhibit the gene that triggers cancer cells to grow; however, there is no scientific evidence to support these claims.

What does it involve?
A healthy diet that includes meat and vegetables containing lipoic acid is the best source of this nutrient. The body also produces lipoic acid naturally. As a person ages, his or her body produces less lipoic acid.

Supplements are available in health food stores and on the Internet, but high doses of any antioxidant supplement may actually cause cell damage. A safe and effective dosage of this supplement has not been established.

What is the history behind it?
In 1937, scientists found certain bacteria contained a compound that was later characterized as lipoic acid. The value of lipoic acid as an antioxidant has been known and studied since 1939. In 1957, lipoic acid was isolated and characterized as a compound found in yeast extracts.

What is the evidence?
In a recent review article, researchers reported that a number of experimental studies and clinical trials over the past five years have found alpha-lipoic acid to be useful in treating nerve problems in diabetics and can improve insulin sensitivity in people with type-2 diabetes. They also suggested that it might be useful in liver disease as well. Laboratory and animal studies have found that alpha-lipoic acid is beneficial in treating stroke, cataract formation, HIV infection, nerve degeneration, and radiation injury. There are no scientific studies, however, showing that lipoic acid supplements will directly prevent the development or progression of cancer.

Are there any possible problems or complications?

Lipoic acid found naturally in foods is safe. Research has shown that 300-600 mg of lipoic acid a day may be safely taken with no side effects. Extremely high doses of lipoic acid supplements, however, may damage cells and should be avoided.

References
Ames BN. Micronutrients prevent cancer and delay aging. *Toxicol Lett.* 1998;102-103:5-18.

Bustamante J, Lodge JK, Marcocci L, Tritschler HJ, Packer L, Rihn BH. Alpha-lipoic acid in liver metabolism and disease. *Free Radic Biol Med.* 1998;24:1023-1039.

Carper J. The 5 most important antioxidants. Start taking these supplements when you're young and healthy-and stay that way! *USA Weekend (Final Edition).* April 4, 1999;8.

Fremerman S. Alpha-lipoic acid. *Natural Health.* 1998;27:151.

Han D, Sen CK, Roy S, Kobayashi MS, Tritschler HJ, Packer L. Protection against glutamate-induced cytotoxicity in C6 glial cells by thiol antioxidants. *Am J Physiol.* 1997;273:R1771-1778.

Packer L, Witt EH, Tritschler HJ. alpha-Lipoic acid as a biological antioxidant. *Free Radic Biol Med.* 1995;19:227-250.

Liver Flush

Other common name(s)	Scientific/medical name(s)
None	None

DESCRIPTION / OVERVIEW

This method is used by alternative medicine practitioners to detoxify or drive "harmful" chemicals out of the liver. A liver flush involves eating or drinking a combination of specially selected herbs, enzymes, juices, and oils. Liver flush formulas vary widely by practitioner and are also available commercially. Some practitioners advise combining liver flushes with fasting (see Fasting). Proponents claim that liver flushing rids the organ of unwanted food by-products, fats, and toxins, therefore inhibiting the formation of diseases, including cancer. They also claim that because the liver is an important hormone regulator, cleansing it will aid conditions caused by hormone imbalances. There is no scientific evidence to support any of the claims made for liver flushes. Individual components of the herbal mixtures used in a liver flush may present health hazards. Relying on this type of treatment alone, and avoiding conventional medical care, may have serious health consequences.

Livingston-Wheeler Therapy

Other common name(s)	Scientific/medical name(s)
None	None

DESCRIPTION

Livingston-Wheeler therapy is an alternative cancer method that includes vaccines, antibiotics, vitamin and mineral supplements, digestive enzymes, cleansing enemas, and a vegetarian diet (see Colon Therapy, Enzyme Therapy, Vegetarianism, and the Chapter on Herbs, Vitamins, and Minerals).

OVERVIEW

There is no scientific evidence that Livingston-Wheeler therapy is effective in treating cancer or any other disease.

How is it promoted for use?

Livingston-Wheeler therapy is promoted primarily for use in the treatment of cancer but it is also used to treat lupus, arthritis, and other chronic conditions. In the case of cancer, proponents believe that when the body's immune system weakens, it allows the spread of a bacterium named *Progenitor cryptocides* to cause cancer. Because practitioners claim Livingston-Wheeler therapy is a form of immunotherapy (a treatment that stimulates a person's immune system), they claim it can boost the immune system to help a person fight off serious illnesses like cancer. There is no evidence to support these claims.

What does it involve?

Livingston-Wheeler therapy is administered only at one facility in the United States. Patients enter a 10-day treatment program, which can be very expensive and requires home treatment as well. Follow-up visits to the clinic are also encouraged.

At the clinic, patients are evaluated and given standard blood and urine tests. Special hormone, liver function, and tumor marker tests are also done. The patient's immune system is also tested in order to design a personalized immune-enhancement vaccine. In addition to the vaccine, the patient may be given antibiotics, nutritional supplements, digestive enzymes, bile salts, enemas, laxatives, and blood transfusions. A strict vegetarian diet is enforced and the patient participates in group or support therapy (see Support Groups).

What is the history behind it?

During the 1950s, Virginia Livingston, MD (who later remarried and became Livingston-Wheeler), developed a theory that cancer was caused by a bacterium (*Progenitor cryptocides*) that becomes activated in the body when the immune system is weakened or under great stress. Based on her theory, she designed a complex treatment to reduce the amount of bacteria in the body so the immune system could fight the cancer. She and her husband, Dr. A.M. Livingston, opened the Livingston Clinic in San Diego in 1969. Following her husband's death, she married Dr. Owen Wheeler, one of her former cancer patients. The clinic was renamed the Livingston-Wheeler clinic in 1976. From 1969 to 1984, it is estimated that more than 10,000 people were treated at the clinic. While the clinic specializes in cancer treatment, the therapy has been expanded to treat arthritis, lupus, allergies, and AIDS.

The clinic may be in violation of the 1959 California Cancer Act which makes it unlawful to prescribe, or administer, any medicine for the treatment of cancer unless it has been approved by the FDA or the California Health Department. Currently, the clinic has not applied for FDA approval.

In 1990, the California Department of Health Services ordered the clinic to stop administering the vaccine used as part of the treatment program which was made from the patient's own urine or blood. Dr. Livingston-Wheeler died the same year. Today, the clinic is still in operation, and it is estimated that about 500 patients with cancer and other problems receive treatment there annually.

What is the evidence?

Based on the studies and research currently available, there is no evidence that Livingston-Wheeler therapy has any beneficial effects for people with cancer. Few studies have evaluated the Livingston-Wheeler therapy. One investigation involving seriously ill cancer patients found no difference in survival between patients receiving conventional treatment and those undergoing Livingston-Wheeler therapy. However, those patients receiving Livingston-Wheeler seemed to experience a lower quality of life.

One report on the bacteria *Progenitor cryptocides*, which Dr. Livingston-Wheeler claimed caused cancer, found that the bacteria does not exist but is actually a mixture of several different types of bacteria which Dr. Livingston-Wheeler labeled as one. The other components of her therapy have also been criticized for lack of scientific evidence.

Are there any possible problems or complications?

The safety of Livingston-Wheeler therapy has never been firmly established. Some reported reactions to the vaccine given in the therapy include aching, slight fever, and tenderness at the injection site.

References

American Cancer Society. Unproven methods of cancer management: Livingston-Wheeler therapy. *CA Cancer J Clin.* 1991;41:A7-A12.

Cassileth B, Lusk EJ, Guerry D, et al. Survival and quality of life among patients receiving unproven as compared with conventional cancer therapy. *N Engl J Med.* 1991;324:1180-1185.

University of Texas Center for Alternative Medicine Research in Cancer. Livingston-Wheeler summary. University of Texas-Houston Health Science Center Web site. Available at: http://www.sph.uth.tmc.edu/utcam/therapies/livingston.htm. Accessed May 10, 2000.

Lyprinol™

Other common name(s)	Scientific/medical name(s)
Lyprinex™	None

DESCRIPTION / OVERVIEW

Lyprinol™ is a fatty acid extracted from Perna canaliculus, a green-lipped mussel (shellfish) native to New Zealand. Lyprinol is promoted in New Zealand as a dietary supplement that can kill cancer cells and treat arthritis and asthma. Today, the extract is sold in capsule form in pharmacies and supermarkets in New Zealand and over the Internet. The idea that this mussel extract could help maintain good health was based on observations of Maori tribes in New Zealand by Western observers in the 1970s and 1980s.

Based on studies done in a laboratory, a researcher announced to the New Zealand media in 1999 that his data showed mussel extract kills cancer cells. He claimed that Lyprinol inhibits two cell pathways that may cause inflammation and possibly cancer in animals and humans. Within a few days, $2 million worth of Lyprinol was sold in New Zealand. Critics questioned the timing of the announcement, which coincided with the release of a new Lyprinol product on the market. In response to the criticism, the original manufacturer stopped distribution of its product, but other manufacturers continued selling it. At the time of the media announcement, another New Zealand researcher from the Malaghan Institute of Medical Research in Wellington, warned that Lyprinol might, in fact, promote tumor growth rather than kill cancer cells. No human studies have been conducted to support this researcher's claims. Relying on this type of treatment alone, and avoiding conventional medical care, may have serious health consequences.

Melatonin

Other common name(s)	Scientific/medical name(s)
None	None

DESCRIPTION

Melatonin is a hormone produced by the pineal gland, which is located just beneath the center of the brain. Melatonin is also manufactured synthetically and used as a supplement.

OVERVIEW

Research suggests that melatonin, produced by the body, plays a large role in the daily rhythms of sleeping and waking. The melatonin supplement is popular as a sleeping aid but studies documenting safe dosage, risks, and benefits are lacking. There have been mixed study results regarding the use of melatonin in people with cancer in terms of increasing survival and improving quality of life.

How is it promoted for use?

There is evidence that melatonin may have a role in the regulation of circadian rhythms (daily body cycles), sleep patterns, mood, reproduction, tumor growth, and aging. It is promoted primarily as a sleep aid. Melatonin production may decrease with age, which explains why many older people experience insomnia, according to proponents. Melatonin is also promoted to help people adjust to odd or irregular work schedules, and to counter the effects of jet lag because it may restore normal sleeping and waking schedules.

Proponents also claim that melatonin is a powerful antioxidant, a compound that blocks the action of activated oxygen molecules, known as free radicals, that can damage cells. Because of melatonin's suspected antioxidant properties, proponents believe it has the ability to suppress the growth of some types of cancer cells, especially when combined with other anticancer drugs. Some supporters propose that melatonin stimulates natural killer cells (a type of white blood cell) which attack tumors. Others speculate that melatonin levels and cycles are abnormal in some people with cancer, and that

melatonin supplements can help them sleep at night. It has also been proposed that melatonin can decrease the toxic effects of radiation therapy and chemotherapy. Some practitioners also believe that melatonin influences hormones in the body that regulate reproduction, the timing of ovulation, and aging. Many of these claims are currently under investigation.

What does it involve?

Melatonin is sold as a supplement and is available in drugstores, health food stores, and over the Internet. There are no widely accepted recommendations for dosage or duration of use.

Melatonin can also be found in many foods, such as milk, peanuts, almonds, turkey, and chicken, but in such small amounts that someone would have to eat large volumes to obtain a measurable dose. For example, someone would have to eat 72 bananas to get .3 mg of melatonin.

What is the history behind it?

In the 1600s, the French philosopher René Descartes called the pineal gland "the seat of the soul," because many people believed emotions originated there. The connection of the pineal gland to melatonin was first identified in the 1950s. Researchers at Yale University first discovered melatonin in 1958. Its connection to sleep and hormonal influences was not studied, however, until the 1970s and 1980s.

What is the evidence?

There is evidence that melatonin supplements can influence sleep and fatigue. However, the exact connection is not well understood. Research has not yet shown the most effective way to use melatonin supplements, (ie, for patients with sleep disorders or for people with occasional insomnia). Some research shows that melatonin affects not only the speed of falling asleep but also the duration and quality of sleep. Melatonin supplements have also been shown to cause insomnia in some people. According to one report, about 10% of people who took high doses of the hormone experienced insomnia and nightmares.

Numerous studies of melatonin and its effects on cancer have been conducted. Some suggest that melatonin extends survival and improves the quality of life for patients with certain types of untreatable cancers. Melatonin combined with interleukin-2, has been studied as an anticancer treatment.

The results of 32 clinical studies designed to measure the effects of melatonin on cancer were mixed and inconclusive. Some found that melatonin increased survival times, while others indicated that melatonin caused little or no response in tumors. Some studies reported that cancer went into total or partial regression in a small number of patients. A study of melatonin's ability to ease the side effects of chemotherapy drugs found that high doses of the hormone had little effect.

One study of patients with solid tumors concluded that melatonin may increase survival time and quality of life for people with cancer. Another study conducted by the same researcher concluded that melatonin increased disease-free survival in patients who had undergone surgery for melanoma. Most of the studies reporting positive results were small and conducted by the same researcher.

Are there any possible problems or complications?

The effects of long-term use of melatonin and how it interacts with other medications or supplements are unknown. Since melatonin may be have effect on ovulation, women who are trying to conceive, are pregnant, or are breast-feeding should not use this supplement. The National Institute on Aging has also warned that melatonin supplements may lead to high blood pressure, diabetes, and even cancer.

Some practitioners believe that children and people under the age of 40 should not take melatonin because they produce enough of the hormone naturally. They also state that people with immune-system disorders (eg, severe allergies), autoimmune diseases (eg, rheumatoid arthritis), or immune-system cancers (eg, lymphoma) should not take melatonin because it may further stimulate the immune system and worsen these conditions. Practitioners also caution people with severe mental illness and those taking steroid medications against using melatonin.

References

Brzezinski A. Melatonin in humans. *N Engl J Med.* 1997;336:186-195.

Fetrow CW, Avila JR. *Professional's Handbook of Complementary and Alternative Medicines.* Springhouse, Pa: Springhouse Corp; 1999.

Herbert V, Kava R. The miracle of melatonin? Health Care Reality Check Web site. Available at: http://www.hcrc.org/contrib/acsh/articles/melaton.html. Accessed March 27, 2000.

Lissoni P, Barni S, Ardizzoia A, Tancini G, Conti A, Maestroni G. A randomized study with the pineal hormone melatonin versus supportive care alone in patients with brain metastases due to solid neoplasms. *Cancer.* 1994;73:699-701.

Lissoni P, Barni S, Tancini G, et al. A study of the mechanisms involved in the immunostimulatory action of the pineal hormone in cancer patients. *Oncology.* 1993;50:399-402.

University of Texas Center for Alternative Medicine Research in Cancer. Melatonin summary. University of Texas-Houston Health Science Center Web site. Available at: http://www.sph.uth.tmc.edu/utcam/therapies/melatonin.htm. Accessed May 8, 2000.

Oxygen Therapy

Other common name(s)	Scientific/medical name(s)
Hyperoxygenation, Bio-oxidative Therapy, Oxidative Therapy, Ozone Therapy, Oxidology, Oxymedicine	None

DESCRIPTION

Oxygen therapy consists of one or more chemicals that are supposed to release oxygen after they are put into the body. The extra oxygen theoretically increases the body's ability to destroy disease-causing cells. Two of the most common compounds used in oxygen therapy are ozone (a chemically active form of oxygen) and hydrogen peroxide (see Hydrogen Peroxide Therapy). Oxygen therapy, as described here, is very different from hyperbaric oxygen, which involves the use of pressurized oxygen (see Hyperbaric Oxygen Therapy).

OVERVIEW

There is no evidence that oxygen therapy is effective in treating cancer or any other disease. It may even be dangerous. There have been reports of patient deaths from this method.

How is it promoted for use?

Oxygen therapy is promoted as a treatment for more than two dozen diseases, including certain cancers, asthma, emphysema, AIDS, arthritis, cardiovascular disease, and Alzheimer's disease. Some proponents claim that cancer cells, and the microorganisms that cause cancer, thrive in low-oxygen environments. They believe adding oxygen to the body creates an oxygen-rich condition in which cancer cells cannot survive. Oxygen therapy advocates claim that it increases the efficiency of all cells in the body and increases energy production, stimulates the production of antioxidants, and enhances the immune system. There is no scientific evidence to support these claims.

What does it involve?

Ozone gas may be introduced under pressure into the rectum or injected into a muscle. Some practitioners use a special device to force ozone into a pint of blood that has been drawn from the patient. The blood is then returned to the patient's body. For hydrogen peroxide therapy, the liquid is first diluted then given to patients orally, rectally, intravenously, or vaginally. Sometimes less frequently used oxygen therapy compounds are injected into muscles. The frequency of treatments varies widely, from three times a day over several weeks, to once a week for several months.

What is the history behind it?

The history of oxygen therapy follows several tracks. Interest in ozone dates back to Germany in the mid-1800s, where it was claimed to purify blood. During World War I, physicians used ozone to treat wounds, trench foot, and the effects of poison gas. In the 1920s, ozone and hydrogen peroxide were used experimentally to treat the flu.

In 1919, William F. Koch, MD, a Detroit physician, proposed that cancer was caused by a single toxin, and that the disease could be prevented or reversed by eliminating that toxin. To achieve this goal, Dr. Koch claimed he had developed glyoxylide, an oxygen compound injected into patients' muscles. Dr. Koch and his followers claimed that glyoxylide forced cancer cells to absorb oxygen, which helped to rid the body of the cancer-causing toxin. In 1942, the FDA charged Dr. Koch with making false claims about glyoxylide. The courts upheld the accusations, and in 1963 the California Cancer Advisory Council reported that glyoxylide therapy had "no value in the diagnosis, treatment, alleviation, or cure of cancer." Later, researchers were unable to confirm that glyoxylide ever existed.

During the 1930s, Otto Warburg, MD, a Nobel Prize winner, discovered that cancer cells have a lower-than-normal respiration rate compared to normal cells. He reasoned that cancer cells thrived in a low-oxygen environment and that increased oxygen levels would harm and even kill them. Many of the beliefs held by oxygen therapy practitioners are still based on Dr. Warburg's theories, even though they have since been discredited.

What is the evidence?

There is no evidence that "bathing" cancer cells in oxygen will harm or kill the cancer cells. One researcher from the Dominican Republic claimed that he used ozone gas to cure 13 people with cancer. A follow-up investigation found that two of the patients had died of cancer, three couldn't be found, two refused to be interviewed, three were alive but still had cancer, and three had questionable diagnoses of cancer. The medical literature contains several accounts of patient deaths attributed directly to oxygen therapy.

Are there any possible problems or complications?

Large amounts of injected hydrogen peroxide can result in a condition called arterial gas embolism, which can lead to irreversible lung damage and death. Relying on this type of treatment alone, and avoiding conventional medical care, may have serious health consequences.

References

Barrett S. Miraculous recoveries. Quackwatch Web site. Available at: http://www.quackwatch.com. Accessed May 8, 2000.

Cassileth B. *The Alternative Medicine Handbook.* New York, NY: W. W. Norton & Company; 1998.

Leon OS, Menendez S, Merino N, et al. Center for Research and Biological Evaluation. Ozone oxidative preconditioning: a protection against cellular damage by free radicals. *Mediators Inflamm.* 1998;7:289-294.

Green S. Oxygenation therapy: Unproven treatments for cancer and AIDS. Health Care Reality Check Web site. Available at: http://www.hcrc.org/contrib/green/oxther.html. Accessed May 8, 2000.

National Cancer Institute. Koch-synthetic antitoxins (malonide, glyoxylide, and parabenzoquinone). National Cancer Institute Web site. Available at: http://rex.nci.nih.gov/INFO_CANCER/Cancer_facts/Section9/FS9_5.html. Accessed May 8, 2000.

US Congress, Office of Technology Assessment. *Unconventional Cancer Treatments.* Washington, DC: US Government Printing Office; 1990. Publication OTA-H-405.

Pharmacological / Biological

Poly-MVA

Other common name(s)	Scientific/medical name(s)
None	None

DESCRIPTION / OVERVIEW

Poly-MVA is a compound that contains various minerals, vitamins, and amino acids such as lipoic acid, palladium, B_{12}, and other B complex vitamins (see Amino Acids, Lipoic Acid, and Vitamin B Complex). It is promoted as a nutritional supplement that is a nontoxic alternative to chemotherapy. Poly-MVA is a reddish-brown liquid that is mixed with water or juice. It is not licensed for use in the United States.

In 1995, Poly-MVA was patented and promoted as a "metalo-vitamin." The development of Poly-MVA is rooted in the theory that cancer is a systematic disease related to many factors, including irreparable gene damage due to cancer causing substances. Makers of Poly-MVA say that it demonstrates antitumor activity. There are claims that it is effective against tumors in the brain, lung, ovaries, and breast, and that it boosts the immune system, reduces pain, and helps people regain energy and appetite. Some even claim that it can lead to longer survival. According to its manufacturers, the compound attacks cancerous cells and protects DNA and RNA. They contend that the lipoic acid allows the various minerals, vitamins, and amino acids to be easily absorbed into the system where they can kill cancerous cells.

There is no scientific evidence that Poly-MVA is effective in preventing or treating cancer. Most of the reports of successful use of Poly-MVA are anecdotal or represent small studies that have not been published in scientific journals. There have been no well-controlled studies of the compound. The potential risks and side effects are currently unknown.

Pregnenolone

Other common name(s)	Scientific/medical name(s)
None	None

DESCRIPTION / OVERVIEW

Pregnenolone is a steroid the body produces that plays a role in the synthesis of several hormones, such as progesterone and DHEA (see DHEA). It is primarily promoted as an alternative treatment that improves memory and alertness, and reduces stress and fatigue. Some promoters claim it also helps treat a variety of other conditions such as arthritis, cancer, osteoporosis, multiple sclerosis, PMS, and menopause. There is no scientific evidence to support these claims. Pregnenolone supplements are sold in capsule form, and there is no standardized dosage. Very little is known about the safety of the supplements or the effects of long-term use.

Revici's Guided Chemotherapy

Other common name(s)	Scientific/medical name(s)
Revici's Biologically Guided Chemotherapy, Revici Cancer Control, Lipid Therapy, Revici's Method	None

DESCRIPTION

Revici's guided chemotherapy is a chemical therapy promoted as an alternative cancer treatment. The therapy varies for every patient but can include a chemical formulation consisting of lipid alcohols, caffeine, zinc, and iron, or a formulation consisting of fatty acids, selenium, magnesium, and sulfur (see Selenium and Zinc).

OVERVIEW

There is no scientific evidence that Revici's guided chemotherapy is effective in treating cancer or any other disease. It may also cause potentially serious side effects.

How is it promoted for use?

Revici's guided chemotherapy is promoted for the treatment of various cancers, including colon, bone, lung, and brain cancers, as well as Alzheimer's disease, arthritis, AIDS, chronic pain, drug addiction, injury from radiation, and schizophrenia. Emanuel Revici, MD, the inventor of the therapy, claimed that even advanced cancer could be treated with his method.

This therapy is based on a theory that cancer and other diseases result from an imbalance of lipids (fat-soluble molecules) in the body that cause abnormal metabolism. Proponents believe that lipid imbalances can be remedied by formulating nontoxic chemotherapeutic medicines to restore the proper balance of lipids.

What does it involve?

Revici used blood and urine tests to detect lipid imbalances and then developed a chemical formula of lipids and lipid-based substances that were unique to each patient. The substances Revici used included alcohols (such as glycerol, butanol, and octanol), selenium compounds, sterols (such as cholesterol), estrogens (female hormones), iodine, mercury, iron, aminobutanol, and nicotinic acid derivatives.

Revici's guided chemotherapy is administered by mouth or injection in dosages that are tailored to each patient. After the initial treatment, patients are taught to test their urine at home and monitor the lipid imbalance. If there are changes, the patient is given a new formula. This therapy is available at a few clinics started by Revici associates.

What is the history behind it?

Born in Romania in 1896, Emanuel Revici received a medical degree from the University of Bucharest in 1920 and taught internal medicine there. In the 1920s, he began research into lipids and cellular metabolism. From 1936 to 1941, he conducted clinical research and practiced medicine in Paris, and from 1941 to 1946 in Mexico City. He began experimenting with a variety of drugs and compounds to treat cancer in 1941.

In 1947, he moved to Brooklyn, New York, and started the Institute of Applied Medicine to conduct research into cancer and other diseases. In 1955, he moved the Institute to Manhattan along with his medical practice. New York State has challenged Revici's medical license on a number of occasions since 1984, but he was able to keep his license until 1993, when it was finally revoked. From 1981 to 1988, Revici received 17 patents in the United States for chemical formulations he used on patients with a variety of conditions, including cancer, drug addictions, viral diseases, and pregnancy. Revici died in 1998 at the age of 101, however, his therapy is still offered by some of his associates.

What is the evidence?

In his 1961 book, Revici listed a large number of case histories of patients he claimed experienced complete or partial remission of their cancer. Some of his patients also testified at a congressional hearing in New York that Revici's treatment put their cancer in remission.

The only published clinical evaluation of Revici's guided chemotherapy appeared in the *Journal of the American Medical Association* in 1965. It was conducted by a group of nine physicians known as the Clinical Appraisal Group. They studied 33 cancer patients referred to Revici for treatment after conventional therapy failed. Twenty-two of the patients died of cancer while on Revici's therapy, 8 showed no improvement, and the remaining 3 showed signs of cancer progression. The group concluded that Revici's method was without value.

Studies of Revici's chemotherapy are hampered by the fact that each formulation is different. A number of scientists who have offered to evaluate his methods were not able to reach agreement with Revici about a study protocol. However, in 1945, a group of American physicians investigated Revici's treatment methods in Mexico and found no positive evidence to support the value of these preparations in treating malignancy. In 1988, the American Cancer Society requested that Revici provide documentation of his work, but never received a reply.

Are there any possible problems or complications?

Revici's guided chemotherapy for cancer has never been proven to be safe or effective.

Revici himself said that his treatment might cause the area around a cancerous tumor to become inflamed and the tumor itself to grow larger and more painful before it shrank or disappeared. Selenium compounds, sometimes used in this therapy, can be toxic. This treatment should be avoided, especially by women who are pregnant or breast-feeding.

Relying on this type of treatment alone, and avoiding conventional medical care, may have serious health consequences.

References

Alternative Medicine: Expanding Medical Horizons. *A Report to the National Institutes of Health on Alternative Medical Systems and Practices in the United States.* Washington, DC: US Government Printing Office; 1994. NIH publication 94-066.

American Cancer Society. Unproven methods of cancer management: Revici method. *CA Cancer J Clin.* 1989;39:119-122.

Barrett S, Herbert V. Questionable cancer therapies. Quackwatch Web site. Available at: http://www.quackwatch.com. Accessed May 10, 2000.

Lyall D, Schwartz M, Herter FP, et al. Treatment of cancer by the method of Revici. *JAMA.* 1965;194:279-280.

Murphy GP, Morris LB, Lange D. *Informed Decisions: The Complete Book of Cancer Diagnosis, Treatment, and Recovery.* New York, NY: Viking; 1997.

Revici E. *Research in Physiopathology as a Basis of Guided Chemotherapy with Special Application to Cancer.* Princeton, NJ: D Van Nostrand, Inc: 1961.

University of Texas Center for Alternative Medicine Research in Cancer. Revici summary. University of Texas-Houston Health Science Center Web site. Available at: http://www.sph.uth.tmc.edu/utcam/summary/revici.htm. Accessed May 10, 2000.

US Congress, Office of Technology Assessment. *Unconventional Cancer Treatments.* Washington, DC: US Government Printing Office; 1990. Publication OTA-H-405.

Pharmacological / Biological

Sea Cucumber

Other common name(s)	Scientific/medical name(s)
None	*Holothuroidea cucumaria*

DESCRIPTION / OVERVIEW

Sea cucumbers are marine animals that have a soft, dark body with the shape and texture of a cucumber. They range in size from 1 inch to 6 $1/2$ feet long and about $1/2$ inche thick and are found in all oceans, especially the Indian and the western Pacific. Promoters claim sea cucumbers release poisons that fight conditions such as cancer, arthritis, sports injuries, tendonitis, and other inflammatory diseases. There is no scientific evidence to support these claims. Research is currently underway to determine the active ingredients in this substance and evaluate their effectiveness in interfering with cancer progression in animal studies.

Shark Cartilage

Other common name(s)	Scientific/medical name(s)
None	None

DESCRIPTION

Shark cartilage is extracted from the heads and fins of sharks. Cartilage is a type of elastic tissue that is found in the skeletal systems of many animals, including humans. Sharks have no bones, so cartilage is the primary component of their skeletal system. The major compounds in shark cartilage are glycoproteins and calcium salts.

OVERVIEW

There is no scientific evidence that shark cartilage, sold as a food supplement, is an effective treatment for cancer, osteoporosis, or any other disease. Although some laboratory and animal studies have shown that components isolated from shark cartilage possess a modest ability to inhibit the growth of new blood vessels, these effects have not been proven in humans. No well-controlled clinical studies have been published; however, clinical trials are currently underway.

How is it promoted for use?

Proponents believe that shark cartilage supplements or cartilage from other animals, such as cows, slow or stop the growth of cancer (see Bovine Cartilage). Shark cartilage, according to supporters, contains a protein that inhibits angiogenesis, the process of blood vessel development. Tumors require a network of blood vessels to survive and grow, so cutting off the tumor's blood supply starves it of nutrients it needs to live, causing it to shrink or disappear. Some proponents also claim that shark cartilage reverses bone diseases such as osteoporosis, arthritis, psoriasis, and inflammation of the intestinal tract.

What does it involve?

Shark cartilage is available as a capsule, powder, or liquid extract. It can be applied directly to the skin or injected by needle into the bloodstream, under the skin, into the lining of the abdomen, or directly into the muscle. It is also sometimes used as an enema (see Colon Therapy). The dose and length of treatment varies widely. There is no assurance, however, that the supplements sold contain the cartilage or its main compounds.

What is the history behind it?

A physician named John Prudden began investigating the use of cartilage in the early 1950s. He used powdered bovine cartilage to help heal the wounds of surgical patients. Since then, many kinds of cartilage such as pig, sheep, chicken, cow, and shark have been studied. After the 1992 publication of a popular book entitled *Sharks Don't Get Cancer*, written by I. William Lane, PhD, shark cartilage supplements became very popular among people interested in alternative medicine. Scientists have thought that since sharks do not appear to develop as much cancer as humans, there may be something in their systems that protects them from getting cancer.

Interest in shark cartilage increased after a television newsmagazine aired a segment in 1993 that showed a study of patients with advanced cancer in Cuba that had gone into remission after being treated with shark carti-lage. The National Cancer Institute (NCI) later concluded that the results of the Cuban study were "incomplete and unimpressive." In June 2000, the Federal Trade Commission ordered shark cartilage manufacturers to stop making unsubstantiated claims that their products have cancer-fighting abilities, and fined them $1 million for false advertising.

Finding drugs that halt the spread of cancer by inhibiting the growth of blood vessels has been the subject of many serious research studies in recent years. Some researchers believe that the therapy (called antiangiogenesis therapy) holds a great deal of promise for people with certain types of cancer. A number of antiangiogenesis drugs have been developed and are currently under investigation. Some researchers are trying to purify antiangiogenic compounds from cartilage; however, the most promising antiangiogenic substances now in existence are those that have been purified from sources other than cartilage or have been synthesized in laboratories.

What is the evidence?

There is no reliable evidence that shark cartilage is an effective treatment for cancer, osteoporosis, or other conditions. Although studies using bovine and shark cartilage in people with cancer began in the early 1980s, few have been published. The scientific validity of most of these studies is questionable because they do not describe how treatment was administered, how patients were assessed, long-term survival outcomes, or information about cartilage used and its components.

Some laboratory and animal experiments have shown that shark cartilage possesses a modest ability to inhibit the growth of new blood vessels. These effects have not been shown in humans. According to one review, results from nine clinical series of patients receiving shark cartilage were mixed. None of the series were subject to rigorous scientific controls. In one recent clinical trial involving 47 patients, researchers concluded that shark cartilage had no effect on patients with advanced-stage cancers.

Researchers generally agree that the protein molecules in shark cartilage are too large to be absorbed by the digestive track and are simply excreted. However, some scientists have suggested that these substances may be more readily absorbed when taken in a liquid form. One study concluded that orally administered liquid shark cartilage effectively inhibited the growth of new blood vessels in healthy men, suggesting to the study authors that the active ingredients in liquid shark cartilage were available for use by the body's healing systems. The NCI is sponsoring a multicenter phase III controlled trial of a liquid shark cartilage extract for the treatment of lung cancer along with conventional therapies.

Are there any possible problems or complications?

Shark cartilage is not thought to be toxic, although it has been known to cause nausea, indigestion, fatigue, fever, and dizziness in some people. It may also slow down the healing process for people recovering from surgery. People with a low white blood cell count should not take shark cartilage enemas, because there is a risk of life-threatening infection. Children should not take it because it could interfere with body growth and development. Women who are pregnant or breast-feeding should also avoid these supplements. Relying on this type of treatment alone, and avoiding conventional medical care, may have serious health consequences.

References

Alternative Medicine: Expanding Medical Horizons. *A Report to the National Institutes of Health on Alternative Medical Systems and Practices in the United States.* Washington, DC: US Government Printing Office; 1994. NIH publication 94-066.

Berbari P, Thibodeau A, Germain L, et al. Antiangiogenic effects of the oral administration of liquid cartilage extract in humans. *J Surg Res.* 1999;87;108-113.

Cassileth B. Evaluating complementary and alternative therapies for cancer patients. *CA Cancer J Clin.* 1999;49:362-375.

Ernst E, Cassileth B. How useful are unconventional cancer treatments? *Eur J Cancer.* 1999;35:1608-1613.

Miller DR, Anderson GT, Stark JJ, Granick JL, Richardson D. Phase I/II trial of the safety and efficacy of shark cartilage in the treatment of advanced cancer. *J Clin Oncol.* 1998;16:3649-3655.

National Cancer Institute. Complementary/Alternative medicine. Cartilage (PDQ®). National Cancer Institute Cancernet Web site. Available at: http://cancernet.nci.nih.gov/cam/cartilage.htm. Accessed May 10, 2000.

University of Texas Center for Alternative Medicine Research in Cancer. Cartilage summary. University of Texas-Houston Health Science Center Web site. Available at: http://www.sph.uth.tmc.edu/utcam/summary/cartilage.htm. Accessed May 10, 2000.

Pharmacological / Biological

Shark Liver Oil

Other common name(s)	Scientific/medical name(s)
None	None

DESCRIPTION

Shark liver oil is promoted as an alternative form of treatment for cancer and other diseases. Shark liver oil is one of the richest sources of alkylglycerols, natural chemicals formed by the combination of a fatty acid and an alcohol molecule. Alkylglycerols are also found in significant amounts in the liver, spleen, bone marrow, and breast milk (both cow and human).

OVERVIEW

Shark liver oil is widely used in addition to conventional cancer treatment in Europe. There has been no scientific evidence showing the effectiveness of alkylglycerols in humans. More recent research has focused on one component of shark liver oil called squalamine. Laboratory research suggests that it has antitumor effects in animal models; however, its effects in humans are not yet known. Phase I clinical trials are currently being conducted.

How is it promoted for use?

Alkylglycerols, found in shark liver oil, are thought to be beneficial in several ways. They are promoted to fight cancer by killing tumor cells indirectly. Proponents claim they activate the immune system by stimulating macrophages (immune system cells that attack and consume invading organisms) and inhibiting protein kinase A (a protein that is a key regulator of cell growth). Additionally, proponents claim that alkylglycerols reduce the side effects of chemotherapy and radiation treatment. This activity is supposedly due to the ability of alkylglycerols to protect cell membranes from oxidative stress.

Due to their proposed immune stimulatory effect, alkylglycerols are also claimed to be effective against colds, flu, chronic infections, asthma, psoriasis, arthritis, and AIDS. Since macrophages are also a key cell in wound healing, alkylglycerols are said to have healing effects. There is no scientific evidence to support these claims.

Depending on the commercial preparation, shark liver oil may also be rich in omega-3 fatty acids and vitamin A (see Omega-3 Fatty Acids and Vitamin A). Other compounds in shark liver oil, such as squalamine, have also been promoted to have beneficial anticancer effects. Claims regarding squalamine are currently under investigation.

What does it involve?

Shark liver oil is commercially available in capsule and liquid forms. A commonly used dosage is one to two 250 mg capsules daily as a preventative measure and up to six 250 mg capsules per day to prevent some of the side effects of radiation therapy. These supplements are available at health food stores and over the Internet.

What is the history behind it?

Shark liver oil has been used as a folk remedy by people on the coasts of Norway and Sweden for hundreds of years. It was primarily used to promote wound healing and as a general remedy for conditions of the respiratory tract and of the digestive system. In the 1950s, a young Swedish doctor suggested that extracts of bone marrow helped boost the recovery of white blood cells in children undergoing radiation and chemotherapy for leukemia. The active ingredient in the bone marrow extract was identified as alkylglycerols. Shark liver oil was found to be one of the richest sources of alkylglycerols. Around 1986, the first commercially purified shark liver oil with a "standard dose" of alkylglycerols was marketed.

What is the evidence?

Most of the studies on alkylglycerols as a cancer therapy are ten to thirty years old and appear to have involved only a small group of people. Although supporters make great claims for the activities of alkylglycerols, the claims have never been widely accepted. Overall, there does not appear to be any recent clinical research on the benefits of alkylglycerols in preventing or treating cancer.

More recently, research has focused on squalamine, an antimicrobial substance found in shark liver oil that fights bacteria, yeasts, and fungi. Researchers at Johns Hopkins University discovered that squalamine had antitumor effects in multiple animal models. Researchers at the Dana-Farber Cancer Institute found that squalamine decreased the number of lung metastases found in laboratory animals.

Squalamine, which has been extracted from the oil, is being tested in Phase I clinical trials at the Cancer Therapy and Research Center in San Antonio Texas and the Lombardi Cancer Center of Georgetown University in Washington, DC.

Are there any possible problems or complications?

Although many people have taken shark liver oil, the issue of potential toxicity at normal doses has not been well studied. Some mild gastrointestinal disturbances, such as nausea, indigestion, and diarrhea, have been reported to occur with the ingestion of shark liver oil in its liquid form.

References

Pugliese PT, Jordan K, Cederberg H, Brohult J. Some biological actions of alkylglycerols from shark liver oil. *J Altern Complement Med.* 1998;4:87-99.

Sills AK Jr, Williams JI, Tyler BM, et al. Squalamine inhibits angiogenesis and solid tumor growth in vivo and perturbs embryonic vasculature. *Cancer Res.* 1998;58:2784-2792.

Teicher BA, Williams JI, Takeuchi H, Ara G, Herbst RS, Buxton D. Potential of the aminosterol, squalamine in combination therapy in the rat 13,762 mammary carcinoma and the murine Lewis lung carcinoma. *Anticancer Res.* 1998;18:2567-2573.

Wang H, Rajagopal S, Reynolds S, Cederberg H, Chakrabarty S. Differentiation-promoting effect of 1-O (2 methoxy) hexadecyl glycerol in human colon cancer cells. *J Cell Physiol.* 1999;178:173-178.

Urotherapy

Other common name(s)	Scientific/medical name(s)
Urine Therapy, Urea	None

DESCRIPTION

Urotherapy is an alternative method that involves the use of a patient's own urine to treat himself or herself for cancer.

OVERVIEW

There have been no well-controlled studies to support the claims that urotherapy can control or reverse the spread of cancer.

How is it promoted for use?

Advocates of urotherapy propose several ways by which the treatment can slow or stop the growth of cancer. One is that urine can stimulate the body's immune system. Cancer and other diseases release chemicals called antigens into the bloodstream. When the immune system detects them, it responds by producing antibodies to fight the invading disease. Some of the antigens produced by cancer cells appear in the urine, so practitioners have hypothesized that if they give urine to cancer patients, the immune system would react more vigorously by producing a greater number of antibodies, thereby increasing its capacity to kill tumor cells.

Other practitioners have speculated that urine inhibits the ability of cancer cells to crowd together, which disrupts their flow of nutrients and waste excretion. Without any way to nourish themselves or eliminate waste products, the tumor cells die.

One proponent asserts that certain components in urine establish a biochemical defense system that operates independently of the body's immune system. It is claimed that these chemicals don't destroy cancer cells, but "correct" their defects and prevent them from spreading. There is no scientific evidence to support these claims.

What does it involve?

Patients undergoing urotherapy may drink their own urine, use it as an enema, or have it injected directly into the bloodstream or into tumors. In powdered form, urea, the byproduct of protein metabolism and the primary component of urine, has been applied directly to tumors appearing on the skin. Urea may also be packed into capsules or dissolved in a flavored drink. There are no established guidelines for determining how much urine or urea is required for this method.

What is the history behind it?

The thought of drinking urine probably offends the sensibilities of most Westerners, but the fact is that human urine has been considered a healing agent in many cultures for centuries. Even now, some physicians recognize urine's antiseptic properties, and in some cultures it is poured directly on wounds to prevent infection. Others mix it with several ingredients to make a tonic that is drunk to promote health.

In the mid-1950s, a Greek physician named Evangelos Danopolous, MD, professed that he had identified anticancer properties in urea and had used the compound to successfully treat patients with certain types of skin and liver cancers. Dr. Danopolous claimed that his therapy significantly extended patients' lives. Other physicians have also noted urea's anticancer characteristics. One of them, Vincent Speckhart, MD, testified about urea's benefits before a House of Representatives Committee. A breast cancer patient whom Dr. Speckhart treated with urea reportedly recovered from her disease and was alive 10 years after therapy.

What is the evidence?

There are some anecdotal reports of urotherapy's ability to stop cancer growth. However, there is no scientific evidence that shows urotherapy to be an effective cancer treatment. There is no valid evidence that urine or urea administered in any form has any beneficial effect for cancer patients.

Are there any possible problems or complications?

Drinking or injecting urine or applying it directly to the skin is reported anecdotally to be safe and not associated with harmful side effects, but the safety of these practices have not been established by scientific studies.

Reference

Eldor J. Urotherapy for patients with cancer. *Med Hypotheses.* 1997;48:309-315.

714-X

Other common name(s)	Scientific/medical name(s)
None	Trimethylbicyclonitramineoheptane chloride

DESCRIPTION

714-X is a substance containing camphor, nitrogen, ammonium salts, sodium chloride, and ethanol used as an alternative method in North America, Western Europe, and Mexico to treat cancer and AIDS. It is not available in the United States.

OVERVIEW

There is no scientific evidence that 714-X is effective in treating any type of cancer. It has not been proven to be safe or effective for any use.

How is it promoted for use?

According to proponents, people with serious illnesses, such as cancer, carry tiny living particles in their bloodstream called somatids. They claim that disease can be diagnosed and monitored by noting the number and forms of somatids in a person's blood. 714-X is said to cure cancer and AIDS by interfering with the flow of somatids through the bloodstream. This interference is said to cause the immune system to grow stronger and diseases to regress.

It is claimed that cancer cells produce a substance called cocancerogenic K factor (CKF), which protects cancer cells from the immune system. 714-X supposedly strips CKF by supplying the body with nitrogen and leaves tumor cells vulnerable to attack by the immune system. There is no evidence to support these claims.

What does it involve?

714-X is prepared as a sterile solution and injected into a lymph node in the groin. Ice packs are used to cool the area of injection both before and after. A course of treatment involves daily injections for 21 days, followed by 3 days of rest. The cycle is typically repeated a total of 3 times.

In Canada, 714-X is available by prescription under the Emergency Drug Release Program of Health Canada. It is not approved, however, for general therapeutic use. 714-X is not approved for use in the United States.

What is the history behind it?

Early in his career, French-born scientist Gaston Naessens developed the somatoscope, a specialized microscope that he used to examine blood at extremely high magnifications. Using the somatoscope, Naessens claimed to have discovered tiny living organisms called somatids in the blood of people with serious diseases, including cancer. He believed that somatids were responsible for the development of disease and he set out to find a way to eliminate or disable them.

In 1963, after moving to Quebec, Naessens developed 714-X. The drug's name is derived from the alphabetical position of Naessen's initials. "G" is the seventh letter of the alphabet, and "N" is fourteenth in line. The "X" is the 24th letter and represents 1924, the year Naessens was born. Naessens claimed that the drug interfered with somatids and could stop or reverse the growth of tumors.

Naessens has been troubled by legal difficulties throughout his career. In 1956, a French court convicted and fined him for practicing medicine without a license. In the 1980s, while living in Quebec, Naessens was prosecuted for health fraud and threatened with life imprisonment. He was acquitted after testimony from many 714-X users who stated that the drug had helped them.

What is the evidence?

Although many patients have reported beneficial effects after taking 714-X, no scientific evidence supports any claims about the existence of somatids or that 714-X can cure cancer or AIDS. No formal clinical studies have been conducted on 714-X.

One component of 714-X, camphor, is being researched in animals for potential anticancer activity; however, the research is at an early stage. There are also some anecdotal reports of successful treatment with 714-X, however, extensive research is needed in order to substantiate these reports.

Are there any possible problems or complications?

714-X appears to cause few side effects. The injections can result in local redness, tenderness, and swelling at the injection site. The potential side effects are not known.

References

Alternative Medicine: Expanding Medical Horizons. *A Report to the National Institutes of Health on Alternative Medical Systems and Practices in the United States.* Washington, DC: US Government Printing Office; 1994. NIH publication 94-066.

Barrett S. Fanciful claims for 714X. Quackwatch Web site. Available at: http://www.quackwatch.com. Accessed March 27, 2000.

Ernst E, Cassileth B. How useful are unconventional cancer treatments? *Eur J Cancer.* 1999;35:1610-1613.

Kaegi E. Unconventional therapies for cancer: 6. 714-X. Task Force on Alternative Therapeutic of the Canadian Breast Cancer Research Initiative. *CMAJ.* 1998;158:1621-1624.

714-X. Canadian Breast Cancer Research Initiative Web site. Available at: http://www.breast.cancer.ca/english/alt/714/over_ec.htm. Accessed June 13, 2000.

University of Texas Center for Alternative Medicine Research in Cancer. 714-X summary. University of Texas-Houston Health Science Center Web site. Available at: http://www.sph.uth.tmc.edu/utcam/therapies/714X.htm. Accessed June 13, 2000.

Resources

Chapter 10

Resource Guide

Health Information on the Internet

There is a vast amount of information about cancer and unconventional methods on the Internet. Mass communication makes it possible for people to share ideas and information quickly. However, there is much information on the Internet written by promoters of unproven treatments. Since any group or individual can publish on the Internet, it is important to consider the credentials and reputation of the organization providing the information.

The Health on the Net Foundation (HON) established a Code of Conduct for medical and health care related sites, providing guidelines for choosing and creating sites that are ethical and contain reliable information. Sites that adhere to these eight principles are considered to demonstrate ethical behavior.

HON Code of Conduct*

1. Any medical/health advice provided and hosted on the site will only be given by medically/health trained and qualified professionals unless a clear statement is made that a piece of advice offered is from a non-medically/health qualified individual/organization.

2. The information provided on the site is designed to support, not replace, the relationship that exists between a patient/site visitor and his/her existing physician.

3. Confidentiality of data relating to individual patients and visitors to a medical/health Web site, including their identity, is respected by this Web site. The Web site owners undertake to honor or exceed the legal requirements of medical/health information privacy that apply in the country and state where the Web site and mirror sites are located.

4. Where appropriate, information contained on this site will be supported by clear references to source data and, where possible, have specific HTML links to that data. The date when a clinical page was last modified will be clearly displayed (eg, at the bottom of the page).

5. Any claims relating to the benefits/performance of a specific treatment, commercial product or service will be supported by appropriate, balanced evidence in the manner outlined above in Principle 4.

6. The designers of this Web site will seek to provide information in the clearest possible manner and provide contact addresses for visitors that seek further information or support. The Webmaster will display his/her e-mail address clearly throughout the Web site.

7. Support for this Web site will be clearly identified, including the identities of commercial and non-commercial organizations that have contributed funding, services, or material for the site.

8. If advertising is a source of funding it will be clearly stated. A brief description of the advertising policy adopted by the Web site owners will be displayed on the site. Advertising and other promotional material will be presented to viewers in a manner and context that facilitates differentiation between it and the original material created by the institution operating the site.

* *Reprinted with permission from the Health on the Net Foundation. The Health on the Net Foundation (HON: http://www.hon.ch) is a not-for-profit organization headquartered in Geneva, Switzerland. According to its mission statement, HON is dedicated to realizing the benefits of the Internet and related technologies in the fields of health and medicine.*

Listing of Organizations

American Botanical Council (ABC)
http://www.herbalgram.org
512-926-4900
ABC was founded and incorporated in 1988 as a nonprofit research and education organization. They publish a journal called *HerbalGram*, and offer an online herb reference guide, and selections from the Commission E monographs.

American Cancer Society (ACS)
http://www.cancer.org
800-ACS-2345
ACS offers comprehensive, up-to-date cancer information 24 hours a day, 7 days a week. An online daily newsmagazine provides information on recent news events and research. A wide variety of educational programs, services, and referrals are offered, as well as information related to complementary and alternative methods.

Canadian Breast Cancer Research Initiative (CBCRI)
http://www.breast.cancer.ca
416-961-7223
CBCRI is a partnership of seven Canadian breast cancer organizations and governmental bodies that encourages and supports research related to the prevention and treatment of

breast cancer. They offer extensive reviews of scientifically credible and methodologically rigorous research on several unconventional therapies.

CancerNet PDQ®

http://cancernet.nci.nih.gov/

CancerNet is a Web site that provides recent and accurate cancer information from the NCI, which is the US Government's cancer research agency. PDQ contains treatment information on more than 80 types of adult and childhood cancers, and is beginning to include summaries on complementary and alternative medicine.

FDA Center for Food Safety and Applied Nutrition (CFSAN)

http://vm.cfsan.fda.gov
800-FDA-1088

CFSAN is an office of the US Food and Drug Administration. It regulates $240 billion worth of domestic food, $15 billion worth of imported foods, and $15 billion worth of cosmetics sold across state lines. The center promotes and protects public health interest by ensuring that food is safe, nutritious, and wholesome and that it is honestly, accurately, and informatively labeled. They offer information on dietary supplements, and the Special Nutritionals Adverse Monitoring System (see Chapter 2).

Healthscout

http://www.healthscout.com

Healthscout is a general health Web site that provides health care news and medical information, including information about complementary and alternative medicine. Connections to other health resources are also provided.

National Agricultural Library Food and Nutrition Information Center (FNIC)

http://www.nal.usda.gov/fnic
301-504-5719

FNIC is one of several information centers at the National Agricultural Library (NAL), part of the US Department of Agriculture's (USDA) Agricultural Research Service. The NAL is a major international source for agriculture and related information. FNIC provides information on dietary supplements including vitamins, minerals, and herbs.

National Institutes of Health (NIH) National Center for Complementary and Alternative Medicine (NCCAM)

http://nccam.nih.gov

NCCAM evaluates alternative medicine practices to determine their effectiveness, to serve as a public information clearinghouse, and to provide a research-training program. The NCCAM facilitates and conducts research, but does not serve as a referral agency for individual practitioners or treatments.

NIH Office of Dietary Supplements (ODS)

http://odp.od.nih.gov/ods
301-435-2920

This office has an extensive International Bibliographic Information on Dietary Supplements (IBIDS) database. It contains articles and abstracts from scientific journals, information about dietary supplements, and a search engine that allows users to search for specific vitamins, minerals, and herbal products. The information in this database is limited to the top 85 to 100 most popular vitamins, minerals, and herbal ingredients.

OncoLink®

http://www.oncolink.upenn.edu

OncoLink is a Web site that was founded by the University of Pennsylvania in 1994 to help cancer patients, families, health care professionals, and the general public obtain accurate cancer-related information free of charge. OncoLink provides comprehensive information about research advances, specific types of cancer, cancer treatment, and information about complementary and alternative medicine.

Quackwatch

http://www.quackwatch.com

Quackwatch, Inc. is a nonprofit corporation whose purpose is to combat health-related frauds, myths, fads, and fallacies. The Quackwatch Web site is a comprehensive source of information regarding fraudulent claims.

US Pharmacopoeia (USP)

http://www.usp.org
800-822-8772

USP establishes standards for the strength, quality, and purity of drugs and dietary supplements for human and veterinary use. National health care practitioner reporting programs support USP standards and information programs. In addition, USP supports many public service programs.

The University of Texas Center for Alternative Medicine Research in Cancer (UT-CAM)

http://www.sph.uth.tmc.edu/utcam

The UT-CAM Web site provides comprehensive, in-depth summaries of a variety of complementary and alternative therapies. UT-CAM was one of 11 centers established by NCCAM at the NIH to evaluate alternative therapies. It was the only Office of Alternative Medicine center specifically focused on alternative and complementary cancer therapies and was co-funded by NCI. UT-CAM is no longer funded; however, the Web site will be available through December 2000.

Glossary

adjuvant therapy: treatment used in addition to the main treatment. It usually refers to hormonal therapy, chemotherapy, or radiation given after surgery to increase the chances of curing the disease or keeping it in check.

alternative therapy: an unproven therapy that is used instead of conventional (proven) therapy. Some alternative therapies have dangerous or even life-threatening side effects. With others, the main danger is that the patient may lose the opportunity to benefit from proven therapy. The American Cancer Society recommends that patients considering the use of any alternative or complementary therapy discuss this with their health care team. *See complementary therapy and unproven therapy.*

antibiotics: drugs used to kill organisms that cause disease. Since some cancer treatments can reduce the body's ability to fight off infection, antibiotics may be used to treat or prevent these infections.

antibody: a protein produced by immune system cells and released into the blood. Antibodies defend against foreign agents, such as bacteria. These agents contain certain substances called antigens. Each antibody works against a specific antigen. *See antigen.*

antigen: a substance that causes the body's immune system to react. This reaction often involves production of antibodies. For example, the immune system's response to antigens that are part of bacteria and viruses helps people resist infections. Cancer cells have certain antigens that can be found by laboratory tests. They are important in cancer diagnosis and in watching response to treatment. Other cancer cell antigens play a role in immune reactions that may help the body's resistance against cancer.

antioxidants: compounds that block chemical reactions with oxygen (oxidation) and are thought to reduce the risk of some cancers. Examples are vitamins C and E and beta carotene.

asymptomatic: not having any symptoms of a disease. Many cancers can develop and grow without producing symptoms, especially in the early stages. Screening tests such as mammograms help to find these early cancers, when the chances for cure are usually highest. *See screening.*

basic science: laboratory studies that are not aimed at specific problems, but provide the necessary knowledge and background for later applied research.

behavioral research: research into what motivates people to act as they do. The results of such research can be used to help convince people to adopt healthy lifestyles and to follow life-saving screening and treatment guidelines.

benign tumor: an abnormal growth that is not cancerous and does not spread to other areas of the body.

beta carotene: a precursor of vitamin A that is found mainly in yellow and orange vegetables and fruits. It functions as an antioxidant and may play a role in cancer prevention.

biologic response modifiers: substances that boost the body's immune system to fight against cancer; interferon is one example. Also called biologic therapy.

blood count: a count of the number of red blood cells, white blood cells, and platelets in a given sample of blood.

cancer: this is not just one disease but rather a group of diseases. All forms of cancer cause cells in the body to change and grow out of control. Most types of cancer cells form a lump or mass called a tumor. The tumor can invade and destroy healthy tissue. Cells from the tumor can break away and travel to other parts of the body. There they can continue to grow. This spreading process is called metastasis. When cancer spreads, it is still named after the part of the body where it started. For example, if breast cancer spreads to the lungs, it is still breast cancer, not lung cancer. Some cancers, such as blood cancers, do not form a tumor. Not all tumors are cancerous. A tumor that is not cancerous is called benign. Benign tumors do not grow and spread the way cancer does. They are usually not a threat to life. Another word for cancerous is malignant.

cancer care team: the group of health care professionals who work together to find, treat, and care for people with cancer. The cancer care team may include any or all of the following and others: primary care physician, pathologist, oncology specialists (medical oncologist, radiation oncologist), surgeons (including surgical specialists such as urologists, gynecologists, neurosurgeons, etc.), nurses, oncology nurse specialists, oncology social workers. Whether the team is linked formally or informally, there is usually one person who takes the job of coordinating the team.

cancer cell: a cell that divides and reproduces abnormally and has the potential to spread throughout the body, crowding out normal cells and tissue.

cancer vaccine: a vaccine used in the treatment (not prevention) of some cancers. It is made from pieces of tumors and works by causing the immune system to recognize and attack cancer cells.

carcinogen: a substance that causes cancer or helps cancer grow. For example, tobacco smoke contains many carcinogens that greatly increase the risk of lung cancer.

case studies: studies in which researchers compare data on people who have an illness with apparently similar, healthy people matched by age, sex, and other factors to define risk factors for an illness.

cell: the basic unit of which all living things are made. Cells replace themselves by dividing and forming new cells (mitosis). The processes that control the formation of new cells and the death of old cells are disrupted in cancer.

cell cycle: the series of steps that a cell must go through to divide; some chemotherapy drugs act by interfering with the cell cycle.

chemotherapy: treatment with drugs to destroy cancer cells. Chemotherapy is often used with surgery or radiation to treat cancer when the cancer has spread, when it has come back (recurred), or when there is a strong chance that it could recur.

clinical research: studies that involve the observed symptoms, treatment, and course of diseases.

clinical trials: controlled research projects that determine whether new treatments are safe and effective for patients. Before a new treatment is used on people, it is studied in the laboratory. If these studies suggest the treatment will work, the next step is to test its value for patients. The main questions researchers want to answer are the following: Does this treatment work? Does it work better than the one we're now using? What side effects does it cause? Do the benefits outweigh the risks? Which patients are most likely to find this treatment helpful? During the course of treatment, the doctor may suggest looking into a clinical trial. This does not mean that the patient is being asked to be a human "guinea pig." A clinical trial is done only when there is some reason to believe that the treatment being studied may be of value. It does not mean that the case is hopeless and the doctor is suggesting a last-ditch effort. Clinical trials are carried out in steps called phases. Each phase is designed to answer certain questions.

complementary therapy: supportive methods that are used to complement, or in addition to, conventional treatments. Some complementary therapies may help relieve certain symptoms of cancer, relieve side effects of conventional cancer therapy or improve a patient's sense of well being. Examples might include meditation to reduce stress, peppermint tea for nausea, and acupuncture for chronic back pain. Complementary methods are not intended to cure disease, rather they are provided to help control symptoms and improve quality of life. Some methods, such as massage therapy, yoga, and meditation, which are now called complementary, have been previously referred to as "supportive care". *See alternative therapy.*

detection: finding disease. Early detection means that the disease is found at an early stage, before it has increased or spread to other sites. However, many forms of cancer can reach an advanced stage without causing symptoms. Mammography can help to detect breast cancer early, and the prostate-specific antigen blood test is useful in detecting prostate cancer.

diagnosis: identifying a disease by its signs or symptoms, and by using imaging procedures and laboratory findings. The earlier a diagnosis of cancer is made, the better the chance for long-term survival.

drug resistance: the ability of cancer cells to become resistant to the effects of the chemotherapy drugs used to treat cancer.

epidemiologic research: the study of diseases in populations by collecting and analyzing statistical data. In the field of cancer, epidemiologists look at how many people have cancer, who gets specific types of cancer, and what factors (such as environment or personal habits) play a part in the development of cancer.

etiology: the cause of a disease. In cancer, there are probably many causes, although research is showing that both genetics and lifestyle are major factors in many cancers.

five-year survival rate: the percentage of people with a given cancer who are expected to survive five years or longer with the disease. Five-year survival rates have some drawbacks. Although the rates are based on the most recent information available, they may include data from patients treated several years earlier. Advances in cancer treatment often occur quickly. These rates, while statistically valid, may not reflect these advances. They should not be seen as a predictor in an individual case.

high risk: the situation in which the chance of developing cancer is greater than that normally seen in the general population. People may be at high risk from many factors, including heredity (such as a family history of breast cancer), personal habits (such as smoking), or the environment (such as overexposure to sunlight).

hormone: a chemical substance released into the body by the endocrine glands such as the thyroid, adrenal, or ovaries. Hormones travel through the bloodstream and sets in motion various body functions. Testosterone and estrogen are examples of male and female hormones.

immune system: the complex system by which the body resists infection by microbes such as bacteria or viruses and rejects transplanted tissues or organs. The immune system may also help the body fight some cancers.

immunology: the study of how the body resists infection and certain other diseases. Knowledge gained in this field is important to those cancer treatments based on the principles of immunology.

investigational therapies: treatments that are being studied in a clinical trial.

in vitro research: studies conducted in an artificial environment outside a living organism (eg, cell cultures).

in vivo research: studies conducted within a living organism (eg, animals or humans).

integrative therapy: the combined use of evidence-based proven therapies and complementary therapies.

invasive cancer: cancer that has spread beyond the layer of cells where it first developed to involve adjacent tissues.

localized cancer: a cancer that is confined to the place where it started; that is, it has not spread to distant parts of the body.

lymph nodes: small bean-shaped collections of immune system tissue, such as lymphocytes, found along lymphatic vessels. They remove cell waste and fluids from lymph. They help fight infections and also have a role in fighting cancer. Also called lymph glands.

malignant tumor: a mass of cancer cells that may invade surrounding tissues or spread (metastasize) to distant areas of the body.

metastasis: the spread of cancer cells to distant areas of the body by way of the lymph system or bloodstream.

nontraditional therapies: unconventional complementary and alternative therapies. These therapies may include remedies that have been used in certain cultures for thousands of years, such as traditional Chinese medicine or Native American medicine. *See unconventional therapies.*

nurse practitioner: a registered nurse with a master's or doctoral degree. Licensed nurse practitioners diagnose and manage illness and disease, usually working closely with a doctor. In many states, they may prescribe medications.

oncologist: a doctor with special training in the diagnosis and treatment of cancer.

oncology: the branch of medicine concerned with the diagnosis and treatment of cancer.

oncology clinical nurse specialist: a registered nurse with a master's degree in oncology nursing who specializes in the care of cancer patients. Oncology nurse specialists may prepare and administer treatments, monitor patients, prescribe and provide supportive care, and teach and counsel patients and their families.

oncology social worker: a person with a master's degree in social work who is an expert in coordinating and providing non-medical care to patients. The oncology social worker provides counseling and assistance to people with cancer and their families, especially in dealing with the non-medical issues that can result from cancer, such as financial problems, housing (when treatments must be taken at a facility away from home), and child care.

palliative treatment: treatment that relieves symptoms, such as pain, but is not expected to cure the disease. The main purpose is to improve the patient's quality of life.

pathologist: a doctor who specializes in diagnosis and classification of diseases by laboratory tests such as examination of tissue and cells under a microscope. The pathologist determines whether a tumor is benign or cancerous and, if cancerous, the exact cell type and grade.

placebo: an inert, inactive substance that may be used in studies (clinical trials) to compare the effects of a given treatment with no treatment. In common speech, a "sugar pill."

population studies: studies in which researchers look at disease incidence and death rates based on an exact amount of a given population in a specific geographic area.

pre-cancerous: *see pre-malignant.*

pre-malignant: changes in cells that may, but do not always, become cancerous. Also called pre-cancerous.

prevention: the reduction of cancer risk by eliminating or reducing contact with carcinogenic agents. A change in lifestyle, such as quitting smoking, for example, reduces the risk of lung and other cancers.

prognosis: a prediction of the course of disease; the outlook for the cure of the patient.

prospective studies: studies in which researchers look at a group of people at a specific point (or points) in time and then wait to see who gets what diseases before making associations between lifestyle and risk of illness.

protein: a large molecule made up of a chain of smaller units called amino acids. Proteins serve many vital functions within and outside of the cell.

protocol: a formal outline or plan, such as a description of what treatments a patient will receive and exactly when each should be given. *See regimen.*

proven treatments: evidence-based, conventional, mainstream, or standard medical treatments that have been tested following a strict set of guidelines and found to be safe and effective. The results of such studies have been published in peer-reviewed journals, meaning that other doctors or scientists in the field evaluate the quality of the research and decide whether the article will be published. These treatments have been approved by the Food and Drug Administration (FDA).

quackery: the promotion of methods claiming to prevent, diagnose, or cure cancers that are known to be false or unproven. These methods are often based on the use of patient testimonials as evidence of their effectiveness and safety. Many times the treatment is claimed to be effective against other diseases as well as cancer.

questionable treatments: unproven or untested therapies.

radiation oncologist: a doctor who specializes in using radiation to treat cancer.

radiation therapy: treatment with radiation to destroy cancer cells. This type of treatment may be used to reduce the size of a cancer before surgery, to destroy any remaining cancer cells after surgery, or, in some cases, as the main treatment.

recurrence: cancer that has come back after treatment. Local recurrence means that the cancer has come back at the same place as the original cancer. Regional recurrence means that the cancer has come back in the lymph nodes near the first site. Distant recurrence is when cancer metastasizes after treatment to organs or tissues (such as the lungs, liver, bone marrow, or brain) farther from the original site than the regional lymph nodes.

regimen: a strict, regulated plan (such as diet, exercise, or other activity) designed to reach certain goals. In cancer treatment, a plan to treat cancer. *See protocol.*

rehabilitation: activities to help a person adjust, heal, and return to a full, productive life after injury or illness. This may involve physical restoration (such as the use of prostheses, exercises, and physical therapy), counseling, and emotional support.

relapse: reappearance of cancer after a disease-free period. *See recurrence.*

research (investigational) treatments: therapies being studied in a clinical trial. Before a drug or other treatment can be used regularly to treat patients, it is studied and carefully tested, first in a laboratory setting (in vitro) and then in animals (in vivo). After these studies are completed and the therapy is found to be safe and promising, it is then tested to see if it helps patients. After careful testing among patients shows the drug or other treatment is safe and effective, the FDA may approve it for regular use. Only then does the treatment become part of the standard, conventional collection of proven therapies used to treat disease in humans.

retrospective studies: studies in which researchers compare people with a disease or other condition with a similar group or people who are not affected and the look back in time to see what differences in their lifestyles might have contributed to the different outcomes in their health status.

review studies (meta-analyses): studies in which researchers analyze the findings of several other studies.

screening: the search for disease, such as cancer, in people without symptoms. For example, screening measures for prostate cancer include digital rectal examination and the prostate-specific antigen blood test; for breast cancer, mammography and clinical breast examinations. Screening may refer to coordinated programs in large populations.

side effects: unwanted effects of treatment such as hair loss caused by chemotherapy, and fatigue caused by radiation therapy.

staging: the process of finding out whether cancer has spread and if so, how far. There is more than one system for staging. The TNM system, described below, is one used often. The TNM system for staging provides three key pieces of information: T refers to the size of the Tumor; N describes how far the cancer has spread to nearby Nodes; and M shows whether the cancer has spread (Metastasized) to other organs of the body. Letters or numbers after the T, N, and M give more details about each of these factors. To make this information somewhat clearer, the TNM descriptions can be grouped together into a simpler set of stages, labeled with Roman numerals. In general, the lower the number, the less the cancer has spread. A higher number means a more serious cancer.

surgeon: a doctor who performs operations.

survival rate: the percentage of survivors with no trace of disease within a certain period of time after diagnosis or treatment. For cancer, a five-year survival rate is often given. This does not mean that people cannot live more than five years, or that those who live for five years are necessarily permanently cured.

therapy: any of the measures taken to treat a disease. See alternative therapy, complementary therapy, unproven therapy, proven treatments, unconventional therapies, and investigational therapies.

tumor: an abnormal lump or mass of tissue. Tumors can be benign (not cancerous) or malignant (cancerous).

unconventional therapies: all types of complementary and alternative treatments that fall outside the definition of conventional (proven) therapies.

unproven (untested) therapy: any therapy that has not been scientifically tested and approved. It may also refer to treatments or tests that are under investigation. In general, adequate scientific evidence is not available to support the use of unproven or untested treatments.

Appendix

American Cancer Society Operational Statement on Complementary and Alternative Methods of Cancer Management

(Developed by the ACS Advisory Group on Complementary and Alternative Methods and reviewed by the ACS Medical Affairs Committee August 12, 1999)

The American Cancer Society realizes that there are many definitions for the terms "alternative" and "complementary" methods and makes the following distinction between these categories. Alternative methods are defined as unproved or disproved methods, rather than evidence-based or proven methods to prevent, diagnose, and treat cancer. "Complementary" methods are defined as supportive methods used to complement evidence-based treatment. Complementary therapies do not replace mainstream cancer treatment and are not promoted to cure disease. Rather, they control symptoms and improve well being and quality of life. This distinction separates methods based on how they are promoted and used.

The Society is sensitive to the growing public interest, in particular, those living with cancer, in information about alternative and complementary methods. The Society acknowledges that more research is needed regarding the safety and effectiveness of many of these methods. The Society advocates for peer-reviewed scientific evidence of the safety and efficacy of these methods. All cancer interventions must withstand the scrutiny of peer-reviewed scientific evaluation before they can be recommended for the prevention, diagnosis, or treatment of cancer.

The Society realizes the need to balance access to alternative and complementary therapies while protecting patients against methods that might be harmful to them. The Society supports patient access, but strongly encourages more oversight and accountability by governmental, public, and private entities to protect the public from harm as they seek therapies to complement mainstream cancer care. Harmful drug interactions may occur and must be recognized. Unnecessary delays and interruptions in standard therapies are detrimental to the success of cancer treatment.

The Society supports the right of individuals with cancer to decide what treatment is best for them. But we encourage people to discuss all treatments they may be considering with their physician and other health care providers. We also encourage people with cancer to consider using methods that have been proved effective or those that are currently under study in clinical trials. We also encourage health care professionals to ask their patients about their use of alternative and complementary methods. Health care professionals should listen and know how to communicate with their patients. Open, trusting, non-critical dialogue is essential in this important area.

1999 COMMITTEE LISTING

David Rosenthal, MD, Committee Chair
Director, Harvard University Health Services
Medical Director, Zakim Center for Integrative
     Medicine, Dana-Farber / Harvard Cancer Center
Boston, MA

Abby S. Bloch, PhD, RD
Nutrition Consultant in Private Practice
New York, NY

Barrie R. Cassileth, PhD
Chief, Integrative Medicine Service
Memorial Solan-Kettering Cancer Center
New York, NY

Freddie Ann Hoffman, MD
(Formerly of the US Food and Drug Administration)
Senior Director, Medical and Clinical Affairs –
    Complementary Medicine
Consumer Healthcare Research & Development,
Warner- Lambert, Co.
Morris Plains, NJ

Richard H. Lange, MD, FACP
Honorary Attending Staff, Ellis Hospital
Schenectady, NY

Michael Lerner, PhD
President, Commonwealth
Bolinas, CA

John J. Lynch, MD, FACP
Associate Medical Director
Washington Cancer Institute & Washington
    Hospital Center
Washington, DC

Saar A. Porrath, MD
Beverly Hills, CA

John H. Renner, MD
Consumer Health Information
Research Institute
Independence, MO

Wallace Sampson, MD
Clinical Professor of Medicine
Stanford University
Associate Chief of Hematology/Oncology
Santa Clara Valley Medical Center
San Jose, CA

Ralph B. Vance, MD
Professor of Medicine
Division of Oncology
University of Mississippi Medical Center
Jackson, MS

David K. Wellisch, PhD
Professor, Department of Psychiatry
UCLA-NPI
Los Angeles, CA

Connie Henke Yarbro, RN, MS, FAAN
Clinical Associate Director
Division of Hematology/Oncology
Adjunct Clinical Assistant Professor
School of Nursing, University of Missouri-Columbia
Columbia, MO

Gabriel Feldman, MD
Former Director of Prostate & Colorectal Cancer
American Cancer Society
Atlanta, GA

CHAIRMAN'S STAFF
Terri Ades, RN, MS, AOCN
Director, Health Content Nursing Staff
American Cancer Society
Atlanta, GA

LaMar McGinnis, MD
Medical Consultant
American Cancer Society
Atlanta, GA

Index

F

Faith healing, 67-68
Family/couples therapy, 91
Fasting, 318-319
FDA Center for Food Safety and Applied Nutrition (CFSAN), 417
Federal Food, Drug, and Cosmetic Act of 1938 (FDC Act), 21
Feldenkrais method, 114-116
Felon herb, 245-246
Feng shui, 69-70
    See also Asian healing therapies
Fire cupping, 125-126
Fish, 342-344, 364-365
Flavonoids, 255-257
Flaxseed, 209-210
Flor essence, 206-207
Flower remedies, 211-212
Folacin, 212-214
Folate, 212-214
Folic acid, 212-214, 287-289
Food
    Good Manufacturing Processes (GMPs) and, 26-27
    labeling, 24-26
    phytochemicals, 255-257
    regulation, 24-26
    sample label, 25f
    sample servings of, 42f
    See also Nutrition
Fragrances
    See Aromatherapy
Fraudulent products, signs of possible, 129
Freedom of choice, 29-30
Fresh cell therapy, 360-362
Fu-tzu, 164
Fu Zhen therapy, 214

G

Gamma linolenic acid, 375-376
Gan cao, 235-236
Garlic, 319-321
Germanium, 214-215
Gerson therapy, 321-323
Ginger, 216-217
Ginkgo biloba, 218-219
Ginseng, 219-221
GLA
    See Gamma linolenic acid
Glucarate, 377-378
Glutamine, 308-309
Glycine, 308-309
Glycine soja, 346-348
Glycyrrhiza glabra, 235-236
Goatweed, 272-274

Gold book tea, 271
Golden bough, 241-243
Goldenseal, 222-223
Goldsiegel, 222-223
Gonzalez treatment, 336-338
Good Manufacturing Processes (GMPs), 26-27
Gotu kola, 189-190
Grapefruits, 338-339, 377-378
Grapes, 323-325
Grass, 237-239
Greasewood, 193-195
Greek cancer cure, 378-379
Green algae, 198-199
Green mint, 253-254
Green tea, 224-225
Grifola frondosa, 334-335
Ground raspberry, 222-223
Group psychotherapy, 99-101
Group therapy, 91, 99-101
Guided imagery, 76-77

H

Hackmatack, 278-279
Hansi, 226
Hatha yoga, 104-105
HBOT
    See Hyperbaric oxygen therapy
Health Maintenance Organizations (HMOs), 46-47
Health on the Net Foundation (HON), 415-416
Healthscout, 417
Heat therapy, 131-132
Hemp, 237-239
Herbal essence, 206-207
Herbal therapies, 18, 31-36
    Chinese, 195-197
    drug interactions with, 33-34
Herbs, 26
    See also Herbs, Vitamins, and Minerals
High colonic detoxification therapy, 122-124
High enema, 122-124
High pH therapy, 190-191
Histidine, 308-309
Hochu-ekki-to, 230-231
Hog apple, 339-341
Holism, 70-72
Holistic aromatherapy, 52-53
Holistic medicine, 18, 70-72
    See also Spiritual healing
Holothuroidea cucumaria, 405
Holy thistle, 239-241
Homeopathy, 380-381
Horn method, 125-126
Hot pepper, 183-185
Hoxsey herbal treatment, 226-228
Huang ch'i, 169-170

Rauwolfia, 229-230
Red clover, 264-265
Red pepper, 183-185
Red valerian, 279-281
Reflexology, 153-155
　　See also Asian healing therapies; Relaxation methods
Regulation, food, 24-26
Reiki, 155-156
　　See also Asian healing therapies; Relaxation methods
Relaxation methods
　　See Biofeedback; Breathwork; Hypnosis; Imagery; Massage; Myotherapy; Polarity therapy; Reflexology; Reiki
Religion, 97-99
　　See also Spiritual healing; Spirituality and prayer
Remifemin, 176-177
Research, 8
　　epidemiological, 12
　　types of, 11
Reserpine, 229-230
Retinol, 285-287
Retrospective studies, 11
Revici's guided chemotherapy, 403-404
Review studies, 11
Rheumatism root, 296-297
Riboflavin, 287-289
Rife machine, 128-130
Rolfing, 114-116
Rose bay, 247-248
Rosen method, 157
Rubenfeld synergy method, 157
Ruibarbo caribe, 339-341

S

Safety of complementary and alternative methods, 21-36
Sample book entries for methods, 4-5
Saw palmetto, 266-267
Scents, 52-53
Sea cucumber, 405
Selected vegetable soup, 344
Selenium, 268-269
Semivegetarian, 348-350
Serenoa repens, 266-267
Serine, 308-309
Serpentwood, 229-230
Sesame seeds, 326-327
714-X, 411-412
Shadow boxing, 102-103
Shamanism, 95-97
Sharks
　　cartilage, 405-407
　　liver oil, 408-409

Shellfish, 397
Sheridan's formula, 358-359
Shiatsu massage, 114-116
Shiitake mushroom, 345-346
Sho-saiko, 230-231
Siberian ginseng, 270-271
Silybum marianum, 239-241
Silymarin, 239-241
Six flavor tea, 271
Slippery root, 201-202
Smoking and cancer prevention, 44
Snakeroot, 229-230
Somatostatin, 370-371
Sonopuncture, 158
Sound therapy, 82-83
Soybean, 346-348, 364-365
Special Nutritionals Adverse Event Monitoring System, 36
Spinach, 364-365, 393-394
Spinal manipulation, 120-121
Spiritual healing, 67-68
　　curanderismo, 63-65
　　faith healing, 67-68
　　Native American healing, 84-86
　　prayer and religion, 97-99
　　shamanism, 95-97
　　See also Holistic medicine
St. John's plant, 245-246
St. John's wort, 272-274
Standardization of products, 32-33
Steroids, 368-369
Strawberries, 316-317
Strychnos nux-vomica, 274-275
Strychnos seed, 274-275
Sulfides, 255-257
Sun chlorella, 198-199
Sun exposure and cancer prevention, 44-45
Sun soup, 344
Support groups, 99-101
SV
　　See Selected vegetable soup
Swamp cedar, 278-279
Sweet root, 235-236
Symphtum officinale, 201-202
Systemic enzyme therapy, 374-375
Syzgium aromaticum, 199-200

T

T-up
　　See Aloe
Tabeuia impetiginosa, 249-251
Taheebo, 249-251
Tahuari, 249-251
Tai chi, 102-103
　　See also Asian healing therapies

Yellow puccoon, 222-223
Yellow root, 222-223
Yocon, 300-301
Yoga, 104-105
  See also Asian healing therapies; Relaxation
  methods
Yohimbe, 300-301
Yohimbine, 300-301
Yohimex, 300-301
Yomax, 300-301

Z

Zapping machine, 128-130
Zen Buddhism
  See Meditation
Zhenjiu, 108-109
Zinc, 302-303
Zingiber officinale, 216-217
Zone therapy, 153-155